1993
YEAR BOOK OF
NEONATAL AND PERINATAL MEDICINE®

Statement of Purpose

The YEAR BOOK Service

The YEAR BOOK series was devised in 1901 by practicing health professionals who observed that the literature of medicine and related disciplines had become so voluminous that no one individual could read and place in perspective every potential advance in a major specialty. In the final decade of the 20th century, this recognition is more acutely true than it was in 1901.

More than merely a series of books, YEAR BOOK volumes are the tangible results of a unique service designed to accomplish the following:

• to *survey* a wide range of journals of proven value

• to *select* from those journals papers representing significant advances and statements of important clinical principles

• to provide *abstracts* of those articles that are readable, convenient summaries of their key points

• to provide *commentary* about those articles to place them in perspective.

These publications grow out of a unique process that calls on the talents of outstanding authorities in clinical and fundamental disciplines, trained literature specialists, and professional writers, all supported by the resources of Mosby, the world's preeminent publisher for the health professions.

The Literature Base

Mosby subscribes to nearly 1,000 journals published worldwide, covering the full range of the health professions. On an annual basis, the publisher examines usage patterns and polls its expert authorities to add new journals to the literature base and to delete journals that are no longer useful as potential YEAR BOOK sources.

The Literature Survey

The publisher's team of literature specialists, all of whom are trained and experienced health professionals, examines every original, peer-reviewed article in each journal issue. More than 250,000 articles per year are scanned systematically, including title, text, illustrations, tables, and references. Each scan is compared, article by article, to the search strategies that the publisher has developed in consultation with the 270 outside experts who form the pool of YEAR BOOK editors. A given article may be reviewed by any number of editors, from one to a dozen or more, regardless of the discipline for which the paper was originally published. In turn, each editor who receives the article reviews it to determine whether or not the article should be included in the YEAR BOOK. This decision is based on the article's inherent quality, its probable usefulness to readers of that YEAR BOOK, and the editor's goal to represent a balanced picture of a given field in each volume of the YEAR BOOK. In addition, the editor indicates when to include figures and tables from the article to help the YEAR BOOK reader better understand the information.

Of the quarter million articles scanned each year, only 5% are selected for detailed analysis within the YEAR BOOK series, thereby assuring readers of the high value of every selection.

The Abstract

The publisher's abstracting staff is headed by a physician-writer and includes individuals with training in the life sciences, medicine, and other areas, plus extensive experience in writing for the health professions and related industries. Each selected article is assigned to a specific writer on this abstracting staff. The abstracter, guided in many cases by notations supplied by the expert editor, writes a structured, condensed summary designed so that the reader can rapidly acquire the essential information contained in the article.

The Commentary

The YEAR BOOK editorial boards, sometimes assisted by guest commentators, write comments that place each article in perspective for the reader. This provides the reader with the equivalent of a personal consultation with a leading international authority—an opportunity to better understand the value of the article and to benefit from the authority's thought processes in assessing the article.

Additional Editorial Features

The editorial boards of each YEAR BOOK organize the abstracts and comments to provide a logical and satisfying sequence of information. To enhance the organization, editors also provide introductions to sections or individual chapters, comments linking a number of abstracts, citations to additional literature, and other features.

The published YEAR BOOK contains enhanced bibliographic citations for each selected article, including extended listings of multiple authors and identification of author affiliations. Each YEAR BOOK contains a Table of Contents specific to that year's volume. From year to year, the Table of Contents for a given YEAR BOOK will vary depending on developments within the field.

Every YEAR BOOK contains a list of the journals from which papers have been selected. This list represents a subset of the nearly 1,000 journals surveyed by the publisher, and occasionally reflects a particularly pertinent article from a journal that is not surveyed on a routine basis.

Finally, each volume contains a comprehensive subject index and an index to authors of each selected paper.

The 1993 Year Book Series

Year Book of Anesthesia and Pain Management: Drs. Miller, Abram, Kirby, Ostheimer, Roizen, and Stoelting

Year Book of Cardiology®: Drs. Schlant, Collins, Engle, Gersh, Kaplan, and Waldo

Year Book of Chiropractic: Drs. Phillips and Adams

Year Book of Critical Care Medicine®: Drs. Rogers and Parrillo

Year Book of Dentistry®: Drs. Meskin, Currier, Kennedy, Leinfelder, Berry, Roser, and Zakariasen

Year Book of Dermatologic Surgery: Drs. Swanson, Salasche, and Glogau

Year Book of Dermatology®: Drs. Sober and Fitzpatrick

Year Book of Diagnostic Radiology®: Drs. Federle, Clark, Gross, Madewell, Maynard, Sackett, and Young

Year Book of Digestive Diseases®: Drs. Greenberger and Moody

Year Book of Drug Therapy®: Drs. Lasagna and Weintraub

Year Book of Emergency Medicine®: Drs. Wagner, Burdick, Davidson, Roberts, and Spivey

Year Book of Endocrinology®: Drs. Bagdade, Braverman, Horton, Kannan, Landsberg, Molitch, Morley, Odell, Rogol, Ryan, and Sherwin

Year Book of Family Practice®: Drs. Berg, Bowman, Davidson, Dietrich, and Scherger

Year Book of Geriatrics and Gerontology®: Drs. Beck, Reuben, Burton, Small, Whitehouse, and Goldstein

Year Book of Hand Surgery®: Drs. Amadio and Hentz

Year Book of Health Care Management: Drs. Heyssel, Brock, Moses, and Steinberg, Ms. Avakian, and Messrs. Berman, Kues, and Rosenberg

Year Book of Hematology®: Drs. Spivak, Bell, Ness, Quesenberry, and Wiernik

Year Book of Infectious Diseases®: Drs. Wolff, Barza, Keusch, Klempner, and Snydman

Year Book of Infertility®: Drs. Mishell, Paulsen, and Lobo

Year Book of Medicine®: Drs. Rogers, Bone, Cline, O'Rourke, Greenberger, Utiger, Epstein, and Malawista

Year Book of Neonatal and Perinatal Medicine®: Drs. Klaus and Fanaroff

Year Book of Nephrology: Drs. Coe, Favus, Henderson, Kashgarian, Luke, Myers, and Curtis

Year Book of Neurology and Neurosurgery®: Drs. Bradley and Crowell

Year Book of Neuroradiology: Drs. Osborn, Eskridge, Harnsberger, and Grossman

Year Book of Nuclear Medicine®: Drs. Hoffer, Gore, Gottschalk, Zaret, and Zubal

Year Book of Obstetrics and Gynecology®: Drs. Mishell, Kirschbaum, and Morrow

Year Book of Occupational and Environmental Medicine: Drs. Emmett, Brooks, Frank, and Hammad

Year Book of Oncology®: Drs. Young, Longo, Ozols, Simone, Steele, and Glatstein

Year Book of Ophthalmology®: Drs. Laibson, Adams, Augsburger, Benson, Cohen, Eagle, Flanagan, Nelson, Rapuano, Reinecke, Sergott, and Wilson

Year Book of Orthopedics®: Drs. Sledge, Poss, Cofield, Frymoyer, Griffin, Hansen, Johnson, Simmons, and Springfield

Year Book of Otolaryngology–Head and Neck Surgery®: Drs. Holt and Paparella

Year Book of Pathology and Clinical Pathology®: Drs. Gardner, Bennett, Cousar, Garvin, and Worsham

Year Book of Pediatrics®: Dr. Stockman

Year Book of Plastic, Reconstructive, and Aesthetic Surgery: Drs. Miller, Cohen, McKinney, Robson, Ruberg, and Whitaker

Year Book of Podiatric Medicine and Surgery®: Dr. Kominsky

Year Book of Psychiatry and Applied Mental Health®: Drs. Talbott, Frances, Freedman, Meltzer, Perry, Schowalter, and Yudofsky

Year Book of Pulmonary Disease®: Drs. Bone and Petty

Year Book of Sports Medicine®: Drs. Shephard, Eichner, Sutton, and Torg, Col. Anderson, and Mr. George

Year Book of Surgery®: Drs. Copeland, Deitch, Eberlein, Howard, Ritchie, Robson, Souba, and Sugarbaker

Year Book of Transplantation®: Drs. Ascher, Hansen, and Strom

Year Book of Ultrasound: Drs. Merritt, Mittelstaedt, Carroll, Babcock, and Goldstein

Year Book of Urology®: Drs. Gillenwater and Howards

Year Book of Vascular Surgery®: Dr. Porter

Roundsmanship® '93–'94: A Student's Survival Guide to Clinical Medicine Using Current Literature: Drs. Dan, Feigin, Quilligan, Schrock, Stein, and Talbott

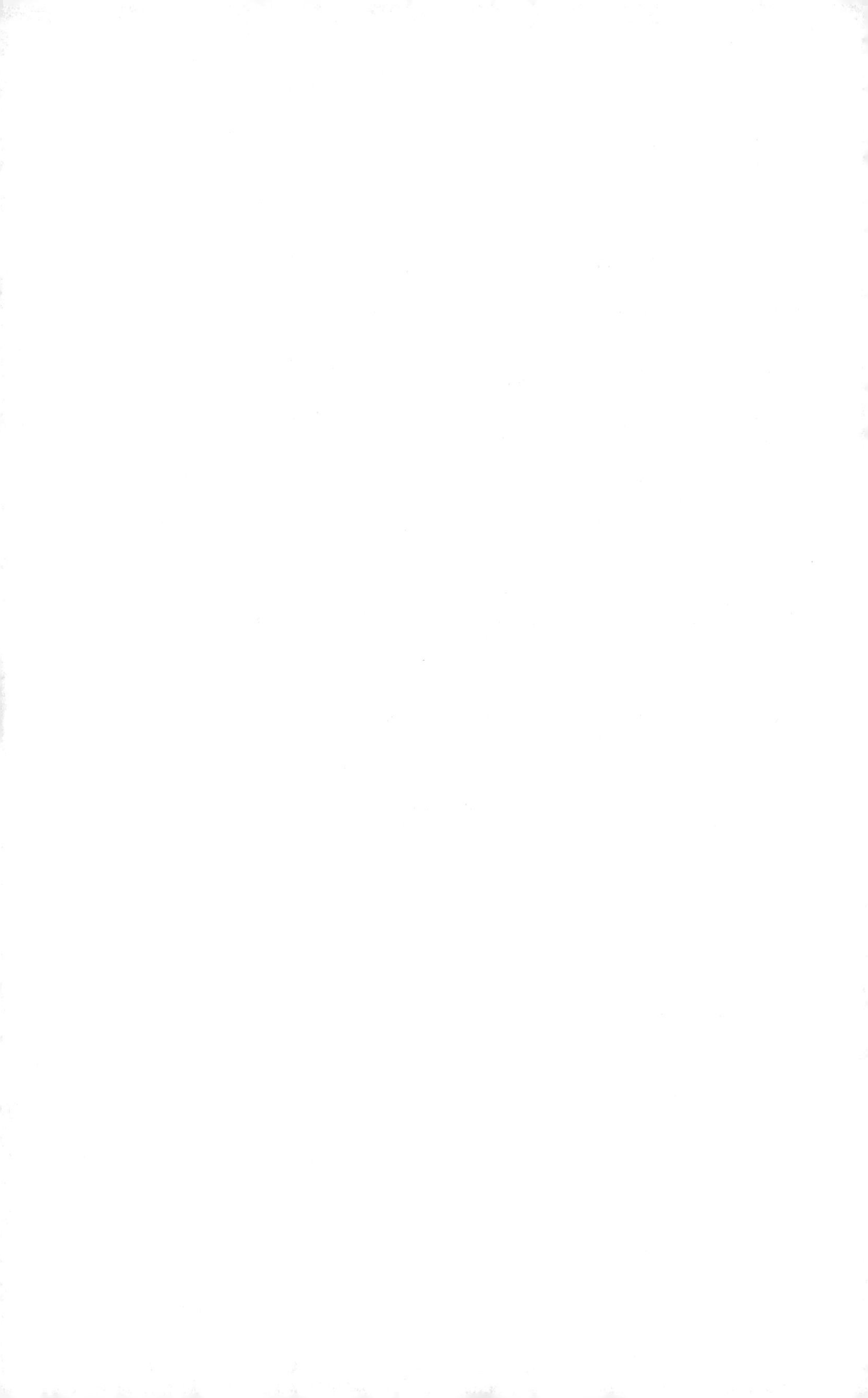

1993 The Year Book of NEONATAL AND PERINATAL MEDICINE®

Editors

Marshall H. Klaus, M.D.

Adjunct Professor of Pediatrics, University of California, San Francisco

Avroy A. Fanaroff, M.B.B.Ch. (Rand), F.R.C.P.E.

Professor, Department of Pediatrics, Case Western Reserve University; Director, Division of Neonatology, Rainbow Babies' and Children's Hospital, Cleveland, Ohio

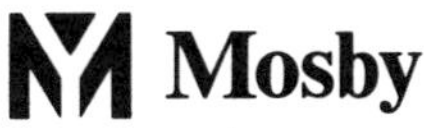

St. Louis Baltimore Boston Chicago London Madrid Philadelphia Sydney Toronto

Vice President and Publisher, Continuity Publishing: Kenneth H. Killion
Sponsoring Editor: Bernadette Buchholz
Illustrations and Permissions Coordinator: Maureen A. Livengood
Manager, Literature Services: Edith M. Podrazik, R.N.
Senior Information Specialist: Terri Santo, R.N.
Information Specialist: Nancy Dunne, R.N.
Senior Medical Writer: David A. Cramer, M.D.
Senior Project Manager: Max F. Perez
Project Supervisor: Tamara L. Smith
Production Editor: Wendi Schnaufer
Senior Production Assistant: Sandra Rogers
Production Assistant: Rebecca Nordbrock
Proofroom Manager: Barbara M. Kelly

1993 EDITION

Printed in the United States of America
Composition by International Computaprint Corporation
Printing/binding by Maple-Vail

Mosby, Inc.
11830 Westline Industrial Drive
St. Louis, MO 63146

Editorial Office:
Mosby, Inc.
200 North LaSalle St.
Chicago, IL 60601

International Standard Serial Number: 1044-4890
International Standard Book Number: 0-8151-5228-0

Table of Contents

Journals Represented

Mosby subscribes to and surveys nearly 1,000 U.S. and foreign medical and allied health journals. From these journals, the Editors select the articles to be abstracted. Journals represented in this YEAR BOOK are listed below.

Acta Neurologica Scandinavica
Acta Obstetricia et Gynecologica Scandinavica
Acta Paediatrica Scandinavica
American Journal of Diseases of Children
American Journal of Epidemiology
American Journal of Human Genetics
American Journal of Hypertension
American Journal of Neuroradiology
American Journal of Obstetrics and Gynecology
American Journal of Perinatology
American Journal of Public Health
American Journal of Roentgenology
Annals of Clinical Biochemistry
Annals of Neurology
Archives of Disease in Childhood
Archives of Internal Medicine
Archives of Ophthalmology
Audiology
Australian and New Zealand Journal of Obstetrics and Gynaecology
Biology of the Neonate
British Journal of Cancer
British Journal of Obstetrics and Gynaecology
British Medical Journal
Cell
Cleft Palate-Craniofacial Journal
Clinical Chemistry
Clinical Pharmacology and Therapeutics
Developmental Medicine and Child Neurology
Developmental Psychology
Diabetes Care
Diabetologia
Diagnostic Microbiology and Infectious Disease
Digestive Diseases and Sciences
Dysphagia
Early Human Development
European Journal of Clinical Pharmacology
European Journal of Obstetrics, Gynecology and Reproductive Biology
European Journal of Pediatric Surgery
Family Planning Perspectives
Gastroenterology
Infection and Immunity
JOGNN: Journal of Obstetric, Gynecologic, and Neonatal Nursing
Journal of Acquired Immune Deficiency Syndromes
Journal of Clinical Endocrinology and Metabolism
Journal of Clinical Investigation
Journal of Developmental and Behavioral Pediatrics
Journal of Family Practice
Journal of Medical Genetics
Journal of Pediatric Gastroenterology and Nutrition
Journal of Pediatric Surgery

Journal of Pediatrics
Journal of Reproductive Medicine
Journal of Thoracic and Cardiovascular Surgery
Journal of Trauma
Journal of Urology
Journal of the American Medical Association
Lancet
Neuropediatrics
New England Journal of Medicine
Ophthalmology
Paediatric and Perinatal Epidemiology
Pediatric Infectious Disease Journal
Pediatric Neurology
Pediatric Pathology
Pediatric Pulmonology
Pediatric Research
Pediatrics
Pharmacotherapy
Prenatal Diagnosis
Radiology
Scandinavian Journal of Work, Environment and Health
Science
Western Journal of Medicine

Standard Abbreviations

The following terms are abbreviated in this edition: acquired immunodeficiency syndrome (AIDS), the central nervous system (CNS), cerebrospinal fluid (CSF), computed tomography (CT), electrocardiography (ECG), human immunodeficiency virus (HIV), and magnetic resonance (MR) imaging (MRI).

Introduction

Choosing the best articles is no science, and it only borders on being an art. There are so many journals and articles that it is extremely difficult for the editors to be able to look at them all, much less judge them. Besides, tastes do and should differ. With that in mind, here are the articles that the editors selected from the abundant number of publications in 1993.

Once again, we have experienced a banner year. The perinatal literature has yielded a plethora of interesting and provocative articles. There has been a steady stream of controlled clinical trials. Although the prevailing hypotheses are not always verified, the scientific foundations for the field of neonatal and perinatal medicine are solidified by these sterling efforts. Multicentered, prospective, randomized trials remain fashionable, and efforts are under way to ensure that they remain cost effective.

The editors have been fascinated and amused by an array of topics. These range from a classic epidemiologic report on third-generation growth impairment after the Dutch famine during World War II to a report on a new primitive reflex. The progress in the Humane Genome Project, the breakthroughs in genetic diagnosis, and the prospects for gene therapy in cystic fibrosis are also highlighted.

Nitric oxide was anointed molecule of the year. Excitement in the academic world has reached a fever pitch as the clinical trials with this gas proceed along a broad frontier. The initial clinical experience is presented. Two fat soluble vitamins, namely E and K, are reevaluated as their potential roles in the clinical arena are defined, and differing views on the use of vitamin K at birth are presented. Furthermore, the role of another vitamin, folic acid, in preventing neural tube defects, is established beyond reasonable doubt by the marvelous study from Hungary. These represent but a few of the many topics that are sure to titillate the reader.

The opening of many new vistas during the past year is testimony to the vitality of the field of neonatal and perinatal medicine. We hope that the readers will share our joy as they peruse the classical studies as well as other topics of interest discovered in some of the obscure journals surveyed during the course of compiling this YEAR BOOK.

We are grateful to Dr. Lois Johnson, Dr. Graham E. Quinn, and Dr. Soraya Abbasi for their opening commentary on and review of vitamin E, the vitamin in constant search of a place in the nursery. Perhaps they will convince you that it has found one. We continue to call liberally on the expertise of our friends and colleagues. Their comments broaden our insight and perspective in their various superspecialized areas of interest. They always respond graciously, if not promptly. We greatly appreciate their efforts.

The staff at Mosby provides superb assistance throughout the process. They greatly facilitate timely completion of the project. We acknowledge

Bernadette Buchholz in particular. The YEAR BOOK OF NEONATAL AND PERINATAL MEDICINE is a labor of love. If and when it becomes a burden, it will be time to pass on the baton.

Avroy A. Fanaroff, M.B.B.Ch. (Rand), F.R.C.P.E.

Marshall H. Klaus, M.D.

Vitamin E and ROP—The Continuous Challenge

Lois H. Johnson, M.D.
Clinical Professor of Pediatrics, University of Pennsylvania School of Medicine; Newborn Pediatrics, Pennsylvania Hospital, Philadelphia

Graham E. Quinn, M.D.
Associate Professor of Ophthalmology, University of Pennsylvania School of Medicine; Children's Hospital of Philadelphia, Philadelphia

Soraya Abbasi, M.D.
Associate Professor of Pediatrics, University of Pennsylvania School of Medicine; Newborn Pediatrics, Pennsylvania Hospital, Philadelphia

In a provocative commentary (1) on the observation that breath pentane, an index of lipid peroxidation, is significantly decreased in normal smoking and nonsmoking subjects who consume supplemental d-α-tocopherol (2, 3), Max Horwitt wrote: ". . . Now that aspirin is realizing acceptance as a beneficial supplement, one wonders whether the tocopherols would achieve greater acceptance if they were called antioxidants rather than vitamins. . . . Obvious signs of a deficiency of vitamin E have not been observed in adults at half the intake of the current RDA, but deficiency is not the condition being evaluated. Rather, the focus of this communication is that there may be an undesirable chronic level of lipid peroxidation occurring in the cellular membranes and other tissue components which can be ameliorated by supplementation with d-alpha-tocopherol, a free radical scavenger." Dr. Horwitt goes on to say that, although the ideal size of the supplement is not known, it appears that serum levels of 1.3 mg of d-α-tocopherol per dL (as opposed to the somewhat less active, commercially available, dl form), would be desirable in adults. He concludes with the challenge, "Let the debate begin."

It is in the spirit of this debate that we offer the following commentary on the need for vitamin E supplementation in the premature infant. It was initially prompted by the 1990 YEAR BOOK OF NEONATAL AND PERINATAL MEDICINE'S abstract (4) of our article on the effect of pharmacologic serum levels of total tocopherol on the incidence and severity of retinopathy of prematurity (ROP), and its misreport of our recommendations for vitamin E supplementation. Its timeliness was later suggested by the findings at long-term follow-up of infants enrolled in the Cryo-ROP Trial (5–7). These have indicated the need for additional treatments to decrease visual compromise after severe (threshold) ROP.

Cryotherapy, as presently recommended, is clearly beneficial, as shown by the multicenter Cryo-ROP trial (5, 8). However, as pointed out by Tasman (9), the 25.7% incidence of unfavorable structural outcome (e.g., retrolental mass, fold through the macula, or posterior retinal detachment) in treated eyes (vs. 47.7% in control eyes) is "unacceptably high." This is even more the case considering the failure rate now being reported for visual function. At the 3.5-year follow-up in the Cryo-ROP Trial (7), an unfavorable visual acuity (low vision, light perception only, or worse) was reported in 51% of treated eyes (vs. 65% of control eyes). Related to this functional outcome is the fact that 34.5% of the treated eyes (vs. 25.6% of the control eyes) showed miscellaneous retinal abnormalities (e.g., macular heterotopia, extramacular fold, or macular pigment scarring) that were not included in the Cryo-ROP Trial's definition of unfavorable structures (5, 6, 8), but which were significantly associated with decreased visual acuity (7, 10). It should be emphasized, however, that not all of the visual dysfunction measured was end organ in nature, because some of the infants also had varying degrees of CNS abnormalities (11). Various strategies have been suggested to improve this outcome (9). We urge further study of the role of vitamin E in the management of this oxidant disease of the avascular, vitamin E-deficient retina.

To begin with, let us briefly review our work with vitamin E and ROP. We began with studies using oral and parenteral E supplements to achieve physiologic serum levels in a vitamin E-deficient premature population (1972–1976). These showed a beneficial effect on the incidence and severity of ROP in an era when survival of infants with birth weights less than 1,000 g was rare (12, 13). The subsequent randomized placebo-controlled clinical trial (CCT) sponsored by the National Eye Institute (1979–1981) used a parenteral investigational drug preparation of the active dl-α-tocopherol (Hoffmann-LaRoche), to target serum E levels of mg/dL for prophylaxis. The classification system (14) used closely resembled the International Classification for Retinopathy of Prematurity (ICROP), which has not yet been published (15). Complete acute-stage ROP data were collected on 755 infants with a birth weight of 2,000 g or less or a gestational age of 36 weeks or less. (The targeted sample size of 1,000 could not be met for budgetary reasons.) This CCT showed a decrease in the incidence of ROP in infants with a birth weight of 2,000 g or less (and in those with a birth weight of 1,500 g or less) by multivariate logistic analysis controlling for birth weight, gestational age, days receiving O_2 and ventilator therapy, and days in the hospital (16). However, pharmacologic prophylaxis was *not recommended,* because most ROP, regardless of the infant's birth weight, is mild and regresses spontaneously, and also because the CCT also demonstrated an increased incidence of sepsis and late-onset necrotizing enterocolitis in infants maintained at serum E levels of 5 ± 1.8 SD mg/dL from birth until completion of retinal vascularization (17). This effect was most obvious in infants with a birth weight of 1,001 g or less. Therefore, the risk/benefit ratio of pharmacologic prophylaxis was unfavorable, because any treatment involving many infants in whom clinically significant disease is unlikely to develop must be completely safe. Rather, *prophylaxis at total tocopherol levels within the physiologic range* (1–3 mg/dL) *was and is recommended* by us (12) and by others (18, 19), using commercially available preparations of vitamin E. Prophylaxis should be started as soon as possible after birth. In infants who receive enteral feedings, the physiologic serum levels of vitamin E can usually be achieved by feeding any of the 3 special premature formulas, all of which have a high vitamin E/polyunsaturated fatty acid ratio. In sick premature infants, they can also be achieved using the pediatric multivitamin infusate (MVI-Pediatric), which became available in 1985.

In our nurseries, we include MVI-Pediatric together with vitamin K in the intravenous fluids started on admission to the intensive care nursery and add MVI to subsequent daily fluid orders at a dose of 65% of vial (or 4 mg per infant per day). In agreement with others, (20, 21) we find that this higher-than-currently-recommended dose (1992 package insert) is needed for the increasingly immature infants being cared for today. Serum vitamin E levels are monitored regularly. After parenteral feedings have been discontinued, a significant number of infants need vitamin E supplements, in addition to those provided by the premature formulas, to maintain serum levels within the physiologic range. This is especially true in infants with a birth weight of 1,000 g or less, in whom zinc deficiency during periods of rapid growth is not uncommon.

A second important finding of the CCT was that of a significantly decreased progression from moderate to severe ROP, which occurred among 3 of 25 (12%) vitamin E-treated infants vs. 9 of 25 (36%) placebo-treated infants (P = .05). Moderate and severe ROP corresponded to the categories of prethreshold and threshold ROP as defined by the Cryo-ROP Trial. One third of the untreated infants with prethreshold ROP (in our study and in the subsequent Cryo-ROP Trial) showed progression to threshold ROP. Therefore, we made the recommendation that serum vitamin E levels be raised and maintained in the upper physiologic range (2.5–3 mg/dL) in infants in whom prethreshold ROP develops (16). Because prethreshold ROP usually is not seen before 6 weeks of age, such serum levels can usually be achieved by oral preparations, such as Aquasol E. However, doses as high as 100 mg/k/day (in aliquots) may be necessary initially. It is important to monitor serum vitamin E levels to be sure they are kept within the targeted upper physiologic range.

The end point of this CCT was the development of threshold ROP or worse. This occurred in only 12 infants with a birth weight of 1,500 g or less (2.8%), 9 of 216 (4.2%) placebo-treated infants vs. 3 of 208 (1.4%) vitamin-treated infants. Because of the small sample size, this difference in treatment groups was not statistically significant (P = .08). However, its probable clinical significance was supported by meta-analysis (16, 22, 23) of the other reported controlled clinical trials of vitamin E for ROP (24–28) if the occurrence of threshold ROP or worse was used as the outcome variable (Mantel-Haenszel technique, P < .02 for infants with a birth weight of 1,500 g or less and P < .05 for those with a birth weight of 1,000 g or less).

As we have pointed out elsewhere (23), threshold or greater-than-threshold ROP (as defined by the Cryo-ROP Trial) or worse is the only appropriate end point for comparison of these disparate clinical trials. Threshold ROP is stage 3 ICROP with plus disease (dilatation and tortuosity of posterior retinal vessels) and 5 or more contiguous or 8 discontiguous clock hours of intravitreal neovascularization (8). It carries a 50%

risk of retinal detachment if untreated. The classification systems used in all of the vitamin E/ROP CCTs adequately defined retinopathy of this severity.

In contrast, others have suggested the use of ≥ stage 3 ICROP without plus disease, as the entry point for meta-analysis (28, 29). Stage 3 ROP without plus disease is associated with an 80% incidence of spontaneous regression (30). Furthermore, ROP of this severity was not clearly defined by all of the classification systems in the other trials, which limits the number of trials suitable for meta-analysis. Unfortunately, stage 3 without plus disease, or worse, has been used on several occasions (23, 29, 31) to represent retinopathy severe enough to define the presence or absence of significant treatment effect. This has added to confusion in the field.

Finally, in our CCT, treatment with parenteral α-tocopherol was given to all infants in whom threshold ROP developed, regardless of original treatment group assignment. This was done because previous data had suggested it might decrease the incidence of blindness (13). This meant that the effect of pharmacologic vitamin E prophylaxis on the cicatricial outcome of ROP could not be accurately assessed because the control infants most likely to have severe sequelae (those with threshold ROP) had received treatment at diagnosis (16). With these qualifications and considering the whole population, there was ($P = .07$) a trend toward decreased cicatricial ROP in the vitamin E-treated group. If only infants with cicatricial residua are considered (13 P, 13 E), the extent of residua in vitamin E-treated infants was significantly less ($P < .025$) than that in placebo-assigned infants (22, 32).

Outcome in the placebo-assigned infants with severe ROP again suggested that pharmacologic vitamin E treatment at diagnosis of disease might be helpful. Threshold ROP usually is not seen until after age 8 to 10 weeks (5, 8, 24, 33), when antibacterial defenses are more mature. In addition, treatment at pharmacologic serum vitamin E levels is only continued until clear signs of regression or progressive scarring are present (usually 2–3 weeks). Therefore, it was believed the risk/benefit ratio of pharmacologic serum levels of vitamin E, used in this way, might be favorable and should be further investigated.

In the 1979–1980 CCT of Hittner et al. in Houston, Texas, (24), the mean serum vitamin E level of infants on admission to the ICN was .3mg/dL (× gestational age of 29.4 ± 2.1 weeks). In control infants, serum E levels remained in the deficient range (≤ .6mg/dL) throughout the course of the study. In vitamin E-treated infants in whom serum levels were raised to a mean of 1.2mg/dL from week 1–8, no threshold ROP was seen. However, in subsequent studies, which enrolled increasingly immature infants and in which vitamin E prophylaxis was given to all infants, treatment did not entirely prevent severe ROP. It did however, decrease severity of disease and delay its onset (19, 34).

Insightful ultrastructural, immunofluorescent and biochemical studies were done on the retinas of infants who died during the clinical trials conducted by the Baylor group (19, 34–38). Interstitial retinol binding protein (IRBP) is secreted by photoreceptor cells that have reached the maturity of stage 2 or greater (35, 36). Interstitial retinol binding protein first appears around the optic disk at 20 weeks' gestation, and it can be detected at the ora serrata by approximately 29 weeks' gestation (37, 38). It is believed to be the carrier protein for vitamin E, as well a vitamin A, in immature retina (35–37). The amount of vitamin E that can be transported to the inner avascular, spindle-cell-populated retina is believed to be related to the amount of IRBP present (35–38).

In the Houston trial, those infants who did not receive increased supplements of oral vitamin E before death (gestational age, 22, 22, 22, 23, 23, 26, 27, 28, and 33 weeks), were found to have a retinal vitamin E content (nanomoles of vitamin E per mg of DNA) within a few days after birth, which was far below that found in adults (by a factor of 8 in the central [vascular] region and by a factor of 20 in the peripheral [avascular] region) (37). However, the vitamin E content of the retina did increase slowly with gestational age, from about .25 nanomoles of vitamin E per mg of DNA at 22–23 weeks' gestation to approximately 2.5 nanomoles of vitamin E per mg of DNA at 34 weeks' gestation. In association with these retinal concentrations of vitamin E in utero, differentiation and vascularization proceed without mishap. However, if this normal pattern of development is interrupted by premature delivery into an oxygen-rich and unstable environment, ROP is apt to develop, especially after very preterm birth.

The retinal vitamin E content of vitamin E-treated infants who died in the Baylor clinical trials was significantly increased compared with that of control infants of the same gestational age. Although the increase in retinal vitamin E was much greater in infants who were born at 28 weeks' gestation or more, a modest increase did occur in more immature infants who had been receiving vitamin E supplements for 1 week or more. It was believed that this suboptimal response explained why threshold ROP could be delayed—but not entirely prevented—in infants less than 28 weeks' gestation (19, 34, 38).

It is noteworthy that, in our clinical trial of pharmacologic prophylaxis, the onset of ROP and age at peak disease were also delayed by at least 1 week in vitamin-treated compared with placebo-treated infants (32, 39). If prophylactic maintenance of serum vitamin E levels within the physiologic range (1.3 mg/dL) in infants of more than 28 weeks' gestation can delay the onset and decrease the severity of threshold ROP, its management (by either surgical or medical means) in these very-high-risk infants would be considerably enhanced (39).

Since 1981, management of ROP in our nurseries has been based on the following guidelines:

1. Monitor serum vitamin E levels weekly by microtechnology in infants with a birth weight of 1,251 g or less or a gestational age less than 31 weeks.

2. As soon as possible after birth, raise and maintain the serum vitamin E levels between 1 and 2.5 mg/dL until peripheral retinal vascular maturity or development of prethreshold ROP.

3. Raise serum vitamin E levels to 2.5–3.5 mg/dL if prethreshold ROP develops.

4. Institute pharmacologic vitamin E treatment and obtain retinal consultation for consideration of cryotherapy or laser therapy if threshold ROP develops. Maintain serum vitamin E levels between 4 and 5 mg/dL until clear signs of regression or retinal detachment are noted, whether or not cryotherapy is used. Monitor vitamin E levels on the basis of individual need (usually every other day). For this aspect of the protocol, a parenteral vitamin E preparation is usually necessary.

5. Maintain serum vitamin E levels between 1.5 and 3 mg/dL until age one year or until complete regression of ROP. (This usually requires no more than monthly monitoring.) If total detachment develops, vitamin E supplementation is stopped.

6. Monitor infants closely for any signs of untoward side effects of physiologic or pharmacologic vitamin E treatment (and of cryotherapy or laser therapy) so that adequate supportive or corrective measures can be promptly instituted and risk/benefit ratios can be estimated.

Using this protocol, we have attempted to assess the feasibility of the following:

1. Maintaining a steady or declining incidence of prethreshold and threshold ROP in spite of increased survival of more and more immature infants (birth weight, 800 g or less; gestational age, 26 weeks or less), using the incidence of disease reported in the Cryo/ROP Trial as a reference.

2. Maintaining a steady or decreasing incidence of unfavorable structural and functional outcome after threshold ROP.

3. Slowing the rate of progression, delaying the age at onset, and decreasing the extent of retinopathy among the neonates in whom threshold ROP develops.

4. Maintaining serum vitamin E levels between 2–3 mg/dL until age one year or until complete regression of ROP. If total detachment develops, vitamin E supplementation is stopped.

5. Following infants with prethreshold and threshold ROP for at least 3 years to assess long-term visual outcome.

Our results for the period from 1981 to 1991 have been reported in abstract form for infants with a birth weight less than 1,251 or a birth weight less than 1,001 g (40–43). They have consistently shown an excellent long-term outcome for both retinal structure and visual acuity. Of a total of 528 Pennsylvania Hospital intensive care nursery admissions (birth weight, less than 1,001 g) from 1981 to 1991 (37% of whom had birth weights between 400 and 750 g), 364 survived (survival rate, 69%). Of these 364, 31 had threshold ROP develop (8.2% of survivors with a birth weight less than 1,001 g. Long-term follow-up has been possible in 30 of the 31. The one infant without follow-up (treated only with vitamin E) was last seen at age 6 months. At that time he had resolving ROP with a suggestion of temporal straightening of the retinal vessels.

Of the 30 infants with follow-up, 10 received only vitamin E therapy: in 9 of these, the severity of plus disease was subsiding when seen by the retinal specialist within 48 hours of diagnosis, and cryotherapy was not considered necessary. In the tenth patient (an Asian child born in 1989), scarring was already beginning only 48 hours after diagnosis, and it was decided that cryotherapy would be of no avail in these circumstances. Seven infants had systemic vitamin E therapy as well as cryotherapy or laser therapy on both eyes. Thirteen infants had systemic vitamin E treatment and cryotherapy for one eye. Overall, an unfavorable structural outcome was found in both eyes of only 4 infants (one, systemic vitamin E treatment only; one, systemic vitamin E treatment plus bilateral cryotherapy; and two, systemic vitamin E treatment with unilateral cryotherapy). Unilateral unfavorable structural outcome was found in 2 other infants. One of able structural outcome was found in 2 other infants. One of these eyes had been treated only with vitamin E, and one had been treated with vitamin E plus cryotherapy.

The incidence of mild to moderate retinal residua of ROP (greater than grade 1 Cic but less than grade 3 Cic) was remarkedly low (table). Such abnormalities occurred in 1 eye each of 2 infants in whom the fellow eye was normal. They occurred in the better eye of 2 infants with unilateral unfavorable structure. In these 2 infants, the better eye showed a favorable visual acuity in one and an unfavorable visual acuity in the other. Therefore, in only 5 of the 30 infants was there unfavorable visual acuity in both eyes (5 of 30, or 16.7%). This outcome compares favorably with that being reported for the Cryo-ROP CCT, which has already been described.

The incidence of CNS deficit in these 30 infants, including grade 3–4 intraventricular hemorrhage, was also very low, especially considering the severity of their illness: x days oxygen therapy 112 ± 40, $\bar{x}$ days on ventilatory support 73 ± 34, $\bar{x}$ BW 718 ± 121, $\bar{x}$ GA 25.7 ± 1.9. All infants had bronchopulmonary dysplasia (oxygen therapy over 28 days).

Finally, in infants with a birth weight less than 1,001 g who were cared for at Pennsylvania Hospital from 1981 to 1991, the median age at onset of threshold disease was 11.8 weeks (range, 8–18 weeks). This is a later age than that reported for onset of threshold ROP in infants with a birth weight less than 1,001 g (33) in the Cryo-ROP CCT (10.8 weeks; range, 7.4–15.3 weeks). The mean number of clock hours of fibrovascular proliferation in our infants with a birth weight less than 1,001 g was 7.5 ± 2.5 SD. This is less than the mean clock hours of fibrovascular prolifera-

Structural Retinal Findings 3 Months After Threshold ROP

	Cryo/ROP Trial BW <1251g	PA Hospital BW <1001g	
	Treated Eye* n = 240 Eyes	Vitamin E ± Cryotherapy n = 30 Babies	
		Worse Eye	Better Eye
Unfavorable Structure	31.5%	20.0%	13.3%
Miscellaneous† Abnormalities	32.9%	6.7%	6.7%
Normal	36.0%	73.3%	80.0%

*Multicenter Trial of Cryotherapy for Retinopathy of Prematurity 3-month outcome. *Arch Opthalmol* 108:195–204, 1990.

†Macular heterotopia, small extramacular fold, retinal pigment scarring under center of macula.

(Courtesy of Drs. Johnson, Quinn, and Abbasi.)

tion (9.7 ± 2 SD) reported for infants with a birth weight less than 1,250 g in the Cryo-ROP CCT (breakdown for infants with a birth weight less than 1,001 g not given) (5, 8). However, the percent of infants with threshold disease in zone 1 was 10% in both studies. This strongly suggests that the infants in our study were of comparable immaturity and risk for sight-threatening disease as infants in the 1986–1987 Cryo-ROP CCT. (Pennsylvania Hospital was a participating hospital in that study.)

In sum, we agree that other modalities in addition to cryotherapy need to be explored to decrease the morbidity from ROP in infants with a birth weight less than 1,001 g. We urge that one of those modalities be vitamin E prophylaxis coupled with pharmacologic vitamin E treatment at diagnosis of prethreshold ROP. Evaluation of this approach by a large CCT would include vitamin E prophylaxis at physiologic serum levels from birth onward, using available commerical preparations, with randomization at diagnosis of prethreshold ROP to pharmacologic serum levels, 4–5 mg/dL) vitamin E treatment or no treatment. A parenteral IND preparation of α-tocopherol-free alcohol is available for this study. In the event that threshold ROP develops in any infant in either arm, retinal consultation would be obtained for consideration of cryo- or laser therapy for (1) both eyes of infants randomized to no additional vitamin E; and (2) for one eye of infants assigned to pharmacologic vitamin E therapy at the onset of prethreshold ROP.

Bibliography

1. Horwitt MK: Supplementation with vitamin E. *Am J Clin Nutr* 47:1088–1109, 1988.
2. Lemoyne M, VanGossum A, Kurian R, et al: Breath pentane analysis as an index of lipid peroxidation: A functional test of vitamin E status. *Am J Clin Nutr* 46:267–272, 1987.
3. Jeejeebhoy KN: In vivo breath alkane as an index of lipid peroxidation. *Free Radic Biol Med* 10:191–193, 1991.
4. 1990 YEAR BOOK OF NEONATAL AND PERINATAL MEDICINE, pp 267–269.
5. Cryotherapy for Retinopathy of Prematurity Cooperative Group: Multicenter trial of cryotherapy for retinopathy of prematurity. One-year outcome. *Arch Ophthalmol* 108:1408–1416, 1990.
6. Palmer EA, for the Cryotherapy for Retinopathy of Prematurity Cooperative Group: Multicenter trial of cryotherapy for retinopathy of prematurity: Fundus outcome 3½ years following treatment. *Invest Ophthalmol Vis Sci* vol 33, 1991.
7. Dobson V, for the CRYO-ROP Cooperative Group: Recognition and resolution acuity results at 42 months in treated vs untreated eyes in the cryotherapy for retinopathy of prematurity (Cryo-ROP) trial. *Invest Ophthalmol Vis Sci* 33:1282, 1992.
8. Cryotherapy for Retinopathy of Prematurity Cooperative Group: Multicenter trial of cryotherapy for retinopathy of prematurity. Three-month outcome. *Arch Ophthalmol* 108:195–204, 1990.
9. Tasman W: Threshold retinopathy of prematurity revisited. *Arch Ophthalmol* 110:623–624, 1992.
10. Gilbert WS, Dobson B, Quinn GE, et al: The correlation of visual function with posterior retinal structure in severe retinopathy of prematurity. *Arch Ophthalmol* 110:625–631, 1992.
11. Dobson V, for the CRYO-ROP Cooperative Group: Multicenter trial of cryotherapy for retinopathy of prematurity. 3½ year outcome: Structure and function. *Arch Ophthalmol,* In press.
12. Johnson L, Quinn GE, Abbasi S, et al: Effect of sustained pharmacologic vitamin E levels on incidence and severity of retinopathy of prematurity: A controlled clinical trial. *J Pediatr* 114:827–838, 1989.
13. Johnson L, Schaffer DB, Boggs TR: Vitamin E deficiency and retrolental fibroplasia. *Am J Clin Nutr* 27:1158–1173, 1974.
14. Johnson L, Schaffer D, Quinn GE, et al: Vitamin E supplementation and the retinopathy of prematurity. *Ann N Y Acad Sci* 393:473–495, 1982.
15. Quinn GE, Schaffer DB, Johnson L: A revised classification of retinopathy of prematurity. *Am J Ophthalmol* 94:744–749, 1982.
16. The Committee for the Classification of Retinopathy of Prematurity. An international classification of retinopathy of prematurity. *Pediatrics* 74:127–133, 1984.
17. Johnson L, Bowen FW, Abbasi S, et al: Relationship of prolonged pharmacologic serum levels of vitamin E to incidence of sepsis and necrotizing enterocolitis in infants with birth weight 1,500 grams or less. *Pediatrics* 75:619–638, 1985.
18. Ehrenkranz RA: Vitamin E and retinopathy of prematurity: Still controversial. *J Pediatr* 114:801–803, 1989.
19. Hittner HM, Godio LB, Speer ME, et al: Retrolental fibroplasia: Further clinical evidence and ultrastructural support for efficacy of vitamin E in the preterm infant. *Pediatrics* 71:423–432, 1983.
20. Tocopherol levels of infants ≤ 1000 grams receiving MVI pediatric. *Pediatrics* 90:992–994, 1992.
21. Gerdes JS, Johnson L, Abbasi S, et al: Vitamin E status in neonates ≤ 1250 g BW on hyperalimentation and transition to enteral feedings. *Pediatr Res* 1993.
22. Schaffer DB, Johnson LH, Quinn GE, et al: Retinopathy of prematurity: Problems and challenges, in Flynn J, Phelps D (eds): *Vitamin E and ROP: The Oph-*

thalmologist's Perspective. March of Dimes Birth Defects Original Article Series, 24:219–235, 1988.

23. Johnson L, Quinn GE, Abbasi S, et al: Vitamin E and retinopathy of prematurity. *Pediatrics* 81:329–331, 1988.
24. Hittner HM, Godio LB, Rudolph AJ, et al: Retrolental fibroplasia: Efficacy of vitamin E in a double-blind clinical study of preterm infants. N *Engl J Med* 305:1365–1371, 1981.
25. Milner RA, Watts JL, Paes B, et al: RLF in 1500 gram neonates: Part of a randomized clinical trial of the effectiveness of vitamin E, in *Retinopathy of Prematurity Conference Syllabus, vol* 2. Washington D.C., December 4–6, 1981, pp 703–716.
26. Finer NN, Schindler RF, Grant G, et al: Effect of intramuscular vitamin E on frequency and severity of retrolental fibroplasia: A controlled trial. *Lancet* 1:1087–1091, 1982.
27. Puklin JE, Simon RM, Ehrenkranz RA: Influence on retrolental fibroplasia of intramuscular vitamin E administration during respiratory distress syndrome. *Ophthalmology* 89:96–102, 1982.
28. Phelps DL, Rosenbaum AL, Isenberg SJ, et al: Tocopherol efficacy and safety for preventing retinopathy of prematurity: A randomized, controlled, double-masked trial. *Pediatrics* 79:489–500, 1987.
29. Phelps DL: Vitamin E in retinopathy of prematurity, in Silverman WA, Flynn FT (eds): *Controversies in Fetal and Neonatal Medicine: Retinopathy of Prematurity.* Boston, Blackwell Scientific Publications, 1985, pp 181–205.
30. Multicenter trial of cryotherapy for retinopathy of prematurity. Commentary. *Pediatrics* 77:428–429, 1986.
31. Sinclar J, Bracken MB (eds): *Retinopathy of Prematurity: Effective Care of the Newborn Infant.* Oxford, England, Oxford Univ Press, 1992, pp 618–638.
32. Quinn GE, Johnson L, Otis C, et al: Incidence, severity and time course of ROP in a randomized clinical trial of vitamin E prophylaxis. *Doc Ophthalmol* 74:223–228, 1990.
33. Palmer EA, Flynn JT, Hardy RJ, et al: Incidence and early course of retinopathy of prematurity. *Ophthalmology* 98:1628–1640, 1991.
34. Hittner HM, Rudolph AJ, Kretzer FL: Suppression of severe retinopathy of prematurity with vitamin E supplementation. Ultrastructural mechanism of clinical efficacy. *Ophthalmology* 91:1512–1523, 1984.
35. Johnson AT, Kretzer FL, Hittner HM, et al: Development of the subretinal space in the preterm human eye: Ultrastructural and immunocytochemical studies. *J Comp Neurol* 233:497–505, 1985.
36. Kretzer FL, McPherson AR, Hittner HM: An interpretation of retinopathy of prematurity in terms of spindle cells: Relationship to vitamin E prophylaxis and cryotherapy. *Graefes Arch Clin Exp Ophthalmol* 224:205–214, 1986.
37. Nielsen JC, Naash MI, Anderson RE: The reginal distribution of vitamins E and C in mature and premature human retinas. *Invest Ophthalmol Vis Sci* 29:22–26, 1987.
38. Kretzer FL, Hittner HM: Retinopathy of prematurity: Clinical implications of retinal development. *Arch Dis Child* 63:1151–1167, 1988.
39. Quinn GE, Johnson L, Abbasi S, et al: Onset of retinopathy of prematurity as related to postnatal and postconceptional age. *Br J Ophthalmol* 76:284–288, 1992.
40. Johnson L, Quinn G, Abbasi S, et al: Treatment modalities for severe retinopathy of prematurity. *Pediatr Res* 27:210A, 1990.
41. Quinn G, Johnson L, Tasman W, et al: Improved outcome of severe ROP with medical as well as surgical Rx. *Pediatr Res* 31:218A, 1992.
42. Johnson L, Quinn G, Abbasi S, et al: Severe retinopathy of prematurity (ROP) in $\leq$ 1000 g birth weight (BW) infants. *Invest Ophthalmol Vis Sci* 33:S1085, 1992.

Featured Abstract

Childhood Cancer, Intramuscular Vitamin K, and Pethidine Given During Labour

Golding J, Greenwood R, Birmingham K, Mott M (Royal Hosp for Sick Children, Bristol, England)

BMJ 305:341–346, 1992

Background.—In a study of a national birth cohort delivered in 1970, an unexpected association was noted between childhood cancer and meperidine given in labor and the prophylactic administration of vitamin K during the neonatal period. To investigate further, all children with a diagnosis of cancer in 1971 to March 1991 and born from 1965 to 1987 in 2 major Bristol maternity hospitals were studied.

Methods.—The odds ratios for cancer in the presence of administration of meperidine or intramuscular vitamin K were obtained for 195 children with cancer and 558 controls, using both logistic regression and Mantel-Haenszel techniques for statistical analyses.

Results.—After adjustment for year of birth and hospital of delivery, the risk of cancer was not increased in children of mothers given meperidine during labor (odds ratio, 1.05; 95% confidence interval, .7–1.5). However, there was an overall significant association between cancer and intramuscular vitamin K administration, with an odds ratio of 1.97 (95% confidence interval, 1.28–3.04) relative to oral vitamin K or no vitamin K administration. There was only minimal difference in risk between oral vitamin K and no vitamin K. The excess risk of cancer associated with intramuscular vitamin K could not be explained by other factors previously associated with administration of vitamin K, such as type of delivery or admission to a special-care nursery.

Discussion.—A similar relation between childhood cancer and intramuscular vitamin K has been reported previously in 2 studies, suggesting that the relation is biologically plausible. Because the potential adverse effects from intramuscular vitamin K far outweigh the prophylactic benefits against hemorrhagic disease, and because oral vitamin K does not carry the same risk of inducing malignancy but provides protection as well, it is prudent to use oral rather than intramuscular vitamin K for prophylaxis.

▶ Frank Greer M.D., Professor of Pediatrics at the University of Wisconsin, has been closely following this vitamin K saga. He was eager to make the following contribution and provide incisive analysis of the current status of vitamin K:

▶ This article by Golding and colleagues from southwestern England has questioned the safety of the routine use of intramuscularly administered vitamin K for the newborn infant, a standard of care that has been present in the United States for more than 30 years. There is no question that intramuscular administration of vitamin K prevents hemorrhagic disease in the newborn, whether it is the classic (early) or late form of the disease. However, in this paper, the authors have produced evidence that the intramuscular administration of vitamin K (as opposed to oral or no vitamin K prophylaxis) has resulted in a significantly increased rate of childhood cancer in infants born in 2 hospitals in Bristol, England.

In the Golding study, 217 infants born between 1965 and 1987 at 2 hospitals were given a diagnosis of cancer between 1971 and 1989. A total of 180 of these infants were compared with a control group of 507 infants born in the 2 hospitals during the same period. Although well done, this epidemiologic study of childhood cancer is weakened by its limited sample size from a very small area of England. There are no statistics supporting an overall increase in childhood cancer cases in England during this period. In fact, there are national data that do not support the Golding conclusion (1). Furthermore, neither hospital had a routine, consistent policy for newborn vitamin K prophylaxis during the years studied. In one of the hospitals, infants with potentially traumatic deliveries (e.g., by cesarean section, forceps, or vacuum extraction) were far more likely to receive intramuscular vitamin K prophylaxis. The authors did rule out a number of potentially complicating variables, including the use of pethidine (meperidine hydrochloride), maternal smoking, maternal x-ray films of the abdomen or pelvis during pregnancy, type of delivery, infant resuscitation, and infant admission to an intensive care unit.

The authors conclude that, in this regional population, the relative risk ratio for acute lymphocytic leukemia in the intramuscular vitamin K group compared with the combined oral and no prophylaxis groups was 2.65 (95% confidence interval, 1.34–5.24). Furthermore, the relative risk ratio for all other forms of childhood cancer and intramuscular administration of vitamin K was 1.72 (95% confidence interval, 1.04–2.84). From these data, the authors arrive at an eye-popping speculation: In a country such as Great Britain, which has 700,000 annual deliveries, the routine use of intramuscular vitamin K prophylaxis would result in 980 extra cases of childhood cancer in these infants before 10 years of age.

Despite these data, is there evidence that vitamin K_1 (phylloquinone) is a human carcinogen? Not surprisingly, there is little basic research evaluating the carcinogenic potential of vitamin K_1. Recent studies implicating vitamin K_1 as an agent that increases sister chromatid exchanges in human and animal lymphocytes are contradictory (2, 3). Sister chromatid exchanges are related to mutagenesis, a process leading up to carcinogenesis. In the Golding study, all of the infants received vitamin K_1. The specific intramuscular preparation used was Konakion (Hoffman-LaRoche, Basel, Switzerland), the vehicle of which includes castor oil, proplylene glycol, and phenol. The possibility that one of the vehicular chemicals is carcinogenic, or in combination with vitamin K_1 is carcinogenic, has not been excluded. It is also puzzling that the Golding study found that vitamin K was associated with an increased incidence of *most* forms of childhood cancer. Such an association of a single agent with a wide variety of cancer types is unprecedented, both in children exposed to ionizing radiation (the atomic bomb) and in adults exposed to various human carcinogens.

Finally, one must address what this study means for newborns routinely receiving intramuscular vitamin K in the United States today. In the first place, there is no alternative oral form of vitamin K available in this country. However, it is likely that one will soon be available for testing. Unfortunately, more than a single oral dose of vitamin K in infancy will be needed as prophylaxis for hemorrhagic disease, especially in those infants who are exclusively breast-fed. Formula-fed infants may need no additional supplementation. In the second place, there is no evidence that the incidence of acute lymphocytic leukemia (ALL) has increased in the United States during the period of near universal use of intramuscular vitamin K prophylaxis. It is true that there is no composite national database for cases of childhood leukemia occurring during the past 30 years; however, regional data compiled during this period in various parts of the country do not show any increased incidence of ALL. In fact, the incidence of ALL in the United States (taken from regional data) indicates that it has remained constant since the late 1940s (4). It must also be pointed out that the most widely used form of vitamin K_1 in the United States is Aquamephyton (Merck & Co, Westpoint, Pennsylvania), which differs from the supplement used in the British study in that it contains a different vehicle (polyoxyethylated fatty acid derivative, dextrose, benzyl alcohol).

The American Academy of Pediatrics ad hoc task force on vitamin K recently published a strong recommendation that vitamin K_1 should continue to be given to all newborns as a single intramuscular injection (5). At present, there seems to be no reason to disagree with this recommendation, considering all the available evidence. More basic research evaluating vitamin K as a carcinogen in the laboratory is needed. In addition, as oral forms of vitamin K become available in the United States, it is likely (for a number of reasons) that its use will increase throughout the newborn population. Therefore, research in the area of the efficacy and bioavailability of oral preparations of vitamin K is needed immediately.—F. Greer, M.D.

References

1. Draper GJ, Stiller CA. Intramuscular vitamin K and childhood cancer, *BMJ* 305:705, 1992.
2. Israels LG, Friesen E, Jansen AH, et al: Vitamin K1 increases sister chromatid exchange in vitro in human leukocytes and in vivo in fetal sheep cells: A possible role for "vitamin K deficiency" in the fetus. *Pediatr Res* 22:405–408, 1987.
3. Cornelissen M, Smeets D, Merx G, et al: Analysis of chromosome aberrations and sister chromatid exchanges in peripheral blood lymphocytes of new borns after vitamin K prophylaxis at birth. *Pediatr Res* 30:550–552, 1991.
4. Devesa SS, Silverman DT, Young JL Jr, et al: Cancer incidence and mortality trends among whites in the United States, 1947–1984. *J Natl Cancer Inst* 79:701–770, 1987.

5. American Academy of Pediatrics Ad Hoc Task Force: Controversies concerning vitamin K and the newborn. *Pediatrics* 1993. In press.

► Also commenting on this featured article is Thomas B. Newman, M.D., M.P.H., Associate Professor of Laboratory Medicine, Pediatrics, Epidemiology, and Biostatistics, University of California, San Francisco:

► In this paper, Professor Golding and colleagues report the results of a case-control study of the association between perinatal intramuscular administration of vitamin K and childhood cancer. The study was performed to confirm the results of 2 unexpected findings in a previous cohort study done by the same investigators: associations between childhood risk of cancer and the receipt of either pethidine (meperidine) or vitamin K. The association with pethidine was not confirmed, but the association between vitamin K and a 10-year risk of cancer was again noted and was statistically significant (odds ratio [OR], approximately 2; $P = .002$). The association was most pronounced for leukemia (OR, 2.65; 95% confidence interval [CI], 1.34–5.24), but it was also significant for other cancers (OR, 1.72; 95% CI, 1.04–2.84)

In discussing the implications of these results, it is helpful to distinguish between *internal validity* and *external validity. Internal validity* addresses the question: Is the association found in the study valid in the study itself? That is, among children born at 2 hospitals in Bristol in the years covered by the study, were those who received intramuscular vitamin K (specifically Konakion, the Hoffman-LaRoche preparation) more likely to have cancer develop? *External validity* addresses how likely it is that the results could be generalized to other times, places, and preparations.

I went over this article at length, but I could not find any significant threats to its internal validity. I also do not believe that any of the letters to the editor regarding this paper contain criticisms of the study design or analysis that would invalidate the results. This is perhaps not surprising given the eminence of the investigators: Jean Golding is the editor of *Paediatric and Perinatal Epidemiology.*

There is always the possibility of confounding in an observational epidemiologic study, but it is hard to come up with a plausible confounder to explain these results. Such a confounder would have to be both a strong cause of childhood cancer and strongly associated with receipt of intramuscular vitamin K. Receipt of intramuscular vitamin K seems to have been determined to a large extent by type of delivery (spontaneous or not), admission to the special care nursery, and by the hospital and year of the infant's birth. However, neither type of delivery nor admission to the special-care nursery was associated with risk of cancer, so these could not be responsible for the association. Also, hospital and year of birth were controlled in the analysis by stratifying: cases with cancer were compared only with controls who were from the same hospital and born the same year. To the extent that the factors determining vitamin K exposure are known to be unrelated to risk of cancer, the strength of causal inference from this study approaches that of a randomized trial.

There is, of course, the possibility that the observed association was a chance finding. This was a fine explanation for the cohort study finding, which the authors themselves refer to as a result of "data trawling." However, the present study was specifically undertaken (and funded by Hoffman-LaRoche) to address the question of cancer risk associated with vitamin K, and the low *P* value in this second study should make us reluctant to cling to chance as an explanation for the findings.

One criticism of the association is that it is not "biologically plausible." For example, vitamin K gives a negative Ames' test for mutagenicity. Although this is a bit reassuring, I don't think it exonerates vitamin K. Nor am I very reassured by the argument that it is not plausible for vitamin K to cause so many different kinds of cancer, because ionizing radiation and cigarette smoke cause plenty of different kinds. The part most difficult for me to believe is that anything as easy as eliminating intramuscularly administered vitamin K could cut childhood cancer in half. This seems too good to be true.

The bottom line for internal validity is that however implausible vitamin K carcinogenicity is, the question remains: Given the results of this study, what else could it be? I have trouble thinking of a more plausible basis than a cause-and-effect relationship for the association in this study.

What about external validity? Here there is at least one important reassuring point. In a letter to the editor (1), Robert Miller notes that there was no increase in the reported incidence of leukemia in 5 surveillance areas in the United States during the period after the adoption of widespread use of intramuscularly administered vitamin K. Perhaps this is because the preparation of vitamin K most commonly used in the United States (Merck's Aquamephyton) is different from that used in the United Kingdom.

How should the results of this study affect clinical practice? One line of argument suggests that the risk of hemorrhagic disease of the newborn is certain and the risk of cancer is not; therefore, we should not change our practice. However, as pointed out in a letter by Lilford and Thornton (2), cancer is so much more common than hemorrhagic disease of the newborn that even a small chance of doubling the risk of cancer may not be worth taking. Using numbers from the paper by Golding et al. and the letters that followed it, use of oral, rather than intramuscular, vitamin K might result in about 1.3 additional cases of late-onset hemorrhagic disease per 100,000. On the other hand, if vitamin K doubled the risk of cancer, it would cause an additional 140 cases of cancer cases per 100,000! Thus, even if there is only a 1% chance that the observed doubling of the risk of cancer associated with intramuscular vitamin K is real, the expected number of cases of cancer caused by vitamin K exceeds the number of cases of hemorrhagic disease prevented. The same is true if there is only a 10% chance of a 10% increase in risk (i.e., a relative risk of 1.1). It is pretty hard to be confident that this is not the case.

A final point, made in part in a letter to the *British Medical Journal* by H.P. Dunn (3), is that the risk associated with intramuscular vitamin K is not just the risk of the vitamin K, nor is it that risk plus the risk of the benzyl alcohol, propylene glycol, phenol, or whatever else it is mixed with. There are also the risks of the injection itself—injection of the wrong substance, infections, sterile abscesses, inadvertent intravenous administration (which a boxed warning in the prescribing information warns can be fatal), and risk of needle sticks to staff.

After discussing all of these issues in a journal club, we decided to begin giving the vitamin K orally. We were concerned both about giving intramuscular vitamin K without informed consent, and about the amount of time and effort that consent process would take. However, we have since reluctantly switched back. Giving the intramuscular preparation by mouth was difficult; the infants spit it out, gagged, and sometimes vomited. Also, with the statement of the American Academy of Pediatrics strongly recommending continued use of intramuscular vitamin K, it became clear that we would need to get informed consent to give the vitamin K orally. With newborn stays often lasting less than 24 hours, we just didn't think it was feasible to go through this issue with parents. We hope that this association is not real in the United States, and we join the American Academy of Pediatrics in urging pharmaceutical companies to develop an oral dosage form.—T.B. Newman, M.D., M.P.H.

References

1. Miller R: *BMJ* 305:1016, 1992.
2. Lilford, Thornton: *BMJ* 305:890, 1992.
3. Dunn HP: *BMJ* 305:710, 1992.

1 The Fetus

Percutaneous Umbilical Blood Sampling: Results From a Multicenter Collaborative Registry

Hickok DE, for the Western Collaborative Perinatal Group (Swedish Hosp Med Ctr, Seattle)

Am J Obstet Gynecol 166:1614–1618, 1992 1–1

Introduction.—The safety of percutaneous umbilical blood sampling for the evaluation of fetal health has been largely established in single centers with extensive experience of only a few operators. The Western Perinatal Collaborative Group maintains a registry of percutaneous umbilical blood sampling at its 13 member institutions. The data from this multicenter collaborative registry were used to assess the safety and effectiveness of percutaneous umbilical blood sampling.

Findings.—From 1986 through 1990, a total of 302 percutaneous umbilical blood samplings were performed between 16 and 39 weeks of gestation. The most frequent indications for the procedure included Rh and non-Rh isoimmunization, intrauterine growth retardation, nonimmune hydrops, fetal anomalies, neural tube defects, and idiopathic

Primary Indication for Percutaneous Umbilical Blood Sampling ($n = 302$)

Indication	*No.*
Rh isoimmunization	65
Intrauterine growth retardation	45
Non-Rh isoimmunization	44
Nonimmune hydrops	31
Multiple anomalies	22
Neural tube defects	21
Idiopathic thrombocytopenic purpura	20
Abnormal amniocentesis	12
Other*	42

*Includes (fewer than 10 each) cardiac malformations, congenital infections, pleural effusions, fetal distress, alloimmune thrombocytopenia, hemoglobinopathies, and metabolic disorder risks.

(Courtesy of Hickok DE, for the Western Collaborative Perinatal Group: *Am J Obstet Gynecol* 166:1614–1618, 1992.)

thrombocytopenia purpura (table). The procedure was successfully performed in 93.7% of cases, most frequently with a 22-gauge needle (81.6%) Samples were obtained from the cord adjacent to the placenta in 89.6%. Immediate procedural complications included transient streaming of blood from the cord in 89.4%, but it persisted for longer than 1 minute in only 10.6% of cases. Fetal heart rate changes were infrequent (7%). There were 6 (2.1%) fetal deaths within 3 days of the procedure; 4 deaths were associated with fetal anomalies and 2 with severe Rh isoimmunization.

Conclusion.—This collaborative multicenter study confirms the safety of percutaneous umbilical blood sampling. The procedure-related complications and intrauterine deaths compare favorably with previous reports.

▶ This represents an interesting collaborative effort. It's a little disconcerting to note that the Western Collaborative Group is composed of 13 member institutions. Only 6 contributed cases and 3 were acknowledged. Was this an oversight, or do some of the contributors wish to remain anonymous? Perhaps the objective was to comply with editorial staff requests to restrict the number of authors.

The spectrum of fetal tissue and blood sampling includes amniocentesis, chorionic villus sampling, percutaneous umbilical blood sampling, and fetal tissue biopsy. The perpetual problem is to weigh the cost/benefit ratio. Whereas it could be argued that the report outlined in this abstract represents an outstanding achievement (success rate, 93.7%) a counter argument would commence with the postprocedural death rate of 2.1%. It is mandatory that strict quality assurance is maintained for all these invasive procedures. Indications for percutaneous umbilical blood sampling have been evolving since the initial reports from Daffos and colleagues appeared.

While one person hesitates because he feels inferior, the other is busy making mistakes and becoming a superior.—Henry C. Link

A.A. Fanaroff, M.B.B.Ch.

Value of Routine Ultrasound Scanning at 19 Weeks: A Four Year Study of 8849 Deliveries

Luck CA (Heatherwood Hosp, Ascot, England)

BMJ 304:1474–1478, 1992 1–2

Introduction.—The effectiveness of routine obstetric ultrasound scanning at 19 weeks' gestation had been evaluated only in major tertiary referral centers. The value of ultrasound scanning at 19 weeks' gestation has now been studied in an unselected population.

Methods.—During a 4-year period, a total of 8,849 mothers attending a general hospital were offered ultrasound scanning, and 8,523 (96%)

accepted. The findings were recorded in close cooperation with obstetricians and pediatricians. Maternal serum levels of α-fetoprotein were also recorded. Cases with fetal cardiac anomalies or certain other complex anomalies were referred to tertiary centers.

Results.—A total of 166 fetal anomalies were recorded at delivery or in the first week of life, and 140 of these were detected by ultrasound at 19 weeks' gestation. The sensitivity of ultrasound at 19 weeks' gestation was 85%, and specificity was 99.9%. Twenty-seven women had fetuses with severely crippling or lethal abnormalities, and 25 requested termination of the pregnancy. Arrangements for early surgical or medical intervention were made for fetuses with less severe anomalies. Counseling was available for all patients.

Conclusion.—Routine ultrasound scanning at 19 weeks' gestation has a relatively high level of accuracy for diagnosing fetal anomalies and also helps reduce perinatal mortality and morbidity. Genetic counseling and pregnancy termination must be made available to all pregnant women.

► Although scanning is available to high-risk pregnant women in many parts of the world, routine scanning is offered to pregnant women at only a few centers. The medical and financial advantages of routine scanning are being closely scrutinized. The prevailing data have shifted opinion in the direction of routine screening because it is apparently cost effective, allegedly harmless, and 90% of malformations occur in fetuses born to mothers who have no recognizable risk factors. This abstracted report further tilts the consensus toward routine screening.

As in the study from Finland (1), compliance was excellent and 96% of eligible women were screened by 2.5 "ultrasound technicians" supported by the author, a radiologist—a modest staff by any measures. The scan at 19 weeks determined fetal growth parameters and consisted of a full fetal anatomy scan and a four-chamber view of the heart. The accuracy was high, and the screening changed obstetric management by altering both the timing and the site of delivery. No screening process is infallible, and according to Dr Luck, "Parents should realise that screening has been performed to detect unknown risks, for the benefit of the mother and the fetus." Her plea for a dedicated counseling room and for the screening to be performed by "trained, experienced ultrasonographers in the right environment with full radiologic, obstetric, and pediatric support" must be heeded for other centers to emulate the high standards achieved in this prospective study.

It is only those who never do anything who never make mistakes.—A. Favre

A.A. Fanaroff, M.B.B.Ch.

Reference

1. 1991 Year Book of Neonatal and Perinatal Medicine, pp 89–90.

Birth of a Normal Girl After In Vitro Fertilization and Preimplantation Diagnostic Testing for Cystic Fibrosis

Handyside AH, Lesko JG, Tarin JJ, Winston RML, Hughes MR (Hammersmith Hosp, London; Methodist Hosp, Houston, Tex)

N Engl J Med 327:905–909, 1992 1–3

Background.—Cystic fibrosis (CF) remains the most common potentially lethal autosomal recessive disease in whites. A majority of cases are caused by a 3-nucleotide deletion (ΔF508) in the CF transmembrane regulator gene. Previously, prenatal diagnosis has entailed chorionic villus sampling or amniocentesis.

Objective.—The first attempts at preimplantation diagnosis of CF after in vitro fertilization were made in 3 couples in which both partners carried the ΔF508 deletion. Each of them had at least 1 affected child. The women were in their mid-30s, and wished to minimize the risk of having to terminate an affected pregnancy.

Methods.—In vitro fertilization was used to recover oocytes and fertilize them with the husband's sperm. Embryos in the cleavage stage were biopsied 3 days after insemination, removing 1 or 2 cells for DNA amplification and analysis. A protocol for nested polymerase chain reaction was used to enhance amplification and minimize nonspecific DNA products.

Results.—In 1 instance, 2 oocytes were fertilized normally; DNA analysis of 1 embryo failed, and CF was diagnosed in the other. Oocytes from each of the other women produced noncarrier, carrier, and affected embryos. In each case, 1 noncarrier embryo and 1 carrier embryo were transferred. One of those women conceived and delivered a girl free of the deletion in both chromosomes, and free of CF.

Conclusion.—When either a single genetic defect has been sequenced or a marker closely linked with the defect has been characterized, the prospect for detecting the defect is encouraging.

▶ The full scope of our abilities to alter "Mother Nature" is vividly illustrated in this report and is, in part, a view of the future. If health-care costs are to be kept at a reasonable level, only a small proportion of parents will be able to control and manipulate the future of their children as these parents have been able to manage.—M.H. Klaus, M.D.

Preconception and Preimplantation Diagnosis for Cystic Fibrosis

Verlinsky Y, Rechitsky S, Evsikov S, White M, Cieslak J, Lifchez A, Valle J, Moise J, Strom CM (Illinois Masonic Med Ctr, Chicago)

Prenat Diagn 12:103–110, 1992 1–4

Background.—Refinements of techniques for embryo handling, in vitro fertilization (IVF), and the polymerase chain reaction (PCR) now permit the use of preconception and preimplantation genetic analysis for human gametes and pre-embryos. This type of analysis provides an alternative for high-risk couples to prenatal diagnosis with termination of affected fetuses. Analysis usually involves the first polar body; however, in some circumstances, blastomere biopsy must also be used. Preimplantation diagnosis for the ΔF508 mutation, which causes most cases of cystic fibrosis, was done on a research basis for 5 couples.

Methods.—The 5 couples who volunteered for preimplantation diagnosis included 4 couples who had had an affected child and 1 with a member who was heterozygous for the ΔF508 mutation. All underwent in vitro fertilization. Removal of the first polar body from oocytes was performed before the oocytes were inseminated. At about 39 hours after insemination, diploid embryos were transferred to the patient if the first polar body was homozygous for the mutation. Other embryos were biopsied, and the blastocysts were frozen. Embryo biopsies were performed at the 4- to 8-cell stage. Blastomeres and polar bodies were tested for the presence of the abnormal gene using PCR.

Results.—Ten patient cycles were compared with those of 40 controls who underwent IVF without polar body removal. No significant differences were found in the fertilization rate, the percentage of embryos entering cleavage, or the percentage of polyspermic embryos. Diagnostic attempts with 22 polar bodies resulted in success in 18 cases. Ultimately, blastomere biopsy resulted in correct diagnosis of 3 additional embryos.

Conclusion.—Preimplantation and preconception diagnosis seems safe and accurate based on preliminary research findings. These techniques should therefore be applied to clinical practice for patients at risk for genetic disorders.

► The frontiers of science are changing at a giddying pace. The latest technologic breakthrough permits preembryonic diagnosis. Preconception and preimplantation genetic diagnosis can be offered to couples who are at high risk for genetic disorders, as indicated above. One of the techniques has been dubbed BABI (*B*lastomere *A*nalysis *B*efore *I*mplantation). In this abstracted report, the oocytes were tested before in vitro fertilization. To paraphrase Verlinsky, "preconception diagnosis by polar body removal has clear advantages over blastomere biopsy as the first polar body has no known function in embryonic development, does not damage the developing embryo and the genetic analysis is complete well within the window of opportunity for implanting the embryo." This preliminary study confirmed the feasibility of preconception and preimplantation diagnosis so that unaffected embryos can be implanted and an undesired genetic disorder can be avoided. No doubt, the techniques will soon be available for sperm in addition to oocytes. In vitro fertilization has brought much joy to infertile couples. The application can now be extended to couples at risk for genetic disorders.

Their future is still in the grip of the past, just as the secret of the oak is folded within the acorn.—Landon Y. Jones

A.A. Fanaroff, M.B.B.Ch.

Fetal Outcome After In Utero Exposure to Cancer Chemotherapy

Zemlickis D, Lishner M, Degendorfer P, Panzarella T, Sutcliffe SB, Koren G
(Univ of Toronto; Princess Margaret Hosp, Toronto)

Arch Intern Med 152:573–576, 1992 1–5

Introduction.—Cancer is the second most frequent cause of death of women in their reproductive years. This historic cohort study examined the fetal effects of chemotherapy in women treated for cancer in 1958–1987.

Methods.—Data on 21 women who were pregnant when given chemotherapy for cancer were compared with those of control women matched for age who were not exposed to teratogens during pregnancy. The most frequent malignancies were breast cancer, Hodgkin's disease, melanoma, and leukemia.

Results.—Of 13 women treated in the first trimester, 4 had spontaneous abortions and 4 others had therapeutic abortion. Two exposed pregnancies resulted in major malformations (hydrocephalus and cardiac anomalies), which were fatal in both patients. Of 4 women treated in the second trimester, 1 had a stillborn infant and 1 had therapeutic abortion. All 4 women receiving chemotherapy in the third trimester had normal infants. Both gestational age and birth weight tended to be lower in the chemotherapy group. Infants of treated women were more likely to be below the 50th birth weight centile.

Conclusion.—Stillbirths and major birth defects are more likely when the mother is given chemotherapy during the time of embryogenesis, but apparently not after the first trimester. Women treated for cancer should be closely monitored to determine the best time for delivery.

▶ The important subject of fetal outcome after chemotherapy has received scant attention. The published reports have been hampered by methodologic problems relating to sample sizes, incomplete records of fetal outcome, and single case descriptions. Over a 30-year period, Zemlick and colleagues have assembled a complete, if somewhat diminutive, series with controls. Overall, there was increased fetal wastage via spontaneous or induced abortion and stillbirth. There also was a greater prevalence of prematurity and malformations. Chemotherapy or radiation therapy during the first trimester poses the biggest hazard to the fetus.

The authors' experience provides some insightful material to guide both perinatal health-care providers and parents who are confronted by a malignancy in pregnancy (1–3). The situation truly represents double jeopardy, because any delay in the diagnosis and institution of therapy may be detrimental to the mother, whereas the aggressive intervention that is mandated can harm the fetus. The first concern should be to ensure timely and appropriate therapy for the mother. Pregnancy in a woman with a malignancy is psychodynamically devastating, because she must simultaneously deal with her own grief and yet attempt to celebrate the forthcoming arrival of a new baby. Breast-feeding may pose another quandary, as some of the chemotherapeutic agents are excreted in breast milk.—A.A. Fanaroff, M.B.B.Ch.

References

1. Doll DC, et al: *Arch Intern Med* 148:2058, 1988.
2. Mulvihill JJ, et al: *Cancer* 60:1143, 1987.
3. Sutton R, et al: *Cancer* 65:847, 1990.

Favourable Outcome in 33 Triplet Pregnancies Managed Between 1985–1990

Boulot P, Hedon B, Pelliccia G, Sarda P, Montoya F, Mares P, Humeau C, Arnal F, Laffargue F, Viala JL (Hopital St Charles, Montpellier, France)
Eur J Obstet Gynecol Reprod Biol 43:123–129, 1992 1–6

Background.—The use of ovulation-inducing agents and in vitro fertilization has resulted in an increased incidence of triplet gestations. Triplet pregnancies are considered "high risk" to both the mother and fetuses, and selective embryonic reduction has been reported in these cases. The management and successful outcome in 33 triplet pregnancies were reviewed.

Method.—The average age of the mother in the 33 triplet pregnancies was 30.1 years. The pregnancies were initiated by in vitro fertilization in 26 cases, by gamete intrafallopian transfer in 1 case, by induction of ovulation in 3 cases, and spontaneously in 3 cases. At the first consultation, patients were informed of the risks of the pregnancy and leave from work and reduction of maternal physical activity was recommended. The women were hospitalized at 28 weeks. Progesterone and β-mimetic drugs were given from 20 weeks until the end of pregnancy and caesarean delivery was performed in all cases.

Outcome.—There were 94 live and 2 dead fetuses delivered. One late abortion occurred at 21 weeks. Perinatal mortality was 4.16%. Birth order is one of the most important factors for neonatal outcome, with the first triplet less vulnerable than the others. The rate of prematurity was 90.6%, with a mean gestational age at delivery of 34.1 weeks. Ninety-one of 92 infants alive after 6 months were healthy; 1 infant had severe mental retardation as a result of prematurity.

Conclusion.—The main problem in triplet pregnancies is the high rate of premature deliveries, but the perinatal mortality in this series of 33 pregnancies was only 4.16%. Careful management is recommended to prolong the pregnancy and to avoid prematurity. Early diagnosis by means of a vaginal scan is important because it allows a reduction in maternal activity. Prolonged hospitalization with ambulatory nursing until

28 weeks and definitive hospitalization for the third trimester appeared efficacious to prevent preterm labor. Progesterone and β-mimetics were used to prevent respiratory distress and prematurity. Only cesarean delivery was permitted. Further research is recommended for assessment of the efficacy of bedrest, progesterone, and β-mimetics used to prevent preterm labor in multiple pregnancies.

▶ Multiple gestations are influenced by race, maternal age, and fertility drugs. In vitro fertilization has resulted in the influx of many multiple gestations (greater than twins) into the neonatal intensive care unit. They present a considerable clinical challenge to the perinatal team. Multiple gestations currently account for almost 20% of low-birth-weight admissions (1) and contribute to perinatal morbidity and mortality disproportionately. According to the National Center for Health Statistics, after reviewing the deliveries from 1972 to 1989, the number of triplets has increased by 156%, quadruplets by 356%, and quintuplets by 182%. The reproductive endocrinologists implant many eggs, which accounts for this quantum leap in the incidence of multiple gestation.

Although the outcome reported by Boulet is spectacular, not all multiple gestations have a happy ending. The mortality is much greater, for example, with monochorionic twins. Determining zygosity is a worthwhile endeavor, because clinical problems can then be anticipated. The process is not that complicated, and it can usually be accomplished by careful examination of the placenta and membranes. The membranes appear translucent when there is a amniotic, monochorionic twin placenta and the amniotic membranes can easily be stripped from the chorion. A monochorionic twin placenta denotes an increased risk for fetal growth discordancy, twin-to-twin transfusion, and other short-term problems. Perhaps of more consequence is the increased risk of neurologic damage (2, 3). The number of fetuses determines the time at which intrauterine growth retardation commences; hence, triplets will manifest growth failure (or intrauterine growth restriction, which is the new terminology) late in the second trimester (4). The survival rates of monochorionic twins do not decrease after 30 weeks' gestation (5). Careful monitoring of the pregnancy and the well-being of the fetuses using ultrasound, physical profile scoring, and the liberal use of bedrest (6), tocolytics, and steroids has improved the outlook for most of these triplet pregnancies.

However, when everything goes smoothly, prematurity is avoided, and the triplets breeze through their nursery stay, the perinatal team transfers the problems to the family. All reproductive endocrinologists should be forced to visit the family at home and attend a follow-up visit involving 2-year-old triplets. The physical and emotional energy needed to care for this instant family is prodigious. I have the greatest admiration for families who endure infancy with triplets.—A.A. Fanaroff, M.B.B.Ch.

References

1. Hack M, et al: *Pediatrics* 87:587, 1991.
2. 1991 Year Book of Neonatal and Perinatal Medicine, pp 162–163.

3. Anderson RL, et al: *Prenat Diagn* 10:513, 1990.
4. Rodis JF, et al: *J Ultrasound Med* 9:443, 1990.
5. Carr SR, et al: *Am J Obstet Gynecol* 163:719, 1990.
6. 1991 YEAR BOOK OF NEONATAL AND PERINATAL MEDICINE, pp 56–57.

β-Endorphin Concentrations in Fetal Blood During the Second Half of Pregnancy

Radunovic N, Lockwood CJ, Alvarez M, Nastic D, Berkowitz RL (Mount Sinai School of Medicine, New York; Univ of Belgrade, Yugoslavia)
Am J Obstet Gynecol 167:740–744, 1992 1–7

Background.—Studies on the role of endogenous opiates in fetal physiologic functions and adaptation to intrauterine stress have been limited by the absence of data on the circulating levels of these substances during fetal life. The availability of percutaneous umbilical blood sampling has provided an opportunity to assess fetal opiate homeostasis in a relatively undisturbed state.

Study Design.—Concentrations of β-endorphin were obtained from uncomplicated, singleton pregnancies that resulted in the delivery of healthy term infants and in which the fetal blood sample was obtained

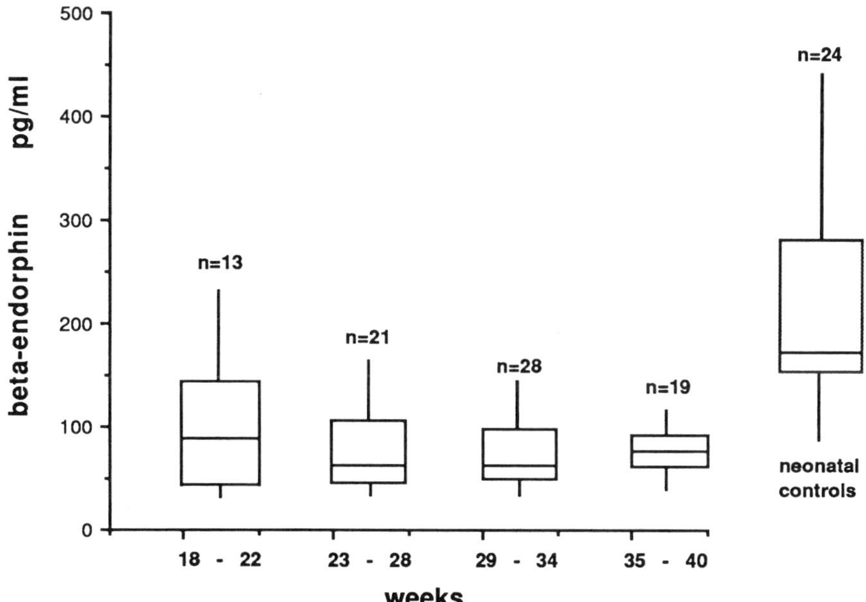

Fig 1–1.—Box-and-whisker plot of serum β-endorphin throughout gestation in 81 fetuses and 12 hours after delivery in 24 neonates. Gestational ages are grouped at 6-week intervals from 18 to 40 weeks. Although values declined between 18 and 28 weeks, no correlation was found with gestational age. (Courtesy of Radunovic N, Lockwood CJ, Alvarez M, et al: *Am J Obstet Gynecol* 167:740–744, 1992.)

without difficulty via a single needle insertion. Eighty-one paired fetal and maternal blood samples were studied. Neonatal cord specimens were also obtained from 24 uncomplicated pregnancies.

Results.—The mean fetal concentrations of β-endorphin were 105.9, 86.4, 89.7, and 85.5 pg/mL at 18–22, 23–28, 29–34, and 35–40 weeks' gestation, respectively. Although the fetal β-endorphin values declined between 18 and 28 weeks' gestation, there was no significant correlation between fetal concentrations of β-endorphin and gestational age. The mean fetal concentration of β-endorphin (90.5 pg/mL) was significantly lower than the mean β-endorphin value in neonates (228.4 pg/mL) (Fig 1–1), but it was significantly higher than the mean maternal value (70.5 pg/mL). However, fetal concentrations of β-endorphin were correlated significantly with maternal values.

Conclusion.—It appears that delivery or fetal adaptation to an extrauterine environment is associated with significant increases in β-endorphin release. The fetal pituitary appears to be the primary source of circulating fetal β-endorphin. Fetal measurements of β-endorphin may be indicated when there is persistent nonreassuring testing in a premature fetus and suspected intrauterine growth retardation.

▶ Although the fetal pituitary contributes to the fetal blood level, maternal and placental contributions are still probable. However, we must ask what their function is. Do they help make fetal life more pleasant, restful, and pain free (1), or are they involved in a special function (such as in a recent animal study of rat pups, where endorphins altered the first acceptance of breast milk)?—M.H. Klaus, M.D.

Reference

1. Smotherman WP, et al: *Behav Neurosci* 106:866, 1992.

2 Genetics and Teratology

In Vivo Transfer of the Human Cystic Fibrosis Transmembrane Conductance Regulator Gene to the Airway Epithelium

Rosenfeld MA, Yoshimura K, Trapnell BC, Yoneyama K, Rosenthal ER, Dalemans W, Fukayama M, Bargon J, Stier LE, Stratford-Perricaudet L, Perricaudet M, Cuggino WB, Pavirani A, Lecocq J-P, Crystal RG (Natl Insts of Health, Bethesda, Md; Transgene SA, Strasbourg, France; Institut Gustave Roussy, Villejuif Cedex, France; et al)

Cell 68:143–155, 1992 2–1

Introduction.—Cystic fibrosis (CF) is a common, lethal, recessive hereditary disorder, the manifestations of which are predominantly abnormalities of the airway epithelial surface. The gene responsible for CF is the CF transmembrane conductance regulator (CFTR) gene, localized on chromosome 7 at q31.

Methods.—Direct transfer of the normal CFTR gene to airway epithelium was studied using a replication-deficient recombinant adenovirus (Ad) vector containing normal human CFTR cDNA (Ad-CFTR).

Results.—In vitro Ad-CFTR–infected CFPAC-1 CF epithelial cells expressed human CFTR messenger RNA and protein. Correction of defective cyclic adenosine monophosphate mediated $C1^-$ permeability was demonstrated. Two days after in vivo intratracheal introduction of Ad-CFTR in cotton rats, human CFTR gene expression in lung epithelium was demonstrated on in situ analysis. Polymerase chain reaction amplification of reverse transcribed lung RNA showed human CFTR transcripts derived from Ad-CFTR. Northern analysis of lung RNA showed human CFTR transcripts for up to 6 weeks. With antihuman CFTR antibody, human CFTR protein was detected in epithelial cells 11–14 days after infection.

Conclusion.—In vivo CFTR gene transfer is a feasible treatment for the pulmonary manifestations of CF. The safety and efficacy of this treatment have yet to be determined.

▶ Pamela B. Davis, M.D., Ph.D., Professor of Pediatrics, Case Western Reserve University School of Medicine, and Director of Pediatric Pulmonology, whose group is at the forefront of the cystic fibrosis gene therapy groups, provided the following comments.

► A colleague of mine has called gene therapy "the Holy Grail" of genetic diseases and, in CF research, the excitement of the quest is running high. The airway epithelium is a tempting target because it is contiguous with the outside environment and therefore is readily accessible. A kind of built-in physical targeting to the cells of the airway epithelium seems possible simply by administering agents via the airway. This paper represents an early attempt to transfer the CF gene to the cells of the airway epithelium in an animal model. The vector selected is a disabled form of adenovirus, a common respiratory pathogen, and it capitalizes on the tropism of this virus for airway epithelium. The choice of the animal model, the cotton rat, was dictated by the propensity of this animal for adenoviral infections in nature. It was possible to transfer the CF gene to the airway cells of the cotton rat both in tissue culture and in vivo, the latter simply by injecting high titers of the vector containing the CF gene down the tracheas of the animals. The CFTR protein was demonstrated in the lungs of these animals 11–14 days after injection, and the messenger RNA was present for at least 6 weeks.

The adenoviral vector used in this case was disabled by removing some of the genes that encode the viral proteins essential for replication. Eliminating these genes served the dual purpose of "making room" in the virus genome for the CF gene and rendering the virus unable to replicate in the animals. The use of any infectious agent, even disabled, as a vehicle for gene therapy raises concern that the vector may be reactivated in vivo and either damage the host or carry the foreign gene to unintended sites. Because infection with adenoviruses is not rare, a naturally acquired adenovirus might complement the missing portion of the vector adenovirus. In this case, the therapeutic gene might be replicated and released and may infect normal individuals in the same way respiratory infections are transmitted. This would be an undesirable result. Also, reactivated adenovirus might become a formidable pathogen in a damaged lung.

Because adenovirus does not promote integration of its DNA into the genome, the CFTR complementary DNA will eventually be lost. Dosing of the therapeutic gene must then be repeated. However, the immunologic response to the first disabled virus may preclude the use of that same vehicle again. Variants must be available. Thus, concerns about safety (release of pathogenic or infectious vector) and permanence must be addressed for this vector before it is pursued in humans.

Other issues must be addressed before gene therapy for CF can be successful in general. The efficacy of gene transfer (the proportion of cells corrected) required for physiologic correction must be able to be achieved in vivo. The level of expression required in each transferred cell must also be ascertained. How much is enough? Is too much deleterious? Is regulation of expression necessary. Are there stem cells in the airway that, once corrected, will continue to produce corrected progeny, or is the cell biology of the airway such that permanent correction is not feasible?

Although there are still many questions to be answered, papers like this, which document pioneering attempts to transfer the CF gene to the appropriate target cells, are critical in framing the questions and finding the answers.—P.B. Davis, M.D., Ph.D.

Rapid Detection of Chromosome Aneuploidies in Uncultured Amniocytes by Using Fluorescence In Situ Hybridization (FISH)

Klinger K, Landes G, Shook D, Harvey R, Lopez L, Locke P, Lerner T, Osathanondh R, Leverone B, Houseal T, Pavelka K, Dackowski W (Integrated Genetics, Framingham, Mass; Brigham and Women's Hosp, Boston)

Am J Hum Genet 51:55–65, 1992 2–2

Objective.—This is the first major prospective comparison of the fluorescence in situ hybridization (FISH) technique and cytogenetic analysis for detecting aneuploidy. Previous limitations of the FISH technique were overcome by constructing DNA probe sets based on chromosome-specific cosmid contigs.

Methods.—Probes were derived from specific subregions of human chromosomes 21, 18, 13, X, and Y, which yielded a single copy-like signal when used in conjunction with suppression hybridization. The signal-to-noise ratio is high, and spatial resolution of the fluorescent signal is acceptable. A total of 526 amniotic fluid samples were analyzed in a blind manner. All 5 probes were used with 117 samples.

Results.—At least 1 hybridization signal was detected in 85% to 95% of cell nuclei. All 21 abnormal samples were correctly identified by the FISH technique. The other samples were correctly identified as disomic for the test chromosomes. Two thirds of the abnormal samples were trisomy 21. Two cases each of trisomy 18 and trisomy 13 were identified, along with 3 sex chromosome aneuploidies. The hybridization patterns of all trisomic samples were clearly different from the pattern seen in normal cells.

Conclusion.—The FISH method is an accurate and efficient means of detecting chromosomal aneuploidies in uncultured cells from amniotic fluid.

▶ Commenting on this article is John Johnson, M.D., Director, Division of Genetics, Children's Hospital, Oakland, California:

▶ This article combines 2 analyses that are relatively new in cytogenetics: interphase chromosomal analysis and fluorescence in situ hybridization (FISH). Interphase (uncultured, unsynchronized) cell cytogenetic analysis would not be possible without FISH. In turn, FISH is a modification of a technique used in the early 1980s—in situ hybridization of DNA probes to fixed chromosomes on a microscope slide. This technique uses DNA hybridization technology to study chromosomes. These analyses have evolved from a series of discoveries and have come to the fore since some technological limitations have been overcome—much as PCR (polymerase chain reaction) was rapidly advanced by the discovery of heat-stable DNA polymerases. A discussion of the background of some of the above advances will clarify the importance of this article and others like it.

The revolution in DNA and molecular biology occurred when it became possible to visualize the hybridization of a DNA "probe" (a sequence of interest) to a sample being investigated. The first applications were Southern blots, named for Dr. Southern; probes were hybridized to DNA samples on a membrane (blot) and were visualized with radioactive labels. Not long after, a technique was developed to hybridize probes to chromosomes. This method allowed for the mapping of DNA probes to specific subregions of chromosomes, which is an essential requirement for the mapping of human genes (such as in the Human Genome Project). However, the technique was hampered by the inefficiency of labeling and hybridization using tritium, with long exposure times and poor spatial resolution with high background.

These problems have recently been overcome with the use of biotin-labeled DNA probes, with visualization using a fluorescent avidin system, or direct labeling and visualization of the probes with modified fluorescent nucleotides. The results are viewed directly through a microscope and photographed. Using multiple probes labeled with different colors, it has been possible to order the derivation of the probes from a given chromosomal subregion. The resolution is certainly equivalent to a chromosomal band. Mapping is much facilitated by these fluorescent techniques (FISH). Other uses include the evaluation of rearranged chromosomes in patients with birth defects or cancer. Chromosome "painting" is used in some of these applications. This is a FISH method applying a cocktail of labeled probes derived from a single chromosome to allow for visualization of most or all of the length of the chromosome. One can detect pieces of the chromosome that have rearranged, especially when they are translocated to another chromosome.

This article uses FISH technology to study chromosomes in cells that generally cannot be used for cytogenetic analysis: interphase cells. By definition, interphase cells do not have discretely visualized condensed chromosomes (as in metaphase). However, DNA probes from a given chromosome can be hybridized in situ to reveal the presence of these chromosomes in the cell. Probes can therefore be used to detect trisomy in these cells (the presence of 3 hybridizing signals instead of 2). There are several advantages of this technique: (1) no culture time to synchronize and cause cells to divide is necessary; (2) cell division is not necessary (this is often a problem in tumor samples); and (3) it is simpler in principle than the complex analysis of a complete karyotype. The disadvantage relates to this latter feature, that this is not a full karyotypic analysis but, rather, one that is focused. In addition, anomalies of hybridization and visualization contribute to the fact that normal cells will occasionally appear trisomic, and trisomic cells will occasionally appear disomic. Statistical analyses must therefore be used to interpret the results.

This article uses this technique to detect 5 of the most common chromosomal anomalies in prenatal samples. Single hybridizations of probes from chromosomes 13, 18, 21, X, and Y were used to detect numerical anomalies of these chromosomes. The advantages of short turnaround time and detection of 90+% of common abnormalities must be compared with the disadvantages of missing a moderate percentage of clinically significant diagnoses in a prenatal diagnosis setting. These will include mosaicism for trisomies of these autosomes and sex chromosomes, partial deletions or duplications of these chromosomes and abnormalities of any other chromosome, including the common deletion syndromes (5p-, cri-du-chat, etc.) or translocations, inversions, and marker fragment chromosomes, all of which can be associated with adverse fetal outcome. Although the approach used by the authors of this article has recently been improved by simultaneous hybridization of all of the probes, this approach to prenatal diagnosis has not been accepted by the genetics community because of the above limitations. In fact, the authors are only using the technique as a quick "screen" with the backup of routine cytogenetic analysis.

However, the use of FISH technology in multiple situations will continue to increase and will allow for more sophisticated genetic diagnoses. The ability to analyze interphase cells allows for direct sample analysis, such as from a buccal scraping or, perhaps, in fetal cells obtained from maternal circulation; it also facilitates analysis of tumors that do not grow or divide well in culture. Perhaps a use of the authors' technique will be in the newborn nursery when an infant is suspected of having a typical trisomy and a rapid confirmation of the clinical diagnosis is required. It may be that considerations relative to medical economics will allow introduction of the authors' approach into standard prenatal practice. However, this is a decision that will have more political support than scientific support.—J. Johnson, M.D.

Maternal Heat Exposure and Neural Tube Defects

Milunsky A, Ulcickas M, Rothman KJ, Willett W, Jick SS, Jick H (Boston Univ; Brigham and Women's Hosp, Boston)

JAMA 268:882–885, 1992 2–3

Background.—Numerous studies in mammalian species have found heat to be a teratogen. The CNS has been reported to be especially vulnerable to heat exposure during pregnancy. The relationship between heat exposure in early pregnancy and subsequent neural tube defects (NTDs) was investigated in a prospective follow-up study.

Methods.—The study cohort consisted of 23,491 women who were part of a larger investigation of pregnancy outcomes. Most were patients at private obstetric practices; all were having serum α-fetoprotein screening or an amniocentesis. The women were asked about their use of a sauna, hot tub, or electric blanket during the first 2 months of pregnancy and whether they had a temperature of 100°F or higher during the first 3 months of pregnancy. Relative risks (RRs) were used to compare the incidence of NTD in those exposed to heat with the incidence among those who were not.

Distribution of Subjects and Relative Risks According to Hot Tub, Sauna, Fever, and Electric Blanket Exposure

	Hot Tub		Sauna		Fever		Electric Blanket	
	Yes	**No**	**Yes**	**No**	**Yes**	**No**	**Yes**	**No**
Neural tube defects								
Yes	7	41	2	47	7	42	7	42
No	1247	21 404	365	22 305	1858	20 719	2876	19 768
Crude RR	2.9	1.0	2.6	1.0	1.9	1.0	1.2	1.0
95% Confidence interval	1.4-6.3	. . .	0.7-10.1	. . .	0.8-4.1	. . .	0.5-2.6	. . .
Adjusted RR*	2.8	1.0	1.8	1.0	1.8	1.0	1.2	1.0
95% Confidence interval	1.2-6.5	. . .	0.4-7.9	. . .	0.8-4.1	. . .	0.5-2.6	. . .

*After controlling for age of mother, folic acid supplements, family history of neural tube defects, and other heat sources.
(Courtesy of Milunsky A, Ulcickas M, Rothman KJ, et al: *JAMA* 268:882–885, 1992.)

Results.—Complete exposure and outcome information was available for 97% of the women. Forty-nine pregnancies ended with an NTD. The RR between any heat exposure and NTD was 1.6; when electric blanket exposure was exluded, the RR increased to 2.2. Multivariate adjusted RRs for individual heat sources were 2.8 for hot tub, 1.8 for sauna, 1.8 for fever and 1.2 for electric blanket (table). When women were exposed to 2 heat sources (excluding an electric blanket), the RR for NTD increased to 6.2.

Conclusion.—Increases in core temperature result from the use of saunas and hot tubs and from episodes of fever. The exposure to these heat sources early during pregnancy is associated with an increased risk for NTD. The use of an electric blanket does not materially increase the risk for NTD.

▶ Although heat is known to be teratogenic in all mammalian species studied, including retrospective studies in humans, this detailed perspective trial adds much to our understanding. Electric blankets are not of great concern, but hot tubs and saunas are off limits for any pregnant woman. It is impressive that exposure to different forms of heat increased the risk sixfold. Unfortunately, the frequency of heat exposure was not available. The Surgeon General should now order every sauna and hot tub to be clearly labeled with a warning that they should not be used by pregnant women.—M.H. Klaus, M.D.

Malformations in Offspring of 305 Epileptic Women: A Prospective Study

Battino D, Binelli S, Caccamo ML, Canevini MP, Canger R, Como ML, Croci D, De Giambattista M, Granata T, Pardi G, Avanzini G (Neurological Inst C Besta, Milan, Italy; Milan Univ; S Paolo Hosp, Milan)

Acta Neurol Scand 85:204–207, 1992 2–4

Objective.—In previous studies, an increased risk for congenital malformations in children of epileptic mothers was reported. More recently, the rate of congenital malformations in the offspring of epileptic mothers was examined, and the possible risk factors were identified.

Patients.—From 1977 to 1989, a total of 305 epileptic women aged 16–42 years were followed prospectively through 318 pregnancies. None of the women had any other chronic illnesses. The patients were seen at least every 4 weeks throughout the pregnancy by a neurologist and an obstetrician, and routine laboratory studies were performed at these visits. Only 9 patients were not taking any antiepileptic drugs (AEDs); 207 were being treated with monotherapy.

Results.—The mean gestational age at delivery was 39.36 weeks. Only 7% of patients had more than 1 convulsive seizure per month during the pregnancy. Malformations were detected at birth in 26 neonates. Three more malformations were detected in utero by ultrasonography, and all 3 women had therapeutic abortions. At birth, minor anomalies were detected in 42 newborns. Statistical analysis revealed that the offspring of mothers treated with valproic acid (VPA) had an increased rate of malformations and minor anomalies. Among women treated with VPA, the mothers of infants with malformations had significantly higher plasma levels of VPA in the first trimester than did mothers of infants without malformations. Omphalocele was detected in utero in 1 woman who was being treated with carbamazepine monotherapy. Four women had a positive family history for major malformations. Neither maternal age, parity, type of epilepsy, seizure frequency during pregnancy, nor gender of the neonate was related to the occurrence of malformations or minor anomalies.

Recommendation.—The need for accurate prenatal ultrasound studies in epileptic women who are being treated with AEDs during pregnancy cannot be overemphasized.

▶ It is disappointing and somewhat disconcerting to reflect on how little information a 12-year prospective observational study can yield. The authors are to be congratulated on their tenacity and the thorough manner in which this trial was conducted. This is a large cohort of pregnant epileptics that, by any standard, is well controlled and extremely compliant. The women all regularly attended for antenatal care and submitted to methodical blood sampling. The inference from the study is that there is an increased risk for malformations in the offspring of epileptics. This is not exactly a revelation—it was anticipated and has been previously documented. Furthermore, establishing VPA as the major villain was also anticipated. The definition of malformations opens a Pandora's box. Inguinal hernia, clinodactyly, or congenital hip dislocations accounted for 10 of 29 malformations.

There is a fine dividing line between minor anomalies and malformations. For example, phimosis (1 case), and clinodactyly (3 cases), to my way of thinking, are minor; also, inguinal hernia (4 cases) and congenital dislocation of the hip (3 cases) are not exactly life-threatening anomalies. Rosa suggested a link between carbamazepine and spina bifida (1). A single case in this series neither supports nor refutes this association. See also References 2–4.—A.A. Fanaroff, M.B.B.Ch.

References

1. 1992 Year Book of Neonatal and Perinatal Medicine, pp 22–23.
2. South J: *Lancet* 2:1154, 1972.
3. Lammer EJ, et al: *Teratology* 35:465, 1987.
4. Jager-Roman E, et al: *J Pediatr* 108:997, 1986.

Prospective Multicentre Study of Pregnancy Outcome After Lithium Exposure During First Trimester

Jacobson SJ, Jones K, Johnson K, Ceolin L, Kaur P, Sahn D, Donnenfeld AE,

Rieder M, Santelli R, Smythe J, Pastuszak A, Einarson T, Koren G (Hosp for Sick Children, Toronto; Univ of California, San Diego; Univ of Pennsylvania, Philadelphia; et al)
Lancet 339:530–533, 1992 2–5

Background.—Lithium carbonate, effective in the treatment of major affective disorders, is used by approximately .1% of pregnant women. Isolated instances of congenital anomalies, especially the rare Ebstein's anomaly, have been linked to lithium exposure during pregnancy. To determine whether lithium is an important human teratogen, effects in 148 women using the drug during the first trimester were evaluated.

Methods.—The women were recruited from 4 teratogen information centers in the United States and Canada. Their mean age was 30 years. All were receiving lithium for major affective disorders (mean daily dose, 927 mg). To rule out cardiac anomalies, all were offered fetal echocardiography at 18 weeks' gestation. The controls were age-matched women seen at one of the centers for counseling about drugs not known or suspected to be teratogenic.

Results.—The 2 groups did not differ significantly in several measures of pregnancy outcomes, including total number of live births, frequency of major anomalies, spontaneous or therapeutic abortions, ectopic pregnancy, and prematurity (table). Birth weight was significantly higher in lithium-exposed infants than in controls. There were 3 major congenital malformations in each group. One woman in the lithium group termi-

Pregnancy Outcome

Outcome	Lithium (n = 138)	Control (n = 148)
Normal live births	105 (76%)	123 (83%)
Full term	99 (72%)	116 (78%)
Premature (< 36 weeks)	6 (4%)	7 (5%)
Congenital defects	3 (3%)	3 (2%)
Spontaneous abortion	13 (9%)	12 (8%)
Therapeutic abortion	15 (10%)	9 (6%)
Stillbirth	1	0
Ectopic pregnancy	1	1
Unknown	10 (7%)	0

Note: Ectopic pregnancies and spontaneous and therapeutic abortions are expressed as percentages of all outcomes (n = 148). Stillbirths and normal live births are expressed as percentages of known outcomes (n = 138). Congenital defects are expressed as a percentage of all live births.

* One therapeutic abortion because of Ebstein's anomaly diagnosed in utero.

(Courtesy of Jacobson SJ, Jones K, Johnson K, et al: *Lancet* 339:530–533, 1992.)

nated pregnancy when a prenatal echocardiogram detected Ebstein's anomaly. That fetus had also been exposed to fluoxetine, trazodone, and L-thyroxine. Infants from the 2 groups available for follow-up showed no differences in attainment of major developmental milestones.

Conclusion.—Although the results of this study cannot rule out an association between lithium and major anomalies, it provides no evidence that the drug is an important human teratogen. Women who require lithium treatment may continue to take the drug during pregnancy as long as level II ultrasound and fetal cardiography are performed.

▶ Commenting on this article is Cynthia Bearer, M.D., Ph.D., Director of Neonatology and Pediatric Environmental Health, Tod Children's Hospital, Youngstown, Ohio, and Associate Professor of Pediatrics, Northeastern Ohio University College of Medicine, Kent, Ohio:

▶ Following a published report from retrospective data indicating that exposure to lithium during first-trimester pregnancies resulted in major congenital anomalies, the authors conducted a prospective study of lithium-exposed pregnancies. As compared to the retrospective study, this prospective study found far fewer major congenital anomalies. However, the initial study found 18 cases of Ebstein's anomaly in 225 exposed infants, whereas this study found 1 case in 148 exposed infants. The background incidence of Ebstein's anomaly is reported to be 1 in 20,000 live births. The authors conclude that lithium is not a "major" human teratogen.

There are several points that need to be addressed in the conclusion reached by the authors. The first point is the comparison between the 2 study populations. Although there are concerns about data derived from retrospective studies, it is not clear from the data in this paper whether the 2 study populations are comparable with respect to drug exposure. In this study, women with minimal exposure to lithium are included in the exposed group. No data are presented as to what proportion of the total study group falls into this category. Although the individual dose of lithium is unlikely to have changed between the 2 studies, the duration of therapy during pregnancy was not investigated. Thus, there could be a very large difference in the exposure of the infants in the retrospective vs. the prospective study.

The second concern is the difference in study population. The first retrospective study was conducted in Denmark, and it included cases from Scandinavia as well as Canada and the United States. The more recent (prospective) study was conducted in Canada and the United States. Many drugs have metabolic pathways for which genetic polymorphisms have been described. The effects of lithium may indeed be dependent on genetic polymorphisms. No information regarding the racial/ethnic background of the study populations is given.

The last point I will address is the meaning of the phrase "major human teratogen." Much of our perception of risk is based on how the risk is expressed. For instance, the content of Alar in apples was estimated to cause 9 excess cancer deaths per million children exposed, thus exceeding the Environmental Protection Agency's tolerable limits. However, expressed differently, Alar increased the probability of dying of cancer from 25% to 25.01%, an apparent negligible increase in risk. The authors of this prospective study suggest that lithium is not a major teratogen, having found only 1 case of Ebstein's anomaly in 148 exposed cases. Yet, given the background rate of Ebstein's anomaly, the data suggest that exposure to lithium in the first trimester may increase the risk of Ebstein's anomaly by more than 100-fold. What is an intolerable risk and what is a major human teratogen? The debate goes on.—C. Bearer, M.D., Ph.D.

Cardiovascular Abnormalities in Infants Prenatally Exposed to Cocaine

Lipshultz SE, Frassica JJ, Orav EJ (Boston City Hosp; Boston Univ; Children's Hosp, Boston; et al)

J Pediatr 118:44–51, 1991 2–6

Introduction.—A recent prospective study suggests an increasing incidence of congenital malformations among infants whose mothers used cocaine during pregnancy. All neonatal urine toxicologic analyses during an 18-month period were reviewed retrospectively to evaluate the relation between maternal cocaine use during pregnancy and the occurrence of congenital cardiovascular abnormalities.

Setting.—Of the 554 neonatal toxicologic screening tests performed between 1988 and 1990, 214 (39%) were positive for cocaine and 340 (61%) showed no detectable cocaine. The numbers of cardiovascular malformations and ECG abnormalities in these 2 groups were compared using matched data from the pediatric cardiology program that included inpatient consultation, outpatient consultations, and ECG.

Results.—Forty-nine patients with neonatal drug screening underwent cardiology examination, 19 had positive results on cocaine metabolite screens, and 30 had negative results. The overall congenital cardiac malformation rate in cocaine-positive patients was significantly higher than in cocaine-negative infants (relative risk, 3.7; 95% confidence interval, 1.4–9.4) and published rates for the general population of infants (relative risk, 7.6; 95% confidence interval, 4.5–13). Structural cardiovascular defects in cocaine-positive infants included peripheral pulmonic stenosis, patent ductus arteriosus, ventricular septal defect with aortic leaflet prolapse through the defect, and ventricular septal defect with an atrial septal defect. In addition, 17 of 19 cocaine-positive patients had abnormal ECG results, including conduction defects, voltage abnormalities compatible with chamber enlargement, and dysrhythmias such as high-grade ventricular ectopy.

Conclusion.—Infants exposed prenatally to cocaine appear to be at risk for development of structural cardiovascular malformations, ECG abnormalities, and, possibly, cardiopulmonary autonomic dysfunction.

► This retrospective study was initiated because "the data on congenital cardiac anomalies in infants of mothers who used cocaine during pregnancy are incomplete, controversial, and largely anecdotal." Analysis of this highly selected group implicates cocaine use during pregnancy in increasing the risk for congenital heart disease. The rates of cardiac disorders may be even greater than first reported, as the control group included women who had used cocaine but had negative neonatal screens. (Two infants with significant heart disease and negative screens during the neonatal period were delivered of women known to have used cocaine during pregnancy.) Furthermore, only the infants referred for cardiac examination at the above institution were included. If a comprehensive cardiac evaluation had been performed on all the infants undergoing toxicologic screening, the rates possibly would have been even greater. Nonetheless, it is disturbing to note that the rate still far exceeds previous published data, the lesions were not trivial, and some major conduction disorders were discovered. The authors were concerned that the infants with peripheral pulmonic stenosis, usually regarded as a benign lesion, had associated right ventricular hypertrophy with ST- and T-wave changes. Reduction in pulmonary blood flow could alter growth of the developing lung.

The cardiac anomalies have been attributed to vascular disruption (1), which may also affect the developing brain (2). Alcohol and HIV also increase the rate of cardiac malformations, but they were not known factors in the above study. It has been rumored that the cocaine epidemic is abating. Like Hurricane Andrew, it is leaving a host of devastation in its path. We can only hope this epidemic is beginning to fade; however, the next recreational drug to reach epidemic proportions in terms of use may be even worse for the fetus.

Every man has the right to be wrong in his opinions. But no man has a right to be wrong about his facts.—Bernard Baruch

A.A. Fanaroff, M.B.B.Ch.

References

1. Hoyme HE, et al: *Pediatrics* 85:743, 1990.
2. Volpe J: *N Engl J Med* 327:399, 1992.

Maternal Occupational Exposure and Congenital Malformations

Cordier S, Ha M-C, Ayme S, Goujard J (Natl Inst for Health and Med Re-

search, Villejuif, Marseille, Paris, France)
Scand J Work Environ Health 18:11–17, 1992 2–7

Objective.—The risk of congenital malformation was related to maternal occupational exposures before and during pregnancy. A total of 325 infants with major malformation were matched with normal infants born just after them in the same ward.

Findings.—Mothers of infants with oral clefts were more often exposed to solvents during pregnancy than mothers of control infants, and they worked more often as cleaners. Digestive anomalies and multiple anomalies also were associated with exposure to solvents at work. The findings persisted after controlling for maternal age, area of residence, and socioeconomic status.

Conclusion.—An association between maternal exposure to solvents at work and an increased risk of oral clefts and digestive malformations was supported.

▶ Commenting on this article is Cynthia Bearer, M.D., Ph.D., Director of Neonatology and Pediatric Environmental Health, Tod Children's Hospital, Youngstown, Ohio, and Associate Professor of Pediatrics, Northeastern Ohio University College of Medicine, Kent, Ohio:

▶ This paper again suggests an association between exposure to organic solvents and specific birth defects, such as oral clefts, digestive anomalies, and multiple anomalies. Of particular note is the method of collecting exposure data. In the study, mothers were asked to estimate their occupational exposures. An industrial hygienist, who was blinded to the case-referent status of the women, then reviewed the mothers' occupational histories and estimated their exposures. There were large discrepancies in the mothers' perception of exposure and the expert's evaluation. Only 31% of the women who were considered highly exposed by the industrial hygienist reported their exposure as high. Why this lack of agreement between the individual being exposed and the expert? Lack of awareness of exposure may lead to greater exposure, which might be prevented. With the data from this and other studies demonstrating an association between solvent exposure and birth defects, worker education, particularly among women of child-bearing age, is necessary. Aspects of this education should include the sources of exposure, how to prevent exposure, and the possible consequences of exposure. In this particular study, a number of the women were from countries other than France. Worker education and warning labels should be available in languages understood by those expected.—C. Bearer, M.D., Ph.D.

Evidence for Decreasing Quality of Semen During Past 50 Years

Carlsen E, Giwercman A, Keiding N, Skakkebæk NE (Rigshospitalet 5064, Copenhagen; Univ of Copenhagen)

BMJ 305:609–613, 1992 2–8

Introduction.—Some studies have reported a relationship between environmental changes of the past 50 years and a decline in the quality of human semen. The international literature on semen analysis since the 1930s was systematically reviewed to determine whether the reported decrease in sperm count reflects a biological phenomenon or methodological errors.

Methods.—Publications were selected from the *Cumulated Index Medicus or Current List* (1930–1965) and the MEDLINE Silver Platter database (1966–August 1991). The analysis was based on 61 articles that included data on 14,947 men. In 39 studies, the subjects were of proved fertility; the men were unselected with respect to fertility in the remaining 22. The mean sperm densities and seminal volumes were analyzed with linear regression weighted by the number of subjects included in the individual reports.

Results.—Forty-six of the publications reported mean seminal volume. Linear regression analysis revealed a marginally significant decrease between 1940 and 1990, from 3.40 to 2.75 mL. There was a significant decrease, however, in mean sperm concentration, from 113 $\times$ 10^6/mL in 1940 to 66 $\times$ 10^6/mL in 1990 (Fig 2–1). The combined effect of the

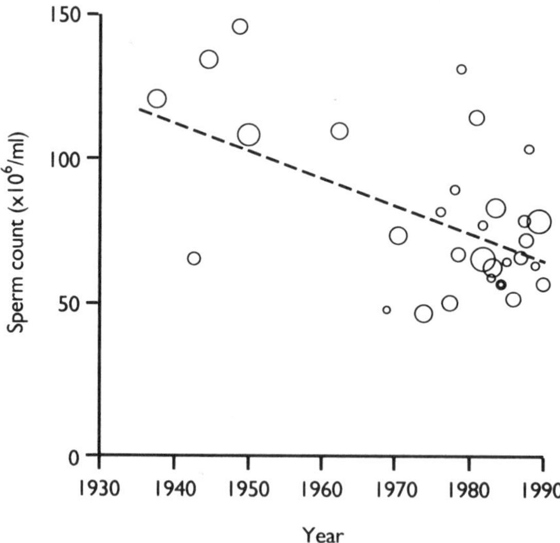

Fig 2–1.—Linear regression of mean sperm density reported in 61 publications (represented by circles whose area is proportional to the logarithm of the number of subjects in study), each weighted according to number of subjects, 1938–1990. (Courtesy of Carlsen E, Giwercman A, Keiding N, et al: *BMJ* 305:609–613, 1992.)

changes in both mean seminal volume and mean sperm concentration indicate an even greater decrease in total sperm count. There was no trend of sperm count with age in the 35 articles that reported the mean age of the subjects.

Conclusion.—The reported declines in mean sperm count and mean seminal volume during the past 50 years appear to be genuine and may reflect an overall reduction in male fertility. During the same period, the incidence of some genitourinary abnormalities, including testicular cancer, has increased. These findings suggest that environmental or endogenous factors are having serious effects on male gonadal function.

▶ Commenting on this article is Cynthia Bearer, M.D., Ph.D., Director of Neonatology and Pediatric Environmental Health, Tod Children's Hospital, Youngstown, Ohio, and Associate Professor of Pediatrics, Northeastern Ohio University College of Medicine, Kent, Ohio:

▶ This paper is a very interesting study on the decline of mean sperm count and seminal volume during the past 50 years. Data were obtained from published accounts of sperm count and seminal volume during the 50-year span. The authors found a significant decline in mean sperm count, from 113 $\times$ 10^6/mL in 1940 to 66 $\times$ 10^6/mL in 1990. Concomitantly, seminal volume has decreased from 3.40 mL to 2.75 mL in the same period. The methods used to perform this study are quite novel, and they allow good longitudinal study of these sensitive parameters of male reproductive health. Of concern are the factors involved in the decline of these parameters. Given the short period over which the effect is observable, the authors postulate that environmental, rather than genetic, factors are important. Other studies that would seem to substantiate this effect of the environment included the increasing incidence of childhood cancers and the increasing incidence of asthma. There may be subtle indicators of increasing neurotoxicity that could be studied in the same way, such as the average age of attaining milestones or the number of geniuses in our society. Our increasing awareness of the link between environmental health and human health will only serve to protect us and the environment.—C. Bearer, M.D., Ph.D.

Correlation Between Omphalocele Contents and Karyotypic Abnormalities: Sonographic Study in 37 Cases
Getachew MM, Goldstein RB, Edge V, Goldberg JD, Filly RA (Univ of California, San Francisco)
AJR 158:133–136, 1991 2–9

Objective.—Previous findings suggest that fetuses whose omphaloceles contain only bowel and not liver have a particularly high proportion of karyotypic abnormalities. This claim was tested by reviewing 37 fetuses who were sonographically found to have an omphalocele in 1984–1990.

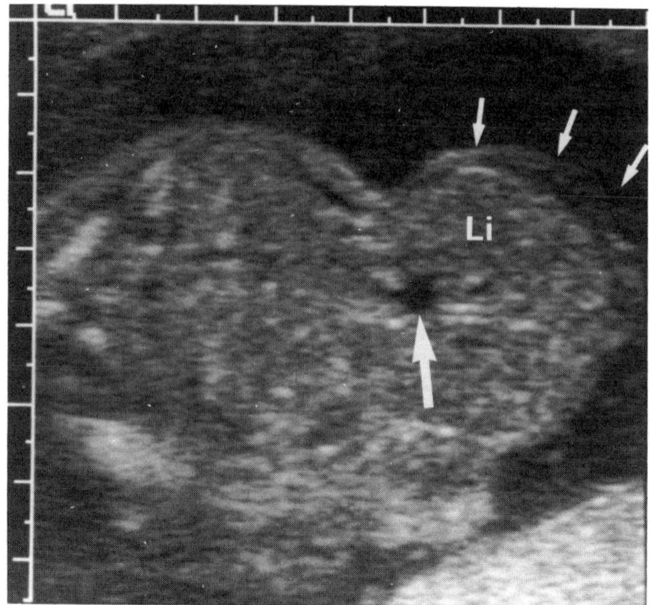

Fig 2–2.—Sonogram shows a liver-containing omphalocele. The lesion is covered by a membrane (*small arrows*). Portal vessel (*large arrow*) confirms that the mass within the omphalocele is liver (*Li*). (Courtesy of Getachew MM, Goldstein RB, Edge V, et al: *AJR* 158:133–136, 1991.)

Observations.—Nine fetuses had morphologic findings of amniotic band syndrome. In 22 of the other fetuses, liver was exteriorized (Fig 2–2), whereas in 6 cases the sac contained only bowel (Fig 2–3). Karyotyping was abnormal in 1 of the 16 fetuses tested that had liver exteriorized. In contrast, 4 of the 6 whose sacs contained only bowel had abnormal karyotypic findings. The latter fetuses all had morphologic abnormalities other than omphalocele; the 2 with normal karyotypes had no other abnormality.

Conclusion.—A small omphalocele or one containing only bowel should not be a source of reassurance. Karyotypic abnormalities are far more prevalent when liver is absent from the sac than when it is present.

▶ The spectrum of anterior abdominal wall defects includes omphalocele, gastroschisis, and the amniotic band syndrome or limb body wall complex. The outcome is dependent, in many instances, on the associated anomalies. An omphalocele affects 1 in 4,000 live births, yet it remains the most commonly observed wall defect in fetal autopsy series (1). Several practical issues arise from Getachew et al.'s series. Foremost is the emerging evidence that the contents of the omphalocele are more significant than its size. The presence of bowel only mandates a fetal karyotype, as the combined literature presents an 87% (26/30) incidence of abnormal karyotypes and multiple other lesions with only bowel in the omphalocele. If the liver is in the om-

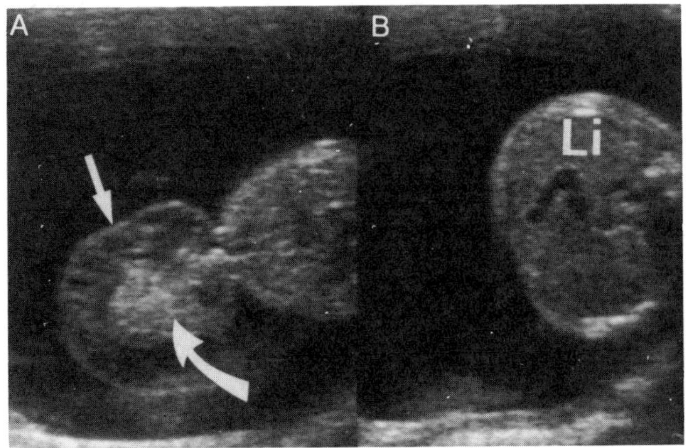

Fig 2–3.—Sonograms of a fetus with trisomy 18 show an omphalocele that contained bowel only. **A,** omphalocele is covered by a membrane (*straight arrow*) and contains collapsed segments of bowel (*curved arrow*). **B,** liver (*Li*) is within the fetal abdomen and is not exteriorized. This fetus also had a lumbosacral myelomeningocele (not shown). (Courtesy of Getachew MM, Goldstein RB, Edge V, et al: *AJR* 158:133–136, 1991.)

phalocele, the likelihood of an abnormal karyotype diminishes to 90% and the outcome brightens. However, many families chose to terminate pregnancy.

It was surprising to learn how infrequently these lesions were connected with abnormalities in amniotic fluid volume or α-fetoprotein. Of the 37 mothers, 32 were referred because of abnormal sonograms and only 5 were referred because of elevated AFP. We are not told why the ultrasound was done, but the skeptics about routine ultrasound in pregnancy have retreated so that their backs are against the wall. For more information on routine ultrasound scanning, see Abstract 1–2.

See everything, overlook a great deal; correct a little.—Pope John XXIII

A.A. Fanaroff, M.B.B.Ch.

Reference

1. Baird PA, MacDonald EC: *Am J Hum Genet* 33:470, 1981.

A Genetic Etiology for DiGeorge Syndrome: Consistent Deletions and Microdeletions of 22q11

Driscoll DA, Budarf ML, Emanuel BS (Univ of Pennsylvania, Philadelphia; Children's Hosp, Philadelphia)

Am J Hum Genet 50:924–933, 1992 2–10

Background.—DiGeorge syndrome (DGS) is a developmental field defect of the third and fourth pharyngeal pouches, characterized by aplasia or hypoplasia of the thymus and parathyroid glands and by conotruncal cardiac malformations. Cytogenetic studies have shown the presence of a DGS critical region (DGCR) in band 22q11. The results of cytogenetic and molecular studies of 14 patients with DGS were reported.

Results.—Cytogenetic analysis, using high-resolution banding techniques, demonstrated interstitial deletions of 22q11 in 5 probands and possible cytogenetic deletions in 3; the other 6 probands had normal karyotypes. In contrast, molecular studies with probes from the DGCR detected DNA deletions in all 14 probands. Two of the 10 loci tested, D22S75 and D22S259, were detected in all 14 patients; a third, D22S66, was deleted in the 8 probands tested. Physical mapping using somatic cell hybrids showed that D22S66 appeared to lie between D22S75 and D22S259, suggesting that it should be deleted in the other 6 probands. The origin of the de novo deletions was studied in 5 informative families. Four probands failed to inherit a maternal allele, and 1 did not inherit the paternal allele. On the basis of this information and previous reports of 6 maternally and 5 paternally derived unbalanced translocations in DGS probands, it appears that neither parent of origin nor imprinting effect plays a vital role in the pathogenesis of DGS.

Conclusion.—These findings confirm a genetic etiology for DGS. The identification of deletions of the same 3 loci in all 14 DGS probands, regardless of the cytogenetic status, suggests that submicroscopic deletions of 22q11 occur in most cases.

▶ This is the first study to evaluate families using restriction fragment length polymorphism and dosage analysis to determine the origin of de novo deletion of loci in the DGCR. For the uninitiated or newly initiated, manuscripts on the new genetics do not make easy reading. They should only be tackled by the alert reader. Otherwise, the abbreviations and loci numbers will be confusing. This report on the microdeletion on chromosome 22 in patients with DGS represents the ultimate in biological detective work. As stated by the authors, "molecular studies with probes from the DGCR are clearly more sensitive than the high-resolution cytogenetic analysis," and so it should be.

It is fascinating to watch the human genum unfold and to observe the revelations from the gene probes. Not only is the lesion on the chromosome precisely located, but the parent from whom the problem arose is identified. The genetic counselors are going to have to deal with finger pointing as the "perfect parents" spawn imperfect offspring.

The known is finite, the unknown infinite. Intellectually, we stand on an islet in the midst of an illimitable ocean of inexplicability. Our business in every generation is to reclaim a little more land, to add something to the extent and solidity of our possessions.—Thomas Henry Huxley

A.A. Fanaroff, M.B.B.Ch.

The Meiotic Stage of Nondisjunction in Trisomy 21: Determination by Using DNA Polymorphisms

Antonarakis SE, Petersen MB, McInnis MG, Adelsberger PA, Schinzel AA, Binkert F, Pangalos C, Raoul O, Slaugenhaupt SA, Hafez M, Cohen MM, Roulson D, Schwartz S, Mikkelsen M, Tranebjaerg L, Greenberg F, Hoar DI, Rudd NL, Warren AC, Metaxotou C, Bartsocas C, Chakravarti A (Johns Hopkins Univ, Baltimore, Md; Univ of Maryland, Baltimore; Univ of Switzerland, Zurich; et al)

Am J Hum Genet 50:544–550, 1992 2–11

Background.—Trisomy 21 is the most common human chromosomal abnormality responsible for mental retardation. Recent DNA polymorphism analysis using numerous DNA markers has indicated that paternal origin of the extra chromosome is less frequent than previously reported. The meiotic stage of nondisjunction in 200 families with free trisomy 21 was determined by using pericentromeric DNA polymorphic markers on chromosome 21.

Method.—Each family had a propositus with chromosomally diagnosed free trisomy 21. Both parents, the propositus, and the unaffected siblings were studied with DNA polymorphisms on human chromosome 21. Southern blot analysis and PCR amplification were the DNA polymorphisms used. The genotypes of DNA polymorphisms at loci in the pericentromeric markers on the long arm of the human chromosome 21 were studied. Maintenance of heterozygosity for parental markers in the individual with trisomy 21 was interpreted as resulting from a meiosis I error, whereas reduction to homozygosity was attributed to a meiosis II error.

Findings.—In 188 cases of maternal nondisjunction, meiosis I was responsible for 77.1% and meiosis II for 22.9% of the cases. In the 9 paternal nondisjunctions, the error occurred in meiosis I in 22.2% of the cases and in meiosis II in 77.8% of the cases. Because the distribution of maternal age did not differ significantly between maternal error I and II, it is unlikely that an error at a particular meiotic stage significantly contributes to the increasing incidence of Down syndrome with advancing maternal age.

Conclusion.—Analysis of DNA polymorphisms at the loci in the pericentromeric region on the long arm of chromosome 21 may provide a more accurate understanding of the meiotic stage of nondisjunction. Analysis of the polymorphisms may provide a more accurate understanding of the meiotic stage of nondisjunction in trisomy 21 than previously provided by chromosomal heteromorphisms.

▶ The human genes, so long secretive about their structure and functions, are rapidly revealing their secrets. There is now a good level of understanding of the basic defects at the DNA level, and the biochemical mechanisms of several diseases have been clarified. Several genes have been cloned and characterized so that the list of genetic disorders needs constant revision and updating. This proliferation can be attributed to the progress of the human genome project. As soon as the genes causing a disorder are identified, mutations are studied and the precise location on the gene is established with sophisticated mathematical analysis, using DNA markers from a large number of families with the disorder.

Improved treatment and prevention of respiratory disorders, asphyxia, birth trauma, and infection have vaulted birth defects to the forefront of the perinatal mortality statistics. Birth defects also account for more and more newborns requiring prolonged hospitalization. There has been considerable shuffling of the charts as the etiologies of many of the birth defects have become more apparent. Although chromosomal abnormalities and polygenic disorders remain difficult to address with current technologies, single gene disorders are proving increasingly tractable to the tools of modern biology (1). See also Abstracts 2–10 and 2–12.

Briefly, the principles underlying the use of DNA markers for genetic prediction are as follows: One or more markers that show consistent co-inheritance with the disease in several families are found. It is then possible to predict the inheritance of the disease in subsequent generations by observing the inheritance of the marker. A number of factors must be operative. Thus, the family to be offered the genetic prediction must have the same genetic type of disorder as the families in which the genetic markers were developed; the DNA marker must be close to the locus of the specific abnormal gene; and the family must be "informative" for the DNA marker that is being used. All of these conditions were operative so that the congenital heart locus and its relationship to duodenal stenosis and the facial features could be located on the 21 chromosome.

To date, most of the progress has been with disorders caused by a single gene. As the molecular basis of these disorders unravels, the geneticists are frantically racing to clone the defective genes and find ways of reinserting them into the cells (see Abstract 2–1).—A.A. Fanaroff, M.B.B.Ch.

References

1. Culotta E, Koshland D: *Science* 258:1864, 1992.
2. Antonorakis SE: N *Engl J Med* 320:153, 1989.

Down Syndrome: Molecular Mapping of the Congenital Heart Disease and Duodenal Stenosis

Korenberg JR, Bradley C, Disteche CM (Univ of California, Los Angeles; Univ of Washington, Seattle)

Am J Hum Genet 50:294–302, 1992 2–12

Background.—Individuals with Down syndrome (DS) may have mental retardation, congenital heart disease, abnormalities of the immune system, an increased risk of leukemia, and an Alzheimer-like presenile dementia. Down syndrome is usually caused by trisomy 21; however, a subset of the syndrome characteristics, including the classical facies and mental retardation, may be caused by duplication of band q22. In a family with DS and a chromosome 21 translocation, a region of distal band 21q22.1–q22.3 likely to contain the genes responsible for some of the DS features was previously defined. Further molecular analyses of 1 individual in the family and 1 unrelated individual with DS were undertaken to define the molecular markers for congenital heart disease, duodenal stenosis, and an "overlap" region for the facial and some of the skeletal features of DS.

Methods.—A clinical, cytogenetic, and molecular analysis of the 2 patients was undertaken. Southern blot analysis and DNA sequences unique to chromosome 21 were used.

Findings.—One patient carried a partial duplication of chromosome 21, including the region 21q21.1–q22.13, or proximal q22.2, and DS features including duodenal stenosis. The duplication of chromosome 21 includes the region defined by DNA sequences for amyloid precursor protein, SOD1, D21S47, SF57, D21S17, D21S55, D21S3, and D21S15; it excludes the regions defined by DNA sequences for D21S16, D21S46, D21S1, D21S19, the breast cancer estrogen-inducible gene (D21S39) and D21S44. The other patient is from a family carrying a translocation associated with DS and congenital heart disease. The duplicated region includes DNA sequences for D21S55 and D21S3, and it excludes DNA sequences for D21S47 and D21S17. The molecular overlap region in the 2 patients includes D21S55, D21S3, and D21S15. The phenotypic features shared by the 2 patients include the facial features, wide space between the first and second toes, broad short hands, incurved fifth finger, and lax ligaments.

Conclusion.—The development of higher resolution mapping methods on normal chromosomes will aid in the definitive mapping of the DNA sequences in the overlap region in patients with DS and partial duplications of chromosome 21.

▶ The chromosome countdown is in full swing, and the Human Genome Project is perhaps ahead of schedule—namely in mapping the entire human genome by 1995. Gigantic strides have been made toward the understanding or the structure and function of human genes in the past 3 decades. In the past year, these advances have culminated in the completion of the maps of the Y chromosome and the infamous chromosome 21, which is responsible for DS and contains the Alzheimer gene. The mapping of these genes is a laborious task requiring sophisticated techniques, meticulous mathematics, and a little luck. "Each map is a scientific coup"(1). This report gets down to the nitty gritty or the "trenches in the cells" to determine the etiology of trisomy 21. It is a tribute to the collaboration between the geneticists and molecular biologists that erroneous meiosis can be pinpointed. See also Abstract 2–11.—A.A. Fanaroff, M.B.B.Ch.

Reference

1. Antonorakis SE: N *Engl J Med* 320:153, 1989.

Patterns of Risk of Hereditary Retinoblastoma and Applications to Genetic Counselling

Draper GJ, Sanders BM, Brownbill PA, Hawkins MM (Univ of Oxford, England)

Br J Cancer 66:211–219, 1992 2–13

Objective.—A registry with information on nearly 1,600 cases of retinoblastoma diagnosed in Britain includes a population-based series of 918 cases diagnosed in 1962–1985. Bilateral cases represented 40% of the total. The proportion of cases known to be hereditary is 44%. Selected groups of cases have been followed to estimate the proportions of siblings and offspring who themselves are affected.

Findings.—Where no previous family history of retinoblastoma was apparent, siblings of patients with retinoblastoma had about a 2% chance of having the disease if the proband was bilaterally affected; they had a 1% chance if the proband was unilaterally affected. The risk levels were lower if there were other, unaffected siblings. The risks for siblings of probands when there is a past family history of disease are given in the table. Children of probands had a 1 in 2 chance of carrying the germ cell mutation. Those who were carriers and whose parents had bilateral disease had close to a 90% chance of having retinoblastoma. Children of parents not known to be carriers have an estimated 1% chance of having retinoblastoma.

Implications for Counseling.—The offspring of patients with hereditary retinoblastoma have an overall risk of about 45%. The risk for patients with sporadic unilateral retinoblastoma and their relatives is smaller than previously thought. Gene carriers now can be identified with a high degree of certainty if at least 2 family members are affected. Even in sporadic cases, it may be possible to identify those that are he-

Estimated Probabilities of Retinoblastoma for Siblings of Probands When There is a Previous Family History

Type of proband	*No. of sibs* at risk*	*No. of affected sibs** *Bilateral*	*Unilateral*	*Total*	*Estimated % of sibs developing retinoblastoma by age 6 years (standard error)*
Bilateral	120	47	4	51	44.8 (5.3)
Unilateral	38	4	7	11	30.0 (9.0)

*In families with more than 1 independently ascertained proband, siblings are counted more than once.
(Courtesy of Draper GJ, Sanders BM, Brownbill PA, et al: *Br J Cancer* 66:211–219, 1992.)

reditary by directly identifying point mutations in the retinoblastoma gene and comparing tumor cells with constitutional cells.

► Commenting on this article is John Johnson, M.D., Director, Division of Genetics, Children's Hospital, Oakland, California:

► The genetics of retinoblastoma are exceedingly complex and difficult to understand at first glance. Even with isolation of the Rb-1 gene and excellent clinical studies such as this one, questions remain as to the inheritance of this tumor. However, retinoblastoma has an important place in the evolution of cancer genetics theory. Knudsen developed the "two-hit" hypothesis to explain the origin of this tumor, and some important molecular work by W. Cavenee and others has confirmed this hypothesis. The hypothesis and discovery of "tumor suppressor" genes is based on the genetics of retinoblastoma. The discoveries of genetic and molecular events leading to the development of this tumor serve as a model for the understanding of other cancers.

This article substantially contributes to our knowledge of the epidemiology of retinoblastoma within affected families. The authors have studied a large and complete registry to answer some basic genetic questions. To understand the significance of the article, one must understand the basic assumptions concerning the inheritance of retinoblastoma. All bilateral cases are assumed to develop in patients who have inherited an Rb-1 mutation (termed "old germ cell mutation" when there is a positive family history); a second "hit" has mutated the other gene in the tumor progenitor cells. Therefore, such an individual has a 50% chance to pass the inherited defect to his/her offspring. However, the penetrance of the gene is about 90%, such that 45% of offspring would be affected.

An individual with bilateral disease may have unaffected parents; however, because of the 10% nonpenetrance, a parent might in fact carry a nonexpressed Rb-1 gene mutation. Therefore, there would be some risk in siblings of an affected individual, even with unaffected parents. However, it is also possible that the individual inherited an Rb-1 mutation present only in a single egg or sperm (this is called "new germ cell mutation" in the article); therefore, the sibling risk would be exceedingly low.

The situation is different for unilateral retinoblastoma. The majority of these cases are believed to be sporadic ("sporadic nonhereditary" in the article), resulting from mutations of the Rb-1 gene on both chromosomes (#13) in the tumor. However, patients with an inherited mutation occasionally have only unilateral disease develop. Therefore, a subset of patients with unilateral retinoblastoma will have a risk for affected offspring; because of the penetrance issue, these patients may have a risk for affected siblings as well, even when parents are normal. If there is a positive family history in the parents, the patient is assumed to have inherited an Rb-1 defect ("old mutation"). If the individual does not seem to have inherited a defect from the parents but has affected offspring, then the supposition is that the individual does carry a mutated Rb-1 gene ("new mutation"). The penetrance in this situation is further reduced to 60%, with 30% of offspring affected (usually with unilateral disease).

This article provides new and possibly more reliable numbers for genetic counseling for the above scenarios. First, the penetrance numbers used in the past are supported by the study. However, the numbers have changed in cases with no family history. Because of nonpenetrant gene carriers, the risks for affected siblings of a bilaterally affected patient with normal parents have been quoted at up to 6%. In this study, the risk was found to be 2%. The risk of 1% usually given to a family with a child affected with unilateral retinoblastoma was confirmed in the study. The risk for affected offspring for an individual with unilateral disease was found to be about 1%, with about 2% considered to carry a new mutation. This differs from the often quoted numbers of 6% and approximately 15%, respectively. This means that the individual who has unilateral disease and is the only one affected in the family is significantly less likely to carry a mutation and possibly have affected siblings and offspring than was previously thought.

Finally, the study found a higher proportion of bilateral cases, approximately 40%, compared with other studies, which found a proportion as low as 20%. This means that the overall percentage of inherited retinoblastoma was higher in this study (44%) than in others. However, the most important contributions of the study relate to the improved genetic counseling possible using the newer and potentially more reliable numbers.—J. Johnson, M.D.

Fetal Alcohol Syndrome and Fatty Acid Ethyl Esters

Bearer CF, Gould S, Emerson R, Kinnunen P, Cook CS (Children's Hosp, Oakland Research Inst, Oakland, Calif; Washington Univ, St Louis; Univ of Calfiornia, San Francisco)

Pediatr Res 31:492–495, 1992 2–14

Introduction.—Fetal alcohol syndrome (FAS) is the most prevalent known cause of mental retardation. Growth also is retarded, and those affected have a hypoplastic midface and neurologic dysfunction. The biochemical mechanisms underlying teratogenesis are not understood.

Hypothesis.—Nonoxidative metabolism of ethanol to fatty acid ethyl esters (FAEE) is catalyzed by FAEE synthases. The accumulation of FAEE in various tissues may underly ethanol-induced toxicity in organs lacking alcohol dehydrogenase. Whether nonoxidative ethanol metabolism and accumulation of FAEE take place in the C57BI/6J murine model of FAS, and whether the human placenta contains FAEE synthase activity were determined.

Results.—Human placenta, mouse placenta, heart, and liver all actively catalyzed FAEE formation. Murine placenta and the mouse fetus accumulated significant amounts of FAEE 1 hour after maternal ethanol administration at a gestational age of 2 weeks. Tissues of pregnant animals given ethanol on gestational day 7 exhibited persistent FAEE on gestational day 14.

Conclusion.—The placenta has significant FAEE synthase activity. In mice, maternal ethanol exposure leads to the accumulation of significant amounts of FAEE in the placenta and in fetal tissues. These findings warrant further research into the role of FAEE in the development of FAS.

▶ For 20 years we have known about the abnormalities produced by alcohol; however, we do not understand the mechanism by which they are produced. A key step in the background for this report is the finding several years ago that the organs without the capacity to oxidize alcohol metabolize alcohol to FAEE, which binds to intact mitochondria and uncouples oxydative phosphorylation in vitro. This report is an important step in trying to prove the hypothesis that the accumulation of FAEE may cause or contribute to the embryopathy of FES. The next step, which is most difficult, is to pin down FAEE as the guilty party.—M.H. Klaus, M.D.

Principles and Practicalities of Carrier Screening: Attitudes of Recent Parents

Green JM (Univ of Cambridge, England)

J Med Genet 29:313–319, 1992 2–15

Objective.—Population carrier screening for cystic fibrosis is now feasible, but little is known about the public's attitude toward genetic disease in general, and cystic fibrosis in particular. A questionnaire was sent to 207 couples who had previously responded to a survey of attitudes toward prenatal screening. Responses were received from 104 women and 71 men.

Findings.—Most respondents viewed the decision on carrier screening as one that people should make for themselves, but many noted that the burden should be on people to object if they do not wish to be screened. Among the prominent reasons for screening were to spare parents the trauma of having a handicapped child, to reassure people that they are not carriers, and to provide children with a right not to be born with a handicap. The respondents were not impressed by cost-based arguments. The most popular option was to test all school leavers. Nearly half the sample opted for testing at the start of pregnancy. Almost half the respondents indicated they would make a special trip to be tested.

Implication.—These respondents represent a minority who are prepared to confront the issues raised by population carrier screening. Ensuring that all potential subjects are making a truly informed decision will not be easy.

▶ As we begin to genetically screen patients for a number of diseases, it is useful to survey the population as to their views on what should be studied. In addition, it will be necessary to survey the knowledge base of the sample.

The responses might simply be the result of a misunderstanding. For example, in another study of genetic screening, 5% of the parents whose children were negative for the disease still believed their children might eventually have the condition. Also, the medical personnel taking part in any screening procedure must fully understand all aspects of the testing. In Abstract 4–11, edited by Diane J. Madlon-Kay, family physicians, in part, did not follow through with AFP screening because they did not believe it was important.—M.H. Klaus, M.D.

Prevention of the First Occurrence of Neural-Tube Defects by Periconceptional Vitamin Supplementation

Czeizel AE, Dudás I (Natl Inst of Hygiene, Budapest)

N Engl J Med 327:1832–1835, 1992 2–16

Objective.—Although folic acid or multivitamin supplementation seems to prevent recurrent neural tube defects, 95% of women who deliver an infant with a neural tube defect have not previously delivered infants with these defects. Whether periconceptional vitamin supplements can decrease the incidence of a first occurrence of neural tube defects was investigated in a randomized, controlled study including 7,540 women who were planning a pregnancy, in most cases their first.

Methods.—At their first visit, the women were randomly assigned to receive either a vitamin supplement containing 12 vitamins—including .8 mg of folic acid, 4 minerals, and 3 trace elements—or a trace-element supplement containing copper, manganese, zinc, and a very low dose of vitamin C. The subjects were instructed to take 1 tablet per day for at least 1 month before conception, until at least the date of the second missed menstrual period. Compliance was assessed by counting unused tablets.

Results.—Four thousand seven hundred fifty-three women had a confirmed pregnancy, the outcome of which was known in 2,104 women receiving the vitamin supplement and 2,052 women receiving the trace-element supplement. The rate of congenital malformations was 23 in 1,000 in the trace-element group vs. 13 in 1,000 in the vitamin group. All 6 cases of neural tube defects occurred in women taking the trace-element supplement. The vitamin supplement group had a rate of 2 in 1,000 for cleft lip with or without cleft palate, nearly twice the population-based rate.

Conclusion.—Use of a folic acid-containing vitamin supplement around the time of conception appears to decrease the incidence of a first occurrence of neural tube defects. All women planning pregnancy should receive such a supplement. The finding of an increased rate of cleft lip in women taking the vitamin supplement disagrees with a previous study showing a protective effect.

3 Medical Complications of Pregnancy

An Evaluation of the Impact of Maternity Care Coordination on Medicaid Birth Outcomes in North Carolina

Buescher PA, Roth MS, Williams D, Goforth CM (Dept of Environment, Health, and Natural Resources, Raleigh, NC; Dept of Human Resources, Raleigh, NC)

Am J Public Health 81:1625–1629, 1991 3–1

Introduction.—In response to the state's high infant mortality rate, North Carolina health agencies developed the Baby Love Program. Medicaid eligibility was expanded and maternity care was coordinated to improve birth outcomes among women in poverty. The first 2 years of the program, 1988 and 1989, were evaluated.

Methods.—Data files were linked to birth certificate records for the study period. The birth outcomes of women who received maternity care coordination services were compared with the outcomes of those who did not receive these services. The measures of outcome were birth weight, infant mortality, and newborn medical care costs. Logistic regression analysis was performed to supplement simple comparisons of percentages and rates.

Results.—The infants of women receiving Medicaid who received maternity care coordination services had significantly better outcomes than the newborns of those women who did not receive the services (table). Low birth weight (< 2,500 g) was 21% higher in the latter group, very low birth weight was 62% higher, and the infant mortality rate was 23% higher. There was an average net savings to Medicaid of $140 for each of the women receiving care coordination. It was estimated that Medicaid saved $2.02 in medical costs for each $1.00 spent on maternity care coordination. Women who received the services for more than 3 months had better outcomes than those in the program for less than 3 months.

Conclusion.—In its first 2 years, the Baby Love Program in North Carolina appeared to have a large impact on low birth weight, the single most important factor contributing to infant death and disability.

Outcome Measures for Singleton Medicaid Live Births by Presence of Maternity Care Coordination: North Carolina, 1988–1989 (Births With No Prenatal Care Are Excluded)

Outcome Measures	Received Care Coordination	Did Not Receive Care Coordination	*P* Value for Difference
Total			
Percent under 2500 g	8.67	10.50	<.0001
Percent under 1500 g	1.23	1.99	<.0001
Infant deaths per 1000 live births	9.9	12.2	.02
Percent on prenatal WIC	90.9	66.8	<.0001
Average amount paid by Medicaid for newborn care beginning within 60 days of age	$1694	$1971	<.0001
Number of births	15 526	34 463	
Prenatal Care at Public Health Department			
Percent under 2500 g	8.61	9.95	.0001
Percent under 1500 g	1.16	1.71	.0001
Infant deaths per 1000 live births	9.7	12.5	.03
Percent on prenatal WIC	92.8	84.6	<.0001
Average amount paid by Medicaid for newborn care beginning within 60 days of age	$1674	$1872	<.0001
Number of births	12 842	14 812	
Prenatal Care Not at Public Health Department			
Percent under 2500 g	8.95	10.91	.001
Percent under 1500 g	1.57	2.21	.02
Infant deaths per 1000 live births	10.8	12.0	.58
Percent on prenatal WIC	81.9	53.4	<.0001
Average amount paid by Medicaid for newborn care beginning within 60 days of age	$1790	$2046	.001
Number of births	2684	19 651	

Abbreviation: WIC, (special supplemental food program for) women, infants, and children.
(Courtesy of Buescher PA, Roth MS, Williams D, et al: *Am J Public Health* 81:1625–1629, 1991.)

Women receiving the services were more likely to participate in nutritional programs and to bring their newborns for well baby care.

▶ Exploring this cautious presentation in more detail reveals a most exciting observation regarding a very large sample. Although there was no randomization of the intervention, the group receiving coordinated care contained significantly more high-risk mothers who were more often unmarried, younger than age 18, and less educated than those in the control group. However, the women who received maternity care coordination had better birth outcomes despite a higher level of risk factors. Additional evidence is supported by results indicating that longer participation in the program was associated with better outcomes. Other benefits of coordinated services were noted after delivery: greater family planning (69% vs. 39%), well baby care (65% vs. 25%), and WIC attendance (77% vs. 36%). The coordinator acts as an advocate assisting the pregnant woman to navigate a complex system with confusing applications, etc. They are encouraged to obtain a variety of services for which they are eligible, including Aid to Families with Dependent Children, job training, social work, transportation, food stamps, and housing assistance. These impressive results were observed in a program appropriately called the Baby Love Program.—M.H. Klaus, M.D.

Randomized Controlled Trial of Effect of Fish-Oil Supplementation on Pregnancy Duration

Olsen SF, Sørensen JD, Secher NJ, Hedegaard M, Henriksen TB, Hansen HS, Grant A (Univ of Aarhus, Denmark; Royal Danish School of Pharmacy, Copenhagen; Natl Perinatal Epidemiology Unit, Oxford, England)

Lancet 339:1003–1007, 1992 3–2

Introduction.—Observations of long pregnancies and high birth weights in the Faroe Islands led to proposals that a high intake of fat from fish and whales, which are rich in long-chain n-3 fatty acids, might prolong gestation. These fatty acids might delay cervical ripening by inhibiting the production of prostaglandins, and they also could relax the myometrium by enhancing prostacyclin production.

Methods.—A randomized trial of fish-oil supplementation was undertaken in 533 healthy Danish women at weeks 30 of gestation. The women were assigned to take 4 1-g Pikasol capsules (containing 2.7 g of

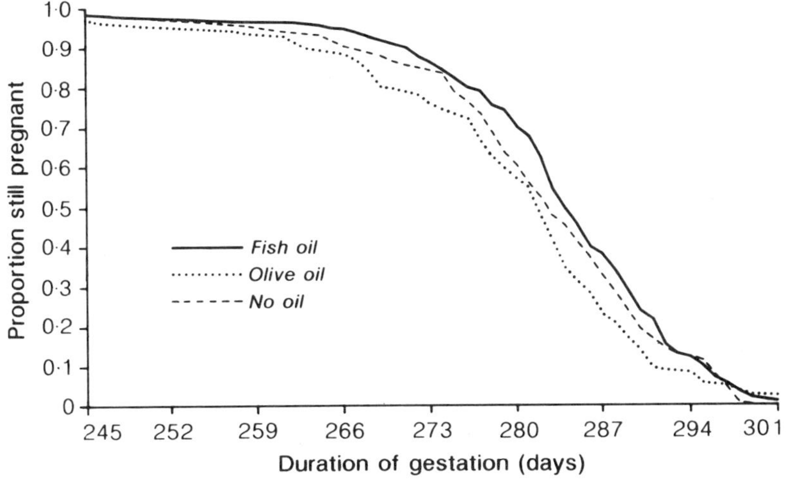

Fig 3–1.—Proportion of women in each group still pregnant at a given duration of gestation. (Courtesy of Olsen SF, Sørensen JD, Secher NJ, et al: *Lancet* 339:1003-1007, 1992.)

n-3 fatty acids) daily; or olive oil capsules; or no supplement. Pikasol consists of eicosapentaenoic acid, docosahexaenoic acid, and tocopherol.

Results.—The average duration of gestation was greater in women given the fish-oil supplement (Fig 3–1), as were birth weights and birth lengths. The difference from women not taking oil was greatest for those who complied with the regimen. Women taking fish oil lost more blood at delivery.

Conclusion.—Fish-oil supplementation in late pregnancy appears to delay delivery without impairing fetal growth or the process of parturition. Whether supplementation will lower the risk of complications from preterm delivery remains to be determined.

▶ Many of our grandmothers would be pleased to read this report on fish oil. This is a most instructive follow-up on a pilot study that we reported in the first YEAR BOOK OF NEONATAL AND PERINATAL MEDICINE 7 years ago. The authors, intrigued by the observation that a diet high in fish oil might explain the long duration of pregnancy and high birth weights in the Faroe Islands, produced this fascinating randomized trial. Several mechanisms could explain this effect of fish oil. The long-chain n-3 fatty acids could delay delivery by inhibiting the production of prostaglandins $F_{2\alpha}$ and E_2, or by relaxing the myometrium by increasing the production of prostacyclins PGI_2 and PGI_3. We await with great interest the results of an ongoing trial to determine whether fish oil reduces the rate of prematurity.—M.H. Klaus, M.D.

Effect of Using Protocols on Medical Care: Randomised Trial of Three Methods of Taking an Antenatal History

Lilford RJ, Kelly M, Baines A, Cameron S, Cave M, Guthrie K, Thornton J (Inst of Epidemiology and Health Services Research, Leeds, England; Univ of Leeds, England; Maternity Hosp, Hull, England)

BMJ 305:1181–1184, 1992 3–3

Background.—Concern about the quality of medical care has prompted more emphasis on quality control by medical audit. However, audit is usually based on retrospective analysis of clinical activity. The effects of different systems were examined in an attempt to prevent errors of omission before they occur.

Methods.—The randomized, controlled trial at an antenatal clinic in a university hospital in England included 2,424 women who came to the clinic for a first visit. Midwives took patient histories using an unstructured paper questionnaire, a structured paper questionnaire including a checklist, or an interactive computerized questionnaire that incorporated 101 clinical reminders. The effects on the quality of obstetric care of these 3 methods of taking an antenatal history were then assessed. The number of clinical responses to factors arising from the antenatal booking history according to a history-taking method was the main outcome measure. Actions were classified as medical and surgical, obstetric, personal, current symptoms and treatment, related to maternal age, and related to cervical smear testing and dental hygiene. The actions were weighted for clinical importance.

Findings.—The unstructured questionnaire prompted 1,063 actions; the structured questionnaire, 1,146; and the computerized questionnaire, 1,122. The unstructured questionnaire had the lowest clinical importance score for the actions prompted. The structured questionnaire was superior to the computerized questionnaire in medical and surgical score, obstetric score, and personal score, but it was inferior in current symptoms score.

Conclusion.—Structured questionnaires, whether on paper or computer, provide more and better information than unstructured questionnaires. The use of the structured questionnaire improves clinical response to risk factors. Computerized systems appear to provide no additional benefit in antenatal clinics.

▶ As we move into the age of computers, both their advantages and disadvantages must be assessed. Although we collect more extensive information on the patient by using structured questionnaires, it is surprising that an interactive computerized questionnaire did not have any advantage. However, some of the most vital and meaningful concerns of the patient are not mentioned when only a structured questionnaire is used. Before beginning any questionnaire, time should be spent listening to the major concerns of the patient using an open-ended process. As David Levy noted many years ago, a major goal of the physician is "to find out where the patient is and take them where they want to go."—M.H. Klaus, M.D.

Clinical Determinants of the Racial Disparity in Very Low Birth Weight

Kempe A, Wise PH, Barkan SE, Sappenfield WM, Sachs B, Gortmaker SL, Sobol AM, First LR, Pursley D, Rinehart H, Kotelchuck M, Cole FS, Gunter N, Stockbauer JW (Harvard Med School, Boston; Harvard School of Public Health, Boston; South Carolina Dept of Health and Environmental Control, Columbia; et al)

N Engl J Med 327:969–973, 1992 3–4

Introduction.—Black infants born in the United States continue to be twice as likely as white infants to die in the first year of life, primarily because of the higher rates of delivery of low-birth-weight (less than 2,500 g) and very-low-birth-weight (less than 1,500 g) infants among black women. The clinical conditions associated with this elevated risk were examined.

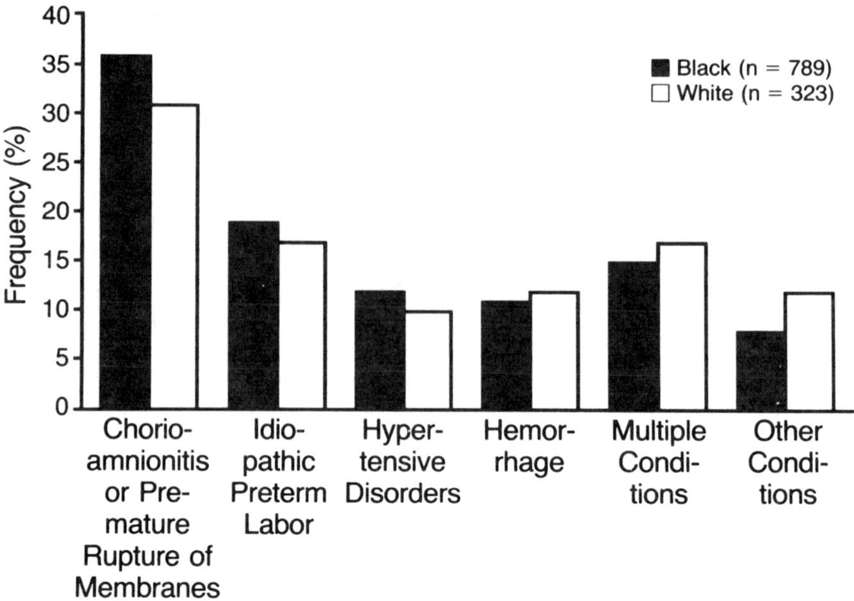

Fig 3–2.—The frequency of maternal conditions associated with delivery of very-low-birth-weight infants among black and white women. The data include all pregnancies in 3 geographic areas. The difference between black and white women in the frequency of other conditions was significant (P = .02). (Courtesy of Kempe A, Wise PH, Barkan SE, et al: *N Engl J Med* 327:969–973, 1992.)

Methods.—The medical records of more than 98% of all infants weighing 5,00 to 1,599 g who were born in Boston from 1980 through 1985 (687 infants), in St. Louis in 1985 and 1986 (397 infants), and in 2 health districts in Mississippi in 1984 and 1985 (215 infants) were examined. The mothers' records were also reviewed for conditions known to precipitate labor and for other relevant medical problems.

Results.—The relative risk of very low birth weight among black infants as compared with white infants ranged from 2.3 to 3.2 in the 3 geographic areas. This finding was related to an elevated risk in black mothers of conditions associated with very low birth weight. Chorioamnionitis or premature rupture of membranes, idiopathic preterm labor, hypertensive disorders, and hemorrhage were all more common among black mothers (Fig 3–2). The most frequent diagnosis in all areas was premature rupture of membranes. Racial differences in maternal age did not account for the distribution of the conditions associated with delivery of a very-low-birth-weight infant.

Conclusion.—These findings raise concerns about the general health status of black women during pregnancy. Comprehensive strategies will be needed to prevent the conditions associated with very low birth weight and the resulting higher rate of infant mortality among blacks.

► Finally, a small step forward in trying to understand the increased mortality of black infants. In a microscopic dissection of the clinical data of infants weighing less than 1,500 g (from a total sample of 81,750 deliveries in the high-risk areas of Boston, St. Louis, and Mississippi), the authors found that two thirds of the excess rate of very low birth weight among black infants was associated with clinical conditions in the mother that precluded the pregnancy. As a result, the authors observe that the largest proportion of the racial disparity is not presently amenable to individual clinical interventions, and any improvement will depend instead on preventive strategies. The next step is to determine how severe social inequities result in an increased incidence of primary chorioamnionitis, premature rupture of the membranes, idiopathic preterm labor, hypertensive disorders, and hemorrhage.—M.H. Klaus, M.D.

Randomized Trial of Comprehensive Prenatal Care for Low-Income Women: Effect on Infant Birth Weight

McLaughlin FJ, Altemeier WA, Christensen MJ, Sherrod KB, Dietrich MS, Stern DT (Vanderbilt Univ, Nashville, Tenn; Metropolitan Nashville Gen Hosp, Tenn)

Pediatrics 89:128–132, 1992 3–5

Objective.—Prenatal health care directed at the behavioral, demographic, and medical variables associated with low birth weight may be the best approach for prevention of low birth weight. In a prospective, randomized study, the effect of comprehensive prenatal care on birth weight was assessed.

Setting.—Two hundred seventeen pregnant women were assigned to comprehensive prenatal care provided by a multidisciplinary team consisting of nurse-midwives, social workers, a nutritionist, paraprofessional home visitors, and a psychologist. The team focused on psychosocial support, education about self-care, and promotion of healthy behaviors during pregnancy. Another 211 pregnant women were assigned to standard prenatal care provided by obstetrics residents in an outpatient prenatal clinic.

Outcome.—Multiple regression analysis using behavioral, demographic, and medical variables for the 308 women with complete data demonstrated a significant relationship between the set of predictors and birth weight; however, for the sample as a whole, there was no significant effect of treatment. Separate multiple regression analyses showed that comprehensive prenatal care was related to higher birth weights among primiparous, but not multiparous, mothers. Similarly, a separate analysis of variance for primiparous and multiparous mothers demonstrated a favorable effect of comprehensive care on birth weight for primiparous, but not for multiparous, mothers.

Conclusion.—Comprehensive prenatal care and psychosocial support appears to favorably affect birth weights of infants born to primiparous low-income women. This may be a function of the primiparas' greater openness to psychosocial intervention.

▶ This randomized trial joins several others that have attempted to improve neonatal outcome by enriching prenatal care. Unfortunately, previous studies of increasing social support during pregnancy have not shown any major effect on the incidence of prematurity, although Olds (1) found that a subset of teenage mothers who enrolled in his intervention before midgestation had infants with higher birth weights than did the control mothers. It should be noted that patients in this sample were at high risk and were chosen because of their increased risk of child maltreatment. We continue to search (to no avail) for an intervention that will magically heal 20 years of social deprivation. We await with interest, however, other outcome measures being studied, including child development and abuse. For more encouraging findings, see Abstract 3–1.—M.H. Klaus, M.D.

Reference

1. Olds DL, et al: *Pediatrics* 77:16, 1986.

Delayed Childbearing and Risk of Adverse Perinatal Outcome: A Population-Based Study

Cnattingius S, Forman MR, Berendes HW, Isotalo L (Natl Inst of Child Health and Human Development, Bethesda, Md; Natl Cancer Inst, Bethesda, Md)
JAMA 268:886–890, 1992 3–6

Introduction.—Increasing maternal age is associated with a greater risk of poor pregnancy outcomes. Although reported increases in risk are modest, the overall impact of delayed childbearing becomes more prominent as it becomes more frequent.

Study Design.—The effects of advancing maternal age on pregnancy outcome were examined in a population-based cohort study of nulliparous Nordic women aged 20 years and older. The 173,715 participants delivered single infants at Swedish hospitals from 1983 through 1987.

Observations.—The risk of late fetal death, very low or moderately low birth weight, very-preterm birth (32 weeks' gestation or earlier), and small-for-gestational-age infants were significantly higher in women aged 30 to 34 years than in those aged 20 to 24 years. The risks of very-preterm birth, low birth weight, and a small-for-gestational-age infant also were increased in women aged 35 years and older.

Conclusion.—The risk of an adverse pregnancy outcome is increased in nulliparous women who delay childbearing, despite an uncomplicated pregnancy.

► Some previous studies of delayed childbirth have reported no increase in infant mortality or low birth weight with advanced maternal age (1, 2). This very large study (173,715) revealed an increased risk in women with uncomplicated pregnancies. It is fortunate that the detailed Swedish records permitted a statistical adjustment for smoking, a history of infertility, and other medical conditions. The authors suggest that a progressive decrease in uteroplacental perfusion with advancing age, secondary to myometrial atherosclerosis, could explain the changes noted. This large study probably gives the best estimate to date of the effects of advancing maternal age on childbearing.—M.H. Klaus, M.D.

References

1. Barkan SE, Bracken M: *Am J Epidemiol* 125:101, 1987.
2. Berkowitz GS, et al: N *Engl J Med* 322:659, 1990.

Parental Cigarette Smoking and the Risk of Spontaneous Abortion

Windham GC, Swan SH, Fenster L (California Dept of Health Services, Berkeley)

Am J Epidemiol 135:1394–1403, 1992 3–7

Introduction.—Smoking is often considered a risk factor for spontaneous abortion, but epidemiologic data are not consistent. The effects of parental cigarette smoking on the risk of spontaneous abortion were evaluated using data from a large case-control study.

Study Design.—Maternal and paternal smoking and maternal passive smoke exposure were studied in 626 women aged 18 years and older who had a spontaneous abortion by 20 weeks' gestation and also in 1,300 control women. The relationship between parental cigarette

Number of Cases With a Spontaneous Abortion and Controls With a Live Birth Who Were Exposed to Environmental Tobacco Smoke

	Cases	Controls	Crude OR*	95% CI*	Adjusted OR†	95% CI
All women						
Exposed ≥1 hour/day	270	466	1.4	1.1–1.7	1.5	1.2–1.9
Unexposed	355	832	1.0	Referent	1.0	Referent
Nonsmokers						
Exposed	178	304	1.4	1.1–1.7	1.6	1.2–2.1
Unexposed	313	738	1.0	Referent	1.0	Referent

Abbreviations: OR, odds ratio; *CI,* confidence interval.
* Crude and adjusted odds ratios among all women and among nonsmokers only, California, 1986–1987.
† Adjusted by multiple logistic regression for maternal age, race, and education; marital status; previous fetal loss; tobacco, alcohol, caffeine, and bottled water consumption; employment; insurance; nausea; and time to interview.
(Courtesy of Windham GC, Swan SH, Fenster L: *Am J Epidemiol* 135:1394–1403, 1992.)

smoking and spontaneous abortion was analyzed while adjusting for confounding variables, including caffeine and alcohol consumption.

Results.—For the women who smoked during the first trimester, the risk of spontaneous abortion among light smokers (1–10 cigarettes/day) was similar to that of nonsmokers. Likewise, there was no excess risk of spontaneous abortion in the 1% of women who smoked heavily (> 20 cigarettes/day). Moderate smokers (11–20 cigarettes/day) had a slightly elevated crude odds ratio of 1.3 that did not persist after adjusting for confounders. The results for paternal smoking were very similar to those for maternal smoking and also disappeared after adjusting for confounders. In contrast, maternal exposure to environmental tobacco smoke for 1 hour or more per day was associated with an increased risk of spontaneous abortion (odds ratio, 1.5), even after adjusting for confounders (table). Furthermore, this association appeared stronger among pregnancies in which the father smoked. The association for maternal direct smoking and environmental smoke exposure appeared to be stronger with second-trimester spontaneous abortion.

Conclusion.—No association between active smoking and spontaneous abortion was found, although a moderate association with passive smoking is evident. However, this does not mean that smoking is safe during pregnancy in view of the previously well-documented adverse effects of smoking on reproductive outcome.

▶ Commenting on this article is Cynthia Bearer, M.D., Ph.D., Director of Neonatology and Pediatric Environmental Health, Tod Children's Hospital, Youngstown, Ohio, and Associate Professor of Pediatrics, Northeastern Ohio University College of Medicine, Kent, Ohio:

▶ Although this careful case-control study failed to find a significant effect of smoking on spontaneous abortions occurring before 20 weeks' gestation, it did find a moderate association of spontaneous abortion and exposure to environmental tobacco smoke (ETS) for 1 hour or more per day. At first this seems implausible: Don't smokers get a much higher dose of the chemicals in tobacco smoke than do passive smokers? However, when one considers the chemical content of ETS vs. mainstream smoke, there may be a difference in the chemicals to which one is being exposed. The amount of ETS per gram of tobacco smoked contains much higher amounts of nitrosamines, carbon monoxide, benzene, and polyaromatic hydrocarbons than does mainstream smoke. This is a result of the lower temperature of combustion, which results in more incomplete products of combustion from the tobacco. The toxic chemicals in tobacco smoke are the products of incomplete combustion. It is very possible that there are chemicals present in ETS that are not present in mainstream smoke. As pointed out by the authors, biomarkers may be useful in determining the dose-response relationships between a number of the chemicals present in ETS and spontaneous abortions. A few biomarkers already available include continine, carboxyhemoglobin, and hydroxyethylvaline adducts of hemoglobin.—C. Bearer, M.D., Ph.D.

Effectiveness of a Pregnancy Smoking Cessation Program

O'Connor AM, Davies BL, Dulberg CS, Buhler PL, Nadon C, McBride BH, Benzie RJ (Univ of Ottawa, Ont, Canada)

J Obstet Gynecol Neonatal Nurs 21:385–392, 1992 3–8

Background.—Fewer than 1 in 5 women stop smoking when learning they are pregnant, although pregnancy appears to be an ideal time to encourage cessation. The most promising results were reported by Windsor et al., who developed a 1-week self-help program for pregnant women, which is provided individually. It is based on a pamphlet describing the hazards of smoking during pregnancy and a guide to ways of analyzing smoking habits keyed to strategies for stopping. How useful this approach is in diverse population groups remains uncertain.

Objective.—New referrals to an antenatal clinic who smoked cigarettes and who were seen before 31 weeks' gestation received either a control intervention (a brief explanation of the hazards of smoking and an invitation to a 2-hour group session using Windsor's cessation program) or an experimental intervention in which women had a choice of when to experience the program and whether to spend 20 minutes or 2 hours. The women in this group also had a choice of individual or group counseling.

Results.—One hundred ninety of 224 women eligible for the study were available for assessment 6 weeks post partum. The cessation rates for those in the experimental group were threefold greater than for those in the control group after 1 month and more than twofold greater at longer term follow-up (table). The experimental program appeared to be most helpful for women who smoked less and those in the first trimester of pregnancy.

Suggestions.—It appears helpful for nurses to provide self-help smoking interventions to pregnant women early in the course of prenatal care. A tailored approach based on individual beliefs about risk and motivation probably will prove most successful.

▶ During the past 7 years, we have included multiple reports on the many deleterious effects of maternal smoking on the fetus. For the first time, we present data comparing 2 methods of stopping smoking in early pregnancy. Sadly, the task is not easy; however, effectiveness increased markedly if the program was begun on the first visit. In several countries, television has been shown to effectively alter health-related behavior. Is it time to use our most popular media?—M.H. Klaus, M.D.

Percentage (Frequencies) of Women Who Quit Smoking, at Each Follow-up, as Function of Cessation Program

	Percentage of quitters in a smoking cessation program			
Follow-up (df = *1)*	*Experimental (quit/total)*	*Control (quit/total)*	*Relative risk (RR) for quitting (95% confidence interval)*	*Chi-square analysis* (p)
1 month postintervention	14.9% (15/101)	5% (5/101)	3.00 (1.20 < RR < 7.50)	5.549 (0.02)
36 weeks' gestation	13.3% (12/90)	6% (5/84)	2.24 (0.85 < RR < 5.89)	2.685 (0.10)
Postpartum	13.8% (13/94)	5.2% (5/96)	2.66 (1.03 < RR < 6.84)	4.116 (0.04)

(Courtesy of O'Connor AM, Davies BL, Dulberg CS, et al: *J Obstet Gynecol Neonatal Nurs* 21:385–392, 1992.)

Blunt Trauma During Pregnancy: Factors Affecting Fetal Outcome
Scorpio RJ, Esposito TJ, Smith LG, Gens DR (Univ of Maryland, Baltimore)
J Trauma 32:213–216, 1992 3–9

Background.—Trauma during pregnancy, although relatively uncommon, is associated with a high rate of fetal loss. In some cases, even minor injuries can result in an adverse outcome. The factors associated with fetal death after blunt maternal trauma were identified.

Methods.—During the period from July 1, 1980 to December 31, 1988, 76 pregnant women who sustained blunt trauma were admitted to a level-I trauma center. Fetal outcome was determined in 59 cases. After excluding 8 patients who underwent elective abortion, there were 51 patients for the retrospective study.

Results.—Thirty-five women (69%) had a successful delivery, which was defined as live birth and survival through the neonatal period (group A). Fetal loss occurred in the remaining (31%) cases (group B). There were no maternal deaths in group A, but 9 of the pregnant women in 16 group B patients died. Except for maternal death, the most significant individual factor associated with fetal outcome was the woman's Injury Severity Score. Another significant factor was admission serum bicarbonate level (table). No other variables influenced fetal outcome.

Regression Analysis of Fetal Outcome and Predictor Variables

Variable	*p* Value
ISS	0.01
Bicarbonate	0.02
Surgery	0.11
GCS Score	0.12
HR	0.17
BP	0.21
DPL	0.27
Gestational age	0.66
pH	0.73
Po_2	0.80
Maternal age	0.93

(Courtesy of Scorpio RJ, Esposito TJ, Smith LG, et al: *J Trauma* 32:213–216, 1992.)

Conclusion.—The severity of maternal anatomical injury and the degree of tissue hypoperfusion and hypoxia are significantly associated with fetal loss. In patients with minor injuries, measurements of serum bicarbonate levels are advisable. Pregnant trauma patients should not have surgery or diagnostic peritoneal lavage withheld, because these factors are not significantly associated with adverse outcome for the fetus.

▶ The effect of trauma on pregnancy is dependent upon a number of variables, including (naturally) the severity of the trauma, the degree of disruption of placental function, and the gestational age of the fetus. Furthermore, trauma to the uterus may initiate uterine contractions by release of arachidonic acid or rupture of the membranes. During the first trimester, the uterus is protected by the bony pelvis; however, later in pregnancy, these bones may directly injure the uterus.

Head injuries and hemorrhagic shock account for most deaths among pregnant women who die as a result of trauma. Abdominal injuries may include rupture of the spleen, retroperitoneal hemorrhage, and the unique injury of rupture of the uterus, which is almost invariably fatal for the fetus. The bowel is reportedly less vulnerable to injury during pregnancy (1). Fetomaternal hemorrhage may also be induced by blunt trauma so that maternal blood should be screened for type and antibodies, and a Kleihauer-Betke acid elution test will reveal the extent of fetomaternal hemorrhage, if present. If the mother is Rh negative, Rhogam should be administered after significant blunt trauma.

Scorpio et al. conclude that the blood gas and, specifically, the maternal bicarbonate were good predictors of the severity of the injury and degree of hypoxia. It is prudent to closely monitor the mother and fetus after any significant injury occurring during pregnancy. Resuscitation of the mother begins with the provision of oxygen and placing her in the left decubitus position if possible. Restoration of circulating blood volume is a high priority. "Maternal resuscitation is the best means of fetal resuscitation, and the stabilization of the vital signs in the mother is the first priority in management after trauma" (1). The fetal heart can then be monitored probably for at least 4 hours. This will signify fetal distress and identify abruptio placentae. Ultrasonography, which is valuable in determining fetal status and size, should be performed.

Trauma during pregnancy renders both the mother and the fetus extremely vulnerable. Both patients should be closely monitored by a skilled team that can anticipate and recognize some of the problems outlined above. They need to prepare for emergency operative delivery and to remain vigilant until both patients have been comprehensively evaluated and fully stabilized.—A.A. Fanaroff, M.B.B.Ch.

Reference

1. Pearlman MD, et al: *N Engl J Med* 323:1609, 1990.

Decreased Birthweights in Infants After Maternal *in utero* Exposure to the Dutch Famine of 1944–1945

Lumey LH (Columbia Univ, New York)

Paediatr Perinat Epidemiol 6:240–253, 1992 3–10

Background.—During the final months of World War II, the western Netherlands was affected by an acute famine as the German occupation forces imposed an embargo on all transport and food supplies. Impaired nutrition in pregnant women caused a sharp drop in their pregnancy weights and a decrease in infant birth weights. The reduction in birth weight was primarily a result of fetal growth retardation, not shorter gestation. The Dutch famine provides an opportunity to study the long-term effects of this environmental exposure; 1 study of adult males with prenatal exposure has been completed. Increased perinatal mortality had been reported in the offspring of women exposed to the famine in utero in 1944 and 1945. The obstetric outcomes in the firstborn offspring of these mothers were studied.

Method.—Using maternity records for births occurring between 1960 and 1984 in Amsterdam, outcomes in 1,808 firstborn singleton offspring of mothers born between 1944 and 1946 in The Netherlands were analyzed. Birth weight and gestational age in first offspring were of special interest. Groupings of the mothers were made according to famine exposure during gestation and early postnatal life.

Findings.—Those mothers who were exposed to famine during their first and second trimester in utero had offspring with lower birth weights than mothers not exposed to famine. Slower fetal growth rate and shorter gestation accounted for the decrease in birth weight. The birth weight of offspring of mothers exposed in their third trimester in utero was not reduced. This effect persisted after control for potential confounding and intervening variables. By contrast, third-trimester exposure to the famine in utero was associated with a reduction in the birth weight of those infants. Paradoxically, a decrease in birth weights was seen in the offspring of mothers born in areas outside the famine-affected cities.

Conclusion.—This is the first report of the clear intergenerational effects in offspring of women exposed in utero to the Dutch famine of 1944 and 1945.

▶ Epidemiology students will exhilarate as they first browse through and then carefully digest this single-authored report. A study of this magnitude could not have been accomplished alone, but by using the word "we" frequently in the manuscript, the author acknowledges that "the final version reflects the comments of several reviewers." Collaborative multicenter trials have forced some editors of medical journals to restrict the number of authors on a single manuscript. This manuscript adds fuel to their flame.

The manuscript is the culmination of the ultimate in longitudinal studies. Therefore, it qualifies as an epidemiologic epic, providing insights into history and medicine simultaneously. The occupation of Holland and the ensuing circumscribed period of famine represented a natural, or unnatural if you prefer, experiment to determine the effects of maternal nutritional deprivation on the fetus. The immediate effects have been well documented. The sequel reported above examines the effect on the next generation of the "famine fetuses." Remarkably, because of the combination of precise record keeping and a stable population, 98% of the eligible pregnancies could be analyzed. That a specific place of birth during the war was unknown in 8% adds credibility to the story. The various cohorts are carefully selected to provide an adequate sample size to test for the critical periods of starvation.

The results speak for themselves and are noncontroversial—with the exception of the inability to explain a decrease in the birth weights of offspring of mothers born in areas outside the famine-affected cities.

Starvation can now be added to radiation and to diethyl-stilbestrol exposure during pregnancy to form a select triad of factors known to affect the third generation. Hopefully, it will not be necessary to expand this notorious list.

Learning is not attained by chance, it must be sought for with ardor and attended to with diligence.—Abigail Adams

A.A. Fanaroff, M.B.B.Ch.

Fetal Surveillance in Pregnancies Complicated by Insulin-Dependent Diabetes Mellitus

Landon MB, Langer O, Gabbe SG, Schick C, Brustman L (Ohio State Univ, Columbus; Albert Einstein College of Medicine, Bronx, NY)

Am J Obstet Gynecol 167:617–621, 1992 3–11

Introduction.—Intensive antepartum fetal surveillance during the third trimester is the standard practice in pregnancies complicated by insulin-dependent diabetes mellitus. It was determined whether maternal vascular disease and/or glycemia control can be related to tests of fetal condition in pregnant women with diabetes.

Study Design.—From 1988 to 1991, 114 women with insulin-dependent diabetes mellitus who used a memory-based glucose reflectance meter were studied prospectively. Nonstress tests (NSTs) were performed weekly at 28–30 weeks and then biweekly at 32 weeks' gestation and thereafter. A nonreactive NST was followed by a biophysical profile.

Results.—Of the 1,676 NSTs performed, 134 (8%) were nonreactive and necessitated a biophysical profile. There were no significant differences in glycemic indices in patients with reactive vs. nonreactive NSTs. Ten patients were delivered because of abnormal test results of fetal condition, including 8 with nephropathy or hypertension. Intervention because of abnormal test results was significantly more common in women with nephropathy or hypertension (40%) compared with women without those risk factors (2.1%). There were no significant differences in glycemic indices in women delivered for suspected fetal jeopardy and those in the nonintervention group. One fetal death occurred; there were no neonatal deaths.

Implications.—Pregnancies complicated by vascular disease should be considered at greatest risk for abnormal results of fetal testing necessitating early delivery. Testing may begin as early as 28 weeks' gestation. In contrast, women without vascular complications and with good glycemic control rarely have fetal compromise, and fetal testing may be initiated at 32 weeks or later.

▶ Satish Kalhan M.D., Professor and Vice Chairman for Research in the Department of Pediatrics at Case Western Reserve University, took time from his sabbatical in Holland to comment as follows:

▶ There are 2 significant findings of the above study:

1. In the presence of an excellent glycemic control in a diabetic subject without vascular disease, the risk to the fetus is low; therefore, these patients can safely undergo follow-up to term gestation.

2. Vascular disease (i.e., chronic hypertension or preeclampsia in a pregnant patient with diabetes mellitus), even in the presence of rigorous metabolic control, is a significant and independent risk factor, necessitating fetal surveillance early in gestation.

It is significant to note that, in the present study, all the indices of glycemic control, i.e., glucose concentration and excursion from median glucose, were similar in the NST reactive and nonreactive groups, suggesting that the alterations in the fetal conditions were primarily related to the maternal vasculopathy, rather than diabetes mellitus or related metabolic decompensation. This study joins others in affirming the practice of nonintervention early in gestation in uncomplicated insulin-dependent diabetic pregnancy. Thus, in the presence of good metabolic control, the majority of such patients should be delivered near term gestation.—S. Kalhan, M.D.

Relationship of Fetal Macrosomia to Maternal Postprandial Glucose Control During Pregnancy

Combs CA, Gavin LA, Gunderson E, Main EK, Kitzmiller JL (Univ of California, San Francisco; Children's Hosp, San Francisco; Univ of Cincinnati, Ohio)

Diabetes Care 15:1251–1257, 1992 3–12

Background.—It is widely accepted that fetal macrosomia is associated with poor glycemic control in diabetic mothers during pregnancy. However, macrosomia has been increasingly noted even when normoglycemia is maintained. The factors that contribute to macrosomia in infants of diabetic mothers were determined in a longitudinal study.

Methods.—During an 8-year period, 111 consecutively seen pregnant women with class B through RF diabetes were studied longitudinally from 13 to 36 weeks' gestation. Pre- and postprandial blood glucose levels, glycosylated hemoglobin, insulin dose, macronutrient intake, and other maternal variables were compared among women who delivered macrosomic infants, defined as birth weight > 99th percentile for sex and gestational age based on California norms, and those who did not.

Results.—Although most women had reasonable glycemic control during pregnancy, macrosomia occurred in 29% of the pregnancies. Maternal age, prepregnant weight, duration of diabetes, White class, macronutrient intake, glycosylated hemoglobin levels, or fasting glucose levels did not differ significantly between women who delivered macrosomic infants and those who did. However, women who delivered macrosomic infants had significantly higher postprandial blood glucose up to 32 weeks' gestation and significantly lower insulin doses from 29 to 36 weeks. Multiple logistic regression analysis showed that macrosomia was significantly associated with postprandial glucose between 29 and 32 weeks' gestation. The incidence of macrosomia increased progressively with increasing postprandial glucose, suggesting that macrosomia could be reduced by keeping postprandial glucose < 7.3 mM (130 mg/dL). However, postprandial glucose values below that level were associated with increasing numbers of small-for-gestational-age infants (18%) compared with values above that level (1%).

Conclusion.—Postprandial glucose measurement should be a part of routine care for diabetes in pregnancy. It appears that a target of 1-hour postprandial glucose value of 7.3 mM (130 mg/dL) may optimally reduce the incidence of macrosomia without increasing the risk of growth retardation.

► Satish Kalhan M.D., Professor and Vice Chairman for Research in the Department of Pediatrics at Case Western Reserve University, took time from his sabbatical in Holland to comment as follows:

► Advances in the regulation of maternal metabolism in diabetic pregnancy, and in obstetric and neonatal care, have resulted in the reduction of perinatal mortality to less than 5%. Thus, in recent years, the major focus of antenatal management has been to decrease perinatal morbidity caused by fetal malformations and macrosomia. Sufficient evidence in the literature suggests that congenital malformations in diabetic pregnancy are related to disordered metabolism in early gestation. In contrast, because macrosomia is considered to be a consequence of metabolic deregulation over a longer period (particularly in the later part of gestation), a significant effort had been placed on the rigorous regulation of maternal metabolism after 20 weeks' gestation.

Until recently, most clinicians had either been monitoring blood glucose concentrations during fasting or measuring HbA_1 concentrations as a measure of metabolic control. The reason for measurement of glucose during fasting was primarily related to standardization in relation to duration of fast after the last meal; thus, one could have a reasonable perspective of adequacy of insulin treatment. However, a number of studies demonstrated that, in spite of "excellent" metabolic control (as measured by fasting blood glucose and by HbA_{1c}), the macrosomia persisted. Thus, investigators began to examine other indices of maternal metabolism as contributors to fetal macrosomia. In this context, this study is significant because it demonstrates that metabolic decompensation after meals was related to fetal macrosomia.

This study confirms the findings of the NIH-sponsored Diabetes in Early Pregnancy Study reported by Jovanovic-Peterson et al. (1), who also observed a correlation between nonfasting glucose value and birth weight. It is significant to note that when the postprandial blood glucose was within the normal range (i.e., less than 7.2 mMol), as in the study by Combs et al., the incidence of macrosomia was similar to that in the non-diabetic population; however, the risk for small-for-gestational-age infants increased significantly. Thus, the clinical management of diabetes in pregnancy involves the fine-tuning of metabolism, both during fasting as well as during the postprandial period, aimed at maintaining the levels of circulating substrates in a narrow range to prevent macrosomia as well as small-for-gestational-age infants. As proposed in this study, a target postprandial glucose value of 7.3 mMol (130 mg/dL) may be the optimal level for such a management.—S. Kalhan, M.D.

Reference

1. Jovanovic-Peterson L, et al: *Am J Obstet Gynecol* 164:103, 1991.

Maternal Phenylketonuria Collaborative Study, Obstetric Aspects and Outcome: The First 6 Years

Platt LD, Koch R, Azen C, Hanley WB, Levy HL, Matalon R, Rouse B, de la Cruz F, Walla CA (Natl Inst of Child Health and Human Development, Bethesda, Md; Children's Hosp, Los Angeles; Children's Hosp, Boston; et al)

Am J Obstet Gynecol 166:1150–1162, 1992 3–13

Background.—Routine newborn screening and early dietary treatment have largely eradicated postnatal phenylketonuria-related brain damage. However, young women who have benefited from this treatment as children and then become pregnant are at high risk for birth defects in their offspring. A preliminary report from the National Maternal Phenylketonuria Collaborative Study, which examined means of assuring a normal fetal outcome in pregnant women with hyperphenylalaninemia (HPA), was reviewed.

Methods.—The study participants were 213 pregnant women with HPA and 78 controls (pregnant women without HPA). Treatment of

Congenital Malformations Observed in Offspring of Women With Hyperphenylalaninemia

	Phenylalanine level					
	≥1200 μmol/L (≥20 mg/dl) (n = 30)		*600 to <1200 μmol/L (10.1 to 19.9 mg/dl) (n = 39)*		*<600 μmol/L (≤10 mg/dl) (n = 32)*	
	No.	*%*	*No.*	*%*	*No.*	*%*
Microcephaly	27	90	19	49	0	0
Intrauterine growth retardation	27	90	4	10	0	0
Facial dysmorphism	29	97	36	92	28	88
Cardiac defects	1	3	5	13	0	0
Ventricular septal defect	0	0	1	3	0	0
Coarctation of aorta	0	0	2	5	0	0
Coarctation, hypoplastic left ventricle	0	0	1	3	0	0
Tetralogy of Fallot	1	3	1	3	0	0
Inguinal hernia	0	0	1	3	1	3
Undescended testes	1	3	1	3	1	3
Hypospadias	1	3	1	3	1	3
Club feet	1	3	1	3	0	0
Syndactyly of finger	0	0	1	3	0	0
Kidney (duplicated collection system)	0	0	0	0	1	3

(Courtesy of Platt LD, Koch R, Azen C, et al: *Am J Obstet Gynecol* 166:1150–1162, 1992.)

women with HPA consisted of adequate nutrition during pregnancy, maintenance of blood concentrations of phenylalanine between 120 and 600 μmol/L, and supplementation with tyrosine and trace elements as needed. Women with HPA were recruited in an attempt to start treatment before conception or as soon after conception as possible.

Results.—The women with HPA were significantly younger than controls, and significantly more were primigravid. Nineteen women in the HPA group did not require dietary treatment, and 31 did not accept it; 36 started special diets before conception, 93 in the first trimester, 32 in the second trimester, and 2 in the third trimester. The HPA group had a fetal loss rate of 37%; approximately half were the result of elective terminations. No spontaneous abortions occurred in women with HPA who did not require dietary treatment. The controls had no fetal loss. In contrast to control pregnancies, 24% of the infants in the HPA group had abnormally small head circumference, 11% had decreased weight, and 11% had decreased length. The number of congenital malformations was related to maternal levels of phenylalanine (table). There was little effect on fetal outcome when diet therapy was delayed until the third trimester.

Conclusion.—These findings illustrate the need for increased involvement by the obstetrics community in maternal phenylketonuria. Dietary management, preferably before conception, is essential for optimal pregnancy outcome. Patients known to have HPA should be counseled about the risks of their pregnancy and the compounding effect of maternal smoking on head size.

▶ The possibility now exists that some 30 years after the identification of phenylketonuria, its therapy with early dietary management, and the virtual elimination of severe mental retardation, a previously very rare devastating problem (i.e., severe fetal damage secondary to untreated maternal hyperphenylalaninemia) may become a major problem. If these women do not follow a strict diet during pregnancy, the incidence of phenylketonuria-related mental retardation could return to the level before screening. It is estimated there may be 5,500 fecund women with phenylketonuria, including those born before neonatal screening or from countries with no screening, who are at risk for delivering an affected infant. If we are to educate the population and attempt to eliminate this problem, it would be helpful to combine this disease with other maternal conditions that require close control before and during pregnancy, such as maternal diabetes. Although preventive measures are less glamorous, they certainly are effective.—M.H. Klaus, M.D.

Effects of Iodine on Thyroid Status of Fetus *Versus* Mother in Treatment of Graves' Disease Complicated by Pregnancy

Momotani N, Hisaoka T, Noh J, Ishikawa N, Ito K (Ito Hosp, Tokyo)

J Clin Endocrinol Metab 75:738–744, 1992 3–14

Purpose.—It is commonly accepted that maternal ingestion of iodine poses a greater risk of fetal hypothyroidism than do thionamides. However, no controlled investigations have been conducted to support this concept. To address this, thyroid function was evaluated in the fetus and mothers during maternal iodine therapy for Graves' disease during pregnancy.

Study Design.—Serum free thyroxine (FT_4) and thyroid stimulating hormone (TSH) levels were measured in cord and maternal sera obtained at delivery in 35 women with Graves' disease who were treated with iodine alone during pregnancy. Iodine dose was 6–40 mg. Severely thyrotoxic mothers were excluded from the study.

Results.—At the initiation of iodine therapy, the maternal FT_4 levels ranged from 28.3 pmol.L to 65.8 pmol/L. At delivery, maternal FT_4 levels ranged from 9.3 pmol/L to 42 pmol/L, being slightly above normal values in 22 and normal in the remaining 13. The fetal FT_4 levels ranged from 11.7 pmol/L to 24.3 pmol/L. High FT_4 levels were significantly less frequent in fetuses than in mothers. However, in the 13 mothers with normal FT_4 levels, cord FT_4 levels were normal, and only 1 fetus had TSH levels above normal. There was a significant correlation between fetal and maternal FT_4 levels, and the correlation was even closer after excluding 12 cases in which maternal FT_4 levels increased after a transient fall. There was no correlation between the dose of iodine and the duration of iodine therapy with fetal or maternal thyroid function. Fetal TSH-binding inhibitory antibody values (TBIAb) strongly correlated with maternal TBIAb values.

Discussion.—Maternal iodine therapy for Graves' disease during pregnancy seldom, if ever, exposes the fetus to the risk of hypothyroidism. The stimulatory and inhibitory factors that affect maternal thyroid function likewise affect fetal thyroid function. However, escape from the inhibitory effects of iodine occurs less often in fetuses, accounting in part for the lower thyroid status in the fetus than in the mother.

► No issue of the YEAR BOOK OF NEONATAL AND PERINATAL MEDICINE can be considered complete without at least one peek at the effect of a maternal thyroid disorder on the fetus. This study by Momotani et al. tackles the treatment of Graves' disease during pregnancy with iodine. The series of 35 patients meeting criteria for Graves' disease, including "1) elevated free thyroid hormone levels, 2) suppressed TSH levels, and 3) diffuse goiter with the presence of ophthalmopathy and/or a positive test for antibodies that inhibit TSH binding (TBIAb)," are prospectively assigned to an oral dose of iodine. Those patients who were severely thyrotoxic were excluded. Maternal bloods are followed sequentially and compared and correlated with cord blood determinations. There follows a comprehensive discussion on the pros and cons of using iodine with and without thionamides. The bottom line is that iodine alone appears to be safe and effective for the treatment of pregnant women with mild hyperthyroidism.

No data were presented with regard to neonatal hyperthyroidism; however, there is much speculation on the etiology of goiters in the newborn. We are reminded that topical iodine preparations may inhibit neonatal thyroid function (1) and that there was an increased recall rate for congenital hypothyroidism in breast-fed infants born to iodine-overloaded mothers (2). Rovet addressed the problem of whether breast-feeding protected the infant with hypothyroidism diagnosed by newborn screening (3). For more information on thyroid hormones, see Reference 4.—A.A. Fanaroff, M.B.B.Ch.

References

1. 1990 Year Book of Neonatal and Perinatal Medicine, p 248.
2. Chanoine JP, et al: *Arch Dis Child* 63:1207, 1988.
3. 1991 Year Book of Neonatal and Perinatal Medicine, pp 196–197.
4. 1992 Year Book of Neonatal and Perinatal Medicine, pp 274–275.

The Effects of Chronic Maternal Hypotension During Pregnancy
Ng PH, Walters WAW (John Hunter Hosp, Newcastle, Australia)
Aust N Z J Obstet Gynaecol 32:14–16, 1992 3–15

Objective.—The effects of chronic maternal hypotension on obstetric outcome were studied in a retrospective review. The records of newborn infants who had complications before their mothers were discharged from the hospital were also reviewed.

Subjects.—Over a 1-year period, 134 women with singleton pregnancies were seen with blood pressure (BP) at or below 110/70 during at least 3 antenatal visits (hypotensive group). Another 134 pregnant women with BP above 110/70 served as controls. Except for the lower maternal age and weight in the hypotensive group, no other differences were noted between the 2 groups.

Outcome.—The hypotensive group had significantly higher risks of (1) delivery before the 38th week of gestation, (2) lower birth weight of infants for gestational age, and (3) postpartum complications than the control group (table). Furthermore, the rates of preterm delivery, birth weight of less than 2,500 g, and significant meconium-staining of the amniotic fluid were higher in the hypotensive group, although these differences were not statistically significant.

Conclusion.—These findings suggest a correlation between chronic maternal hypotension and adverse obstetric outcome. Larger prospective studies are necessary to define this relationship.

▶ This report raises the question of a critical blood pressure for the placenta to function efficiently, ensuring appropriate fetal growth and well-being. There are a number of limitations to this study (apparent to the authors) that preclude any substantial conclusions. The bottom line is that "hypotensive pregnant women deliver smaller babies at an earlier gestation" (this reaffirms findings in earlier publications). However, the definition of hypotension requires clarification. If a diastolic pressure of 60 mm Hg had been selected, would a clearer pattern have emerged? What if a hypotensive woman weighed less and was younger? What if they had been matched for age and weight? The infants weighed 160 g less but were also delivered earlier, and

Fetal Outcome

Variable	Patients: Group A (hypotensive) (n = 134)	Group B (normotensive) (n = 134)	P value	Significance
Birth-weight (mean, g)	3281	3444	0.035 ‡	S
Gestation at delivery (mean, weeks)	38.7	39.2	0.017 §	S
Apgar score at (1 minute) <7	9 (6.7%)	11 (8.2%)	0.94 †	NS
Sex of fetus (male)	60 (44.8%)	75 (56.0%)	0.15 †	NS
Birth-weight <2,500 g	11 (8.2%)	6 (4.5%)	0.50 †	NS
Neonatal intensive care unit admission	5 (3.7%)	3 (2.2%)	0.80 †	NS
Perinatal mortality	4 (3.0%)	3 (2.2%)	0.9*	NS

Abbreviations: S, significant; *NS,* not significant.
* Chi-square test with Yates' correction.
† Chi-square test.
‡ Two samples, 1 test.
§ Mann-Whitney U test.
(Courtesy of Ng PH, Walters WAW: *Aust N Z J Obstet Gynaecol* 32:14–16, 1992.)

there are no data concerning maternal diet, smoking, or socioeconomic status. We must conclude the chronic hypertensive pregnancy is, indeed, worthy of further study—a rather lame conclusion, you will agree.

It may be that the race is not always to the swift, nor the battle to the strong—but that is the way to bet.—Damon Runyon

A.A. Fanaroff, M.B.B.Ch.

The Effect of Magnesium on Maternal Blood Pressure in Pregnancy-Induced Hypertension: A Randomized Double-Blind Placebo-Controlled Trial

Rudnicki M, Frölich A, Rasmussen WF, McNair P (Univ of Copenhagen)

Acta Obstet Gynecol Scand 70:445–450, 1991 3–16

Objective.—The effects of prolonged oral magnesium supplementation on maternal blood pressure in women with pregnancy-induced hypertension were evaluated in a randomized, double-blind, placebo-controlled trial.

Treatment.—Magnesium or placebo was administered intravenously for 48 hours, followed by daily oral intake until 1 day after delivery. Twenty-seven patients received magnesium and 31 received placebo. The groups were comparable regarding maternal age, gestational age at inclusion, and pretreatment mean arterial blood pressure (MAP). Twenty patients in each group were nulliparas.

Results.—Magnesium supplementation significantly reduced MAP, although there was no reduction in the need for antihypertensive medication in the magnesium-supplemented women. The gestational age at delivery was the same for both groups, but the relative birth weight was significantly less in the placebo group, especially among nulliparas. Unbalanced analysis of variance suggested a positive influence of magnesium on the relative birth weight. There were no adverse effects from magnesium supplementation.

Implications.—Magnesium supplementation can reduce MAP in women with pregnancy-induced hypertension without adverse effects on the infants. Further studies are warranted to evaluate the beneficial effects of magnesium on birth weight.

► Magnesium sulfate has long been the obstetrician's standby drug for use in preventing convulsions in women with preeclampsia. The term pregnancy-induced hypertension (PIH) has replaced preeclampsia to denote the syndrome that occurs predominantly during the first pregnancy in 6% to 8% of pregnancies (1). The goal is to detect the onset of PIH disorders early so that intervention can minimize the severe complications for the mother and fetus. Preliminary reports with the use of newer therapies to prevent eclampsia have been encouraging. Calcium supplementation was noted to prevent hypertensive disorders in pregnancy (2, 3). This small, controlled trial presents evidence that magnesium sulphate significantly reduced the blood pressure of hypertensive pregnant women, with no adverse effects on the offspring. Although magnesium reduced blood pressure in the hypertensive women, it did not reduce the need for supplementary hypertensive medication in those women already receiving medication for the elevated blood pressure. It has been postulated that magnesium reduces blood pressure by affecting angiotensin-converting enzyme and other vasoactive substances (4).

In selecting an agent to treat hypertension in pregnancy, it is necessary to answer a number of questions. What agents are available? Is this woman truly hypertensive? What are the side effects of the medication, and what harm can it do to the fetus? What, if any, are the benefits of treatment, and which is the best regimen for the agent? Over the years, magnesium sulphate has appeared safe for the fetus and may even prolong gestation. Further studies are required to define its role in the treatment of PIH.

Antihypertensive drugs may be used in pregnancy; however, delivery is the only cure for established PIH. If antihypertensive agents are used, both the mother and the fetus require close supervision and monitoring. If the hypertension persists after delivery, then the underlying cause should be sought.

I don't believe in pessimism. If something doesn't come up the way you want, forge ahead. If you think it's going to rain, it will.—Clint Eastwood

A.A. Fanaroff, M.B.B.Ch.

References

1. Zuspan FP, et al: *Am J Obstet Gynecol* 163:1689, 1990.
2. 1992 Year Book of Neonatal and Perinatal Medicine, pp 33–34.
3. 1991 Year Book of Neonatal and Perinatal Medicine, pp 64–65.
4. Fuentes A, Goldkrand JW: *Am J Obstet Gynecol* 156:1375, 1987.

Infection and Labor: VII. Microbial Invasion of the Amniotic Cavity in Spontaneous Rupture of Membranes at Term

Romero R, Mazor M, Morrotti R, Avila C, Oyarzun E, Insunza A, Parra M, Behnke E, Montiel F, Cassell GH (Yale Univ, New Haven, Conn; Univ of Alabama, Birmingham)
Am J Obstet Gynecol 166:129–133, 1992 3–17

Introduction.—Microbial infection can occur upon the premature rupture of membranes in preterm deliveries. However, no data exist for the microbial status of the amniotic cavity when the membranes undergo rupture upon reaching full gestation. The prevalence and characterics of microbial invasion after the spontaneous breakage of the membranes at term was measured through transabdominal amniocentesis.

Methods.—An obstetric database provided the retrospective patient sample of women who delivered infants larger than 2,500 grams 48 hours after amniocentesis. The amniotic fluid from these patients underwent culture for both aerobic and anaerobic bacteria using standard methodology, including the limulus amebocyte lysate assay. Patients received antibiotic therapy if they had a positive Gram stain, and labor was induced. Cases of chorioamnionitis and puerperal endometritis were recorded.

Results.—Thirty-two patients were included in the study, 11 of whom demonstrated a positive amniotic fluid culture. The most frequently cultured organisms were *Ureaplasma urealyticum* (10 cases), *Peptostreptococcus* species (4 cases), and *Lactobacillus* species (2 cases). Polymicrobial invasion of the amniotic cavity was 45.4% (5 of 11). One patient had clinical chorioamnionitis, and 3 of the 32 patients (9.4%) had puerperal endometritis. Women delivering vaginally with a positive amniotic fluid culture had significantly more endometritis than did women with negative cultures. Three women, 2 having a positive amniotic fluid culture and 1 with a negative culture, underwent cesarean delivery.

Conclusion.—This is the first published report of microbial invasion of the amniotic fluid in pregnant women who have prematurely ruptured membranes. Endometritis and chorioamnionitis can often occur without any overt signs of either maternal or fetal infection.

▶ Articles are sometimes selected because they provide the unambiguous answer to a problem. More often, the manuscripts will draw attention to the state of the art and specify the unsolved questions, which should serve as a stimulus for the next research phase. This manuscript falls into the latter category, and it is one of a series of ongoing collaborative studies addressing the larger issue of infection and labor. Surprisingly little data have been gathered regarding microbial invasion of the amniotic cavity when membranes rupture at term. As subjects required a transabdominal amniocentesis within 48 hours of delivery at term, the comprehensive database yielded only a small sample. They were in fact acquired by chance, as the amniocentesis was performed with the premise that membranes had ruptured prematurely, but delivery took place within 48 hours and the infants weighed more than 2,500 grams.

This small sample restricts the power of both the results and the conclusions. Nonetheless, it was interesting that the prevalence of microbial invasion of the amniotic cavity in women seen with ruptured membranes at term 11 of 32, or 34.3%, is similar to that found with preterm premature rupture of membranes (28.5%) (1,2). The study reaffirmed how the current definition of clinical chorioamnionitis lacks the sensitivity to indicate microbial invasion of the amniotic cavity.

Future research needs to address the temporal relationship between microbial invasion of the amniotic cavity and rupture of the membranes. Which comes first, rupture of the membranes or invasion by bacteria?, Why does microbial invasion of the amniotic cavity occur in women with rupture of the membranes and not in others?—A.A. Fanaroff, M.B.B.Ch.

References

1. Romero R, et al: *Am J Obstet Gynecol* 159:661, 1988.
2. Romero R, et al: *Contemp Obstet Gynecol* Dec 2, 1988.

Maternal and Foetal Outcome Following Hodgkin's Disease in Pregnancy

Lishner M, Zemlickis D, Degendorfer P, Panzarella T, Sutcliffe SB, Koren G (Hosp for Sick Children, Toronto; Princess Margaret Hosp, Toronto; Univ of Toronto)

Br J Cancer 65:114–117, 1992 3–18

Introduction.—The incidence of Hodgkin's Disease (HD) peaks among people between 20 and 40 years of age, therefore occurring during pregnancy in female patients. An historical cohort of pregnant patients with HD was studied to assess the effects of pregnancy on HD and vice versa.

Methods.—The historical records from 1958 to 1984 were searched for the female patients with histologically confirmed HD and obstetrical information in 1 hospital. Forty-eight women with HD who were pregnant were included in the study. An attempt was made to find 3 matched controls for each pregnant patient with HD. Because of the selective nature of the matching criteria, only 67 matched controls were found for 33 patients.

Results.—The 48 pregnant patients with HD had a mean age of 26.1 years. Two of the 48 had 2 pregnancies each; of these 50 pregnancies, 12 received their HD diagnosis before becoming pregnant, 10 during the pregnancy, and 27 after delivery or the termination of pregnancy. Among the 48 women, 31 received radiotherapy alone, 3 had chemotherapy alone, and 11 had combined radiotherapy and chemotherapy. The 20-year survival rate of the 33 patients was not significantly different from that of their 67 matched controls. Of the 50 pregnancies, 40 resulted in deliveries, including 2 stillbirths, plus 5 miscarriages and 4 therapeutic abortions. The incidence of stillbirth in the patients, with HD did not differ from that occurring in the general population. No differences for birth weight, delivery method, or pregnancy outcome were found between the infants born to the women with HD or to controls.

Conclusion.—Patients with HD who become pregnant experienced no adverse effects from the disease on their survival or infant outcome compared with control subjects. In addition, the pregnancy did not promote the progress of the disease or advance its stage.

▶ This study is the first large, long-term project using a case-control method in which the pregnant women were matched for the known prognostic factors of HD. In contrast to breast cancer, pregnancy in a woman with HD does not appear to delay diagnosis or change the biology of the tumor. In addition, the infants born to these women did not have an increased risk for prematurity or growth failure. The sample, however, was not large enough to define the fetal risk of chemotherapy.—M.H. Klaus, M.D.

Sexual Abuse as a Factor in Adolescent Pregnancy and Child Maltreatment

Boyer D, Fine D (Univ of Washington, Seattle; Washington Alliance Concerned With School Age Parents, Seattle)

Fam Plann Perspect 24:4–11,19, 1992 3–19

Background.—Child abuse merits exploration as a risk factor in the continuing problem of adolescent pregnancy and parenting. Data from an ongoing longitudinal field study in the state of Washington were examined to evaluate the relationship between sexual abuse and adolescent pregnancy among a large and diverse sample of pregnant and parenting teenagers.

Subjects.—A total of 535 young women 21 years old or younger (mean age, 17.6 years) who were 19 or younger at the time of their first pregnancy (mean, 15.7 years) were recruited from public school alternative programs, various human service agencies, and tribal organizations. The subjects completed survey questionnaires that emphasized sexual and physical abuse. A majority of the respondents were parenting (62%) and had been pregnant only once (60%).

Findings.—Sixty-six percent of the young women who became pregnant as adolescents had been sexually victimized: 55% who had been molested, 42% had been victims of attempted rape, and 44% had been raped (table). Sixty-two percent of these women were sexually victimized before their first pregnancy. Compared with adolescent women who became pregnant but had not been abused, sexually victimized subjects began intercourse a year earlier (mean, 13.2 years), were twice as likely to have used drugs or alcohol, and were less likely to practice contraception. Furthermore, victimized subjects were more likely to have experienced other forms of abuse or neglect and had exchanged sex for money, drugs, or a place to stay. The data also showed that victimized subjects were more likely to report that their own children had been abused or taken from them by Child Protective Services.

Discussion.—There is a high prevalence of sexual victimization among pregnant and parenting adolescents. This is a factor that has been overlooked in previous studies of adolescent high-risk sexual behavior and adolescent pregnancy. This is yet another component that needs to be added to the array of services for preventing adolescent pregnancy.

▶ As Donald Winnicott noted, "a mother mothers in a similar fashion to the way she was cared for as a baby." It is not surprising that young adolescent

Number and Percentage of Respondents Who Had Had at Least One Unwanted Sexual Experience, by Type of Experience (n = 535)

Experience	%	N
Any experience	**66.2**	**351**
Contact molestation	**51.4**	**275**
Did someone ever make you touch their body, or touch your body, when you did not want them to?	47.7	254
Did someone ever make you touch their breasts or genitals, or touch yours, when you did not want them to?	46.2	246
Noncontact molestation	**35.5**	**190**
Did someone ever make you look at them naked, or look at you naked, when you did not want them to?	33.8	180
Did someone ever take sexual photographs of you when you did not want them to?	5.8	31
Attempted Rape	**42.4**	**225**
Has a man ever tried to have sexual intercourse with you when you didn't want to by threatening to use physical force or violence?	27.6	145
Has a man ever tried to have sexual intercourse with you when you didn't want to by using some force (like twisting your arm or holding you down)?	31.3	165
Has a man ever tried to have sexual intercourse with you when you didn't want to by giving you alcohol or drugs?	22.1	116
Rape	**43.6**	**231**
Have you ever given in to sexual intercourse with a man because of his position of authority (teacher, boss, minister)?	4.7	25
Have you ever had sexual intercourse with a man because he threatened you with physical violence?	20.1	106
Have you ever had sexual intercourse because a man used physical force?	29.0	153
Have you ever had sexual intercourse because a man threatened you with a weapon or tied you up?	8.6	45
Have you ever had sexual intercourse with a man when you did not want to because you were affected by drugs or alcohol that he gave you?	19.6	103

Note: All percentages have been adjusted for missing values by excluding nonresponses for specific items from the denominators.

(Courtesy of Boyer D, Fine D: *Fam Plann Perspect* 24:4–11, 19, 1992.)

mothers, who are so frequently molested, will have major difficulties in caring for their own infants. There is now evidence that early and intensive work with the abused women before, during, and immediately after delivery is effective in partially healing their psychic wounds and improving their child caretaking. Every attempt should be made to identify abused teenagers during pregnancy so intensive work can begin as soon as possible. The authors emphasize that "a key factor in the conundrum of adolescent high-risk sexual behavior and pregnancy and repeated pregnancies—sexual victimization and abuse—has been overlooked," or we might say repressed.—M.H. Klaus, M.D.

4 Antepartum Fetal Surveillance

Randomised Trial of Cardiotocography Alone or With ST Waveform Analysis for Intrapartum Monitoring

Westgate J, Harris M, Curnow JSH, Greene KR (Plymouth Gen Hosp, England)

Lancet 340:194–198, 1992 4–1

Purpose.—Cardiotocography (CTG) is widely used during labor, but fetal heart rate and uterine contraction patterns during labor are difficult to interpret. The ST waveform on fetal ECG recorded from the scalp electrode can be used to detect fetal heart rate during labor. Previous studies have suggested that a combination of CTG and ST waveform analysis might improve the predictive value of intrapartum heart rate monitoring. Intervention rates and neonatal outcomes in labors monitored by CTG alone and by CTG plus ST analysis were compared.

Patients.—Of 1,221 women giving birth at 34 weeks' or more gestation, 606 who had a mean age of 26.3 years were randomly allocated to fetal monitoring with CTG alone, and 615 who had a mean age of 25.9 years were monitored by ST plus CTG. Only pregnancies with no gross fetal abnormalities were included in the study. Neonatal outcome was defined by umbilical cord blood gas analysis, Apgar scores, resuscitation needs, and the postnatal course. All tracings were retrospectively re-

Indications for Operative Deliveries

—	CTG (n=606)	ST+CTG (n=615)	p	Odds ratio (95% CI)
Abnormal pH on FBS	8	9	0·98	0·90 (0·35–2·35)
Abnormal trace	50	18	<0·001	2·98 (1·72–5·17)
Deliveries for fetal distress	58	27	<0·001	2·30 (1·44–3·69)
Deliveries for failure to progress	129	125	0·96	1·02 (0·77–1·34)

Abbreviations: FBS, fetal blood sampling: *CTG,* cardiotocography; *ST + CTG,* ST waveform analysis plus CTG.

(Courtesy of Westgate J, Harris M, Curnow JSH, et al: *Lancet* 340:194–198, 1992.)

viewed to verify adherence to the trial protocol by an independent observer who was blinded to the neonatal outcome.

Results.—There were no significant differences between the 2 groups in terms of asphyxia at birth or neonatal outcome. The addition of ECG ST waveform information to CTG monitoring reduced the rate of operative deliveries for fetal distress by 53% with no changes in neonatal outcome (table). However, the additional ST waveform information did not reduce the rate of operative deliveries for other reasons. Although the rate of metabolic acidosis and low 5-minute Apgar scores were lower in the group monitored with CTG plus ST waveform analysis, the difference did not reach statistical significance. Most of the reduction in the operative intervention rate attributable to ST waveform information occurred among patients with normal or intermediate CTG patterns, whereas the additional information did not reduce the operative intervention rate for women with abnormal CTG recordings.

Conclusion.—Monitoring the fetal ECG ST waveform during labor reduces the rate of operative deliveries for fetal distress without affecting neonatal outcome.

▶ Despite widespread use for more than 3 decades, the role of electronic fetal heart rate monitoring remains controversial. There has been inconsistent interpretation of fetal heart rate patterns and unnecessary operative intervention, as evidenced by a vigorous fetus with no evidence of stress or distress at birth. (In fact, there is a growing body of advocates for redefining the terminology, eliminating the term "fetal distress.") Shy (1) found that it performed not better than intermittent auscultation, confirming the results of the meta-analysis of fetal heart rate monitoring (2). Cardiotocography, supplemented by fetal blood gas sampling, improves the specificity; however, it is invasive, costly and, at best, intermittent. Nevertheless, refining CTG by adding an EKG component significantly reduced the need for operative delivery without increasing the rates of neonatal depression or morbidity.

The preliminary studies were performed in animals and, a pilot group of 100 patients permitted personnel training in the technology. The study was well designed, and a rigid protocol with clear definitions and indication for intervention was adhered to. This prospective study eventually yielded results consistent with the hypothesis. Quality control was further insured as all tracings were reviewed by an impartial investigator who was unaware of fetal outcome. Asphyxia was confirmed by measurement of arterial and venous blood gases from the cord blood. The time is opportune to further evaluate this technology. Combining the fetal heart rate pattern with an EKG appears to increase both the sensitivity and specificity of fetal heart rate monitoring, thereby enhancing the science and diminishing the art.

Making the simple complicated is commonplace; making the complicated simple, awesomely simple, that's creativity.—Charles Mingus.

A.A. Fanaroff, M.B.B.Ch.

References

1. 1991 Year Book of Neonatal and Perinatal Medicine, pp 112–113.
2. Chalmers I, et al: *Effective Care in Pregnancy and Childbirth.* Oxford, England, Oxford University Press, 1989, pp 872–873.

Computerized Measurement of Heart Rate Variation in Fetal Anemia Caused by Rhesus Alloimmunization

Economides DL, Selinger M, Ferguson J, Bowell PJ, Dawes GS, Mackenzie IZ (John Radcliffe Hosp, Oxford, England)

Am J Obstet Gynecol 167:689–693, 1992 4–2

Background.—Fetal heart rate (FHR) monitoring is a noninvasive test commonly used in the management of red-cell alloimmunized pregnancies. The FHR pattern is not, however, sufficiently sensitive in predicting mild to moderate anemia. Whether computerized recording and analysis of the variations in FHR could be used to detect anemia before cardiac decompensation develops was investigated.

Methods.—Sixty-five computerized recordings of FHR were obtained in 36 red-cell alloimmunized pregnancies immediately before ultrasonographically guided fetal blood sampling for measurement of fetal hematocrit. The mean gestational age was 30 weeks.

Results.—Even after adjusting for the effect of gestation, short- and long-term variations in FHR were significantly correlated with fetal hematocrit (Fig 4–1). When short-term variation was less than 5 ms or long-term variation was less than 30 ms, the positive predictive values for a fetal hematocrit of less than 30 were 85% and 90%, and the negative predictive values were 56% and 57%, respectively. A weaker correlation existed between the number of accelerations per hour and the degree of fetal anemia. There were no significant correlations between fetal movements per hour or basal heart rate and the degree of fetal anemia.

Conclusion.—A computerized analysis of the patterns of FHR in red-cell alloimmunized pregnancies yielded a strong correlation between variations in FHR and hematocrit. This relationship was best described by a quadratic model. In contrast to previous studies, decelerations were not present in the majority of fetuses with moderate or severe anemia.

▶ Marked observer variability has been a major deterrent to the visual interpretation of FHR patterns and has spurred the obstetrics unit at Oxford to develop a computerized assessment of FHR variations. This method appears to be a significant improvement over visual inspection. For markedly affected infants, short-term FHR variation was reduced to less than half the mean for 7 fetuses that were severely anemic. When short-term variability was moderately reduced (by 50% to 75%), 83% of the fetuses were anemic. However, anemia cannot be excluded when the short-term variation was 75% to 100% of normal, because one fetus in this group was found to be severely

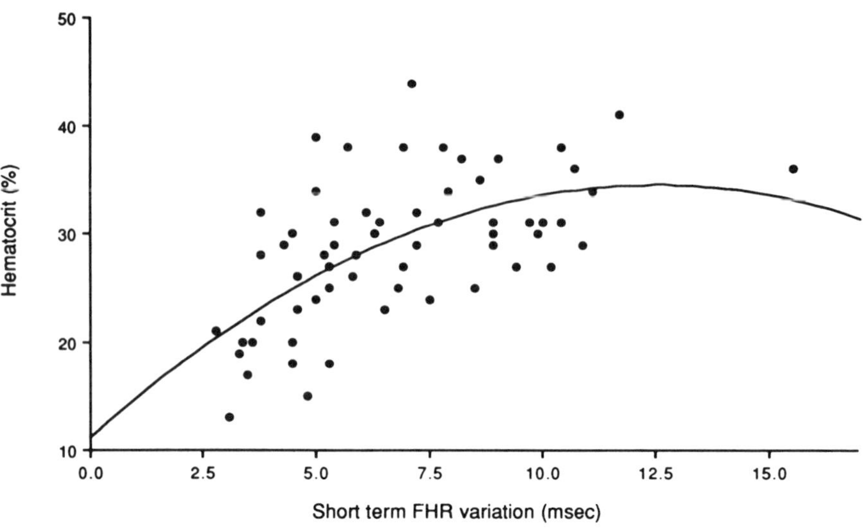

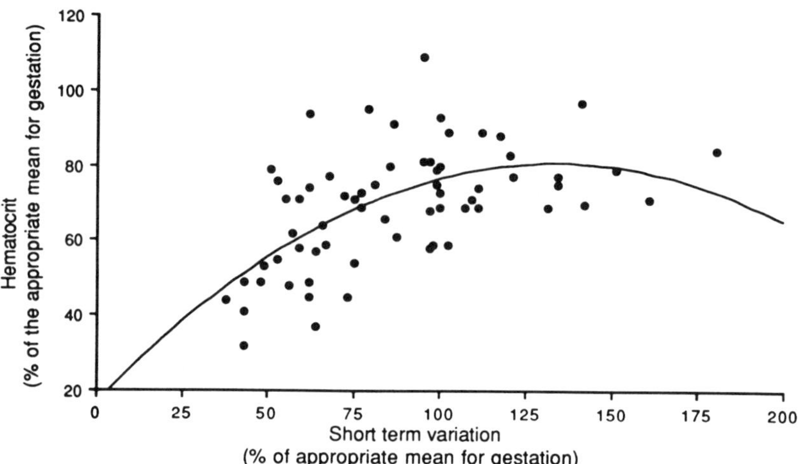

Fig 4–1.—Correlation between short-term FHR variation and fetal hematocrit (r = .60. n = 65, P < .05, $y = 10.99 + 3.752 - .15x^2$). Also shown is correlation between 2 variables expressed as percent of mean for gestational age (r = .60, n = 65, P < .01, $y = 19.264 + .913x - .003x^2$). (Courtesy of Economides DL, Selinger M, Ferguson J, et al: *Am J Obstet Gynecol* 167:689–693, 1992.)

anemic. Further studies are needed to evaluate this new tool.—M.H. Klaus, M.D.

Description, Evaluation and Clinical Decision Making According to Various Fetal Heart Rate Patterns: Inter-Observer and Regional Variability

Lidegaard Ø, Bøttcher LM, Weber T (Univ of Copenhagen)
Acta Obstet Gynecol Scand 71:48–53, 1992 4–3

Objective.—Despite its widespread application, there remains some controversy regarding the sensitivity and specificity of electronic fetal heart rate monitoring for fetal asphyxia. The interobserver and regional variability in the description and evaluation of fetal heart rate patterns was evaluated.

Study Design.—In 10 Danish obstetric departments, 42 senior and 74 junior residents evaluated 11 fetal heart rate patterns on an arbitrary 0% to 100% scale and were given relevant clinical information to form a clinical decision for each case. The 11 traces included 5 antepartum and 6 intrapartum patterns, normal and pathologic patterns, traces from normal and asphyxiated babies.

Findings.—For description of fetal heart rate patterns, the degree of agreement was high for baseline, silent, and sinusoidal patterns (87% to 94%) but low for evaluation of variability and type of deceleration (50% to 72%). These wide differences in the detailed description partly accounted for the low agreement score in the interpretation of heart rate pattern (59%). Senior residents generally interpreted the heart rate changes as being indicative of less serious fetal stress compared with junior residents. This was reflected in their clinical decisions, as junior residents found an indication for cesarean section 30% more often than did senior residents. The interobserver variability between regions ranged from 57% to 63%, and between departments, from 57% to 65%; these differences were not significant.

Implications.—There is still a need for scientific clarification of which specific heart rate changes constitute the best predictors of fetal stress. One promising avenue is the use of artificial intelligence programs for interpreting fetal cardiotocograms and electrocardiographic signals.

▶ Investigators and clinicians alike are finding that fetal heart rate patterns do not reliably predict fetal outcome. Furthermore, as noted by Barrett (1), there are wide interobserver and intraobserver inconsistencies in management decisions in obstetrics. As noted above, the Danish experience confirms these observations. The value of electronic fetal heart rate monitoring continues to be the subject of many reports. None, however, appear to justify the mini-industry that has sprung up to ensure that all patients in labor are electronically monitored. Central monitoring stations have become the norm at many obstetric units and no self-respecting plaintiff's lawyer would appear in court without the monitoring strips and an expert to interpret same.

Murphy (2), after attempting to predict birth asphyxia from the intrapartum cardiotocograph, concluded that "the interpretation of the intrapartum cardiotocograph remains a major problem, and a more objective method of interpretation should be found." Pello (3) postulated that a large randomized trial of fetal heart rate screening in early labor could serve to demonstrate the usefulness of detecting decelerations with reduced variation. However, more than 10,000 patients would be needed to detect benefit in 2 of every 1,000. (Is this what the government panels mean by cost effective?) For those who are dissatisfied with the shortcoming of electronic monitoring to predict early neonatal problems, Shy and colleagues (4) were unable to demonstrate that electronic fetal heart rate monitoring improved the neurologic development of children born prematurely. Periodic auscultation of the fetal heart rate was equally effective. Painter (5) noted that "periods of abnormal FHR patterns continuing for up to 375 minutes in the moderately severe deceleration group and up to 975 minutes in the severe and late deceleration groups were associated with normal outcome at 6–9 years of age." There has been a call for the use of artificial intelligence in interpreting these monitoring strips. It may well provide more consistency, but perhaps we should start believing the results of all the controlled trials and look for other means of documenting fetal jeopardy. The addition of an ECG to electronic fetal heart rate monitoring is discussed in the 1992 YEAR BOOK OF NEONATAL AND PERINATAL MEDICINE. Fetal monitoring with pulse oximetry is also under investigation (6).

These few words of wisdom from *A World Treasury of Folk Wisdom* by Feldman and Voelke should guide us in this dilemma

To ask is a temporary shame; not to ask is an eternal one (Japanese); Doubt is the key to knowledge (Iranian); One who is afraid of asking is ashamed of learning (Danish).

A.A. Fanaroff, M.B.B.Ch.

References

1. 1991 YEAR BOOK OF NEONATAL AND PERINATAL MEDICINE, pp 81–83.
2. 1991 YEAR BOOK OF NEONATAL AND PERINATAL MEDICINE, pp 121–123.
3. Pello LC: *Br J Obstet Gynecol* 95:1128, 1988.
4. 1991 YEAR BOOK OF NEONATAL AND PERINATAL MEDICINE, pp 112–113.
5. Painter MJ: *Am J Obstet Gynecol* 159:854, 1988.
6. 1992 YEAR BOOK OF NEONATAL AND PERINATAL MEDICINE, pp 1–2.

Randomised Controlled Trial of Doppler Ultrasound Screening of Placental Perfusion During Pregnancy

Davies JA, Gallivan S, Spencer JAD (Queen Charlotte's and Chelsea Hosp,

London; Univ College London)
Lancet 340:1299–1303, 1992 4–4

Background.—Screening studies suggest there is little value in routine Doppler ultrasound examinations of all pregnancies, as adverse outcomes are poorly predicted. The effects of primary management and outcomes of routine Doppler ultrasound assessments of the umbilical and uterine arteries in pregnancy were determined in a randomized controlled study.

Methods.—In a 9-month period, 2,600 women were recruited from a general obstetric population for the study. All had singleton pregnancies. Of the 2,475 women delivering in the hospital after 20 weeks' gestation, 1,246 had been randomly assigned to receive standard antenatal care including routine Doppler assessments. The first Doppler ultrasound examination was done at 19–22 weeks of gestation. Thereafter, examinations were done monthly if the pregnancy was considered at high risk or once at 32 weeks if the pregnancy was low risk. The 1,229 women in the control group received standard prenatal care without Doppler ultrasonography.

Findings.—The 2 groups did not differ in number of prenatal admissions or cardiotocographs, gestational age at delivery, delivery method, frequency of deliveries with fetal distress, or the need for resuscitation or admission to the neonatal intensive care unit. There were more perinatal deaths in the Doppler group, with a relative risk of 2.4. However, only 1 of 11 normally formed stillbirths and none of the 4 normally formed neonates who died after 24 weeks' gestation had an abnormal umbilical-artery Doppler examination.

Conclusion.—Routine Doppler ultrasound examinations during pregnancy in an unselected population are not likely to improve management and perinatal outcome. These findings are consistent with findings from previous observational screening studies.

▶ Commenting on this study is Michael Katz, M.D., Associate Professor of Obstetrics and Gynecology of Reproductive Science, University of California, San Francisco, and Chief of Perinatal Service, California Pacific Medical Center:

▶ This study evaluates the possible role of Doppler velocimetry testing as a screening and management tool for the prediction of adverse perinatal outcome in normal pregnancies. The authors correctly conclude that the availability of Doppler velocimetry has no proven advantages for the population studied. Whether a possible reduction (specifically in perinatal mortality) can be achieved in this population could only be demonstrated if a much larger sample were tested. As far as the increased perinatal mortality that was observed in one of the subsets of the Doppler group, no explanation can be found, and this may be a random event. This reviewer believes that it is very possible that what can be detected by Doppler velocimetry is not necessarily associated with the specific conditions responsible for most of the perinatal mortality in unselected populations. Therefore, Doppler testing has no substantial role in either the screening or management of low-risk pregnancies.—M. Katz, M.D.

The Effect of Glucose on Doppler Flow Velocity Waveforms and Heart Rate Pattern in the Human Fetus

Gillis S, Connors G, Potts P, Hunse C, Richardson B (St Joseph's Health Centre, London, Ont, Canada; University of Western Ontario, London, Canada)
Early Hum Dev 30:1–10, 1992 4–5

Introduction.—Analysis of Doppler flow velocity waveforms (DFVW) can help to assess compromises in fetal oxygenation. Other factors, however, can affect waveform indices, including fetal heart rate (FHR), behavioral state, gestational age, and glucose. Researchers studied 24 healthy pregnant women to determine the effect of glucose on the DFVW in fetal cerebral and umbilical arteries.

Methods.—Women with singleton pregnancies between 36 and 40 weeks' gestation were randomized to either a 50-g oral glucose drink or an equivalent amount of water. The DFVW measurements were ob-

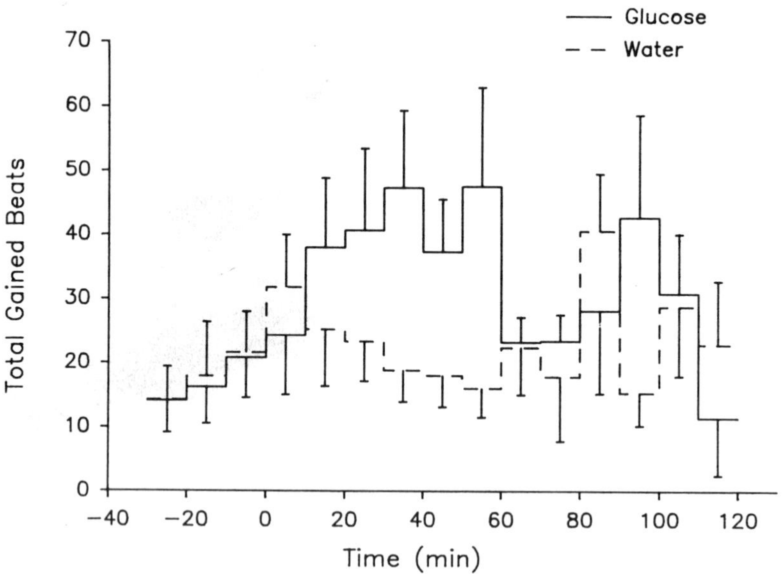

Fig 4–2.—Total gained beats calculated in 10-minute intervals during the control and study periods. The total gained beats were significantly increased 30 to 60 minutes after the glucose drink when compared with the water drink ($P < .05$). (Courtesy of Gillis S, Connors G, Potts P, et al: *Early Hum Dev* 30:1–10, 1992.)

tained before and at 45 and 120 minutes after the drink. At these same periods, blood samples were taken for determination of whole blood glucose concentration. The Resistance Index, as an index of vascular resistance, was calculated for the anterior cerebral, internal carotid, and umbilical arteries. Behavioral state was measured by monitoring the FHR pattern as determined by FHR variability.

Results.—In the mothers receiving glucose, maternal glucose concentrations increased approximately twofold at 45 minutes after the glucose drink. They remained elevated at 120 minutes, but were significantly lower than at 45 minutes. The Resistance Index of both fetal cerebral vessels studied was significantly reduced at 45 minutes after the glucose drink; this effect was still evident at 120 minutes in the anterior cerebral artery. The Resistance Index of the umbilical artery varied little after either drink. The mean minute range as a measure of long-term FHR variability did not significantly differ between the 2 groups up to 30 minutes after and more than 60 minutes after glucose or water. Between 30 and 60 minutes after the drink, a significantly higher mean minute range was observed for the glucose group, indicating a differential effect on FHR pattern. During the same period, the total gained beats and the number of FHR accelerations were significantly higher for the glucose group (Fig 4–2).

Conclusion.—The effect of glucose on the cerebral Doppler waveform indices of the human fetus is an indirect one, mediated through changes in behavioral state. Doppler flow velocity waveform measurements may be done successfully irrespective of maternal meals, provided that FHR pattern is controlled for.

▶ Commenting on this article is Cynthia Bearer, M.D., Ph.D., Director of Neonatology and Pediatric Environmental Health, Tod Children's Hospital, Youngstown, Ohio, and Associate Professor of Pediatrics, Northeastern Ohio University College of Medicine, Kent, Ohio:

▶ The authors of this study provide very logical data to suggest that increases in fetal block glucose decrease cerebral vascular resistance by inducing changes in the behavioral state. They further speculate that this effect of glucose may have an effect on the growth and development of the brain in the perinatal period. This speculation may be the hypothesis for further studies. Certainly, infants of diabetic women who are large for gestational age have been exposed to higher serum glucose levels. Are they at risk for neurobehavioral abnormalities? If the fetal serum glucose level remains elevated, does the effect on behavioral state and, thus, cerebral vascular resistance dampen? The changes in maternal serum glucose levels were from 57 mg/dL to 106 mg/dL. Changes in cerebral vascular resistance and, therefore, behavioral state were seen with these changes. What implications does this observation have for the growth and development of the premature infant brain when glucose values in the intensive-care nursery can vary anywhere from 50 to 180 mg/dL? Should we be much more vigilant over the allowable glucose range in these fragile infants? Perhaps a study of cerebral vascular resistance in these infants at different times (dependent on their serum glucose levels) is indicated.—C. Bearer, M.D., Ph.D.

Comparison of Umbilical-Artery Velocimetry and Cardiotocography for Surveillance of Small-for-Gestational-Age Fetuses

Almström H, Axelsson O, Cnattingius S, Ekman G, Maesel A, Ulmsten U, Årström K, Maršál K (Danderyd's Hosp, Stockholm; Uppsala Univ, Sweden; Malmö Gen Hosp, Sweden; et al)

Lancet 340:936–940, 1992 4–6

Background.—Intrauterine growth retardation is associated with a greater risk of fetal asphyxia and increased perinatal morbidity and death. With ultrasound fetometry, fetuses that are small for gestational age can be detected. Doppler velocimetry of the umbilical artery is a good predictor of fetal distress, but it is unknown whether it could replace cariotocography in antenatal surveillance of small-for-gestational-age fetuses. The 2 methods were compared in a randomized study.

Methods.—Women with fetuses that were small on ultrasound examination at 31 weeks' gestation or later were studied. Four different obstetric departments in Sweden participated. The women were randomly assigned to prenatal surveillance with Doppler velocimetry or cardiotocography. Pregnancies in the Doppler group were managed according to a protocol based on blood-flow classes from a semiquantitative assessment of umbilical-artery velocity waveforms. Antenatal cardiotocography was not done unless the pregnancy was complicated by another disorder.

Findings.—Compared with the cardiotocography group, the Doppler group had fewer monitoring occasions, prenatal hospitalization, inductions of labor, emergent cesarean sections for fetal distress, and admissions to neonatal intensive care. The 2 groups were comparable in mean gestational age at birth, birth weight, Apgar scores, and total number of cesarean deliveries.

Conclusion.—Small-for-gestational-age fetuses in otherwise uncomplicated pregnancies can apparently be monitored prenatally by Doppler velocimetry only. Such a strategy will reduce costs and maternal psychosocial stress. However, when the risk of impaired fetal health is greater, combining the 2 methods is still reasonable.

▶ Commenting on this study is Michael Katz, M.D., Associate Professor of Obstetrics and Gynecology of Reproductive Science, University of California, San Francisco; and Chief of Perinatal Service, California Pacific Medical Center:

▶ This study compared the traditional surveillance technique, i.e., fetal heart rate nonstress (NST) testing in small-for-gestational-age pregnancies with a more recent method using Doppler velocimetry evaluations of the umbilical artery. The results indicated a significantly increased incidence of antepartum and intrapartum interventions in the NST group, including a number of antepartum admissions to the hospital, inductions of labor, and incidence of operative deliveries. In terms of the perinatal-neonatal outcome, no differences were observed between the groups.

Clearly, interventions on behalf of the fetus that are based on fetal heart rate (FHR) monitoring surveillance are not accurate or reliable. Although reassuring FHR patterns are reliable predictors of well-being, the nonreassuring patterns have long been known to be erroneous in approximately 50% of occurrences. Therefore, one should view this study not so much as a big advantage of Doppler velocimetry but, rather, as a weakness of nonreassuring FHR in predicting fetal distress. Whether STSs should be completely abandoned and replaced by doppler velocimetry in small-for-gestational-age pregnancies will require further studies.—M. Katz, M.D.

The Acute Response of the Umbilical Artery Pulsatility Index to Changes in Blood Volume in Fetal Sheep

van Huisseling H, Muijsers GJJM, de Haan J, Hasaart THM (Univ Hosp, Maastricht, The Netherlands)

Eur J Obstet Gynecol Reprod Biol 43:149–155, 1992 4–7

Introduction.—Absent or reversed end-diastolic flow in Doppler umbilical artery waveforms is associated with fetal and neonatal morbidity and mortality. The flow velocity waveform is the result of several interacting factors, and changes in 1 of these factors might influence the flow velocity waveform indices. However, to what extent the changes in any of these factors influence the umbilical artery waveform in vivo is not known. The effects of acute changes in fetal circulating blood volume on the umbilical artery pusatility index (PI) were investigated.

Methods.—Six fetal sheep between 117 and 125 days' gestation were provided with an electromagnetic flowmeter for measurement of the umbilical venous blood flow, catheters for the determination of arterial blood pressure and umbilical venous pressure, and a 5-MHz Doppler transducer placed around 1 umbilical artery for umbilical artery flow velocity analysis. A few days after instrumentation, fetal hypervolemia was induced by infusing 50 mL of maternal blood, and hypovolemia was induced by withdrawing 50 mL of fetal blood.

Results.—Hypervolemia resulted in an increase in arterial pressure and umbilical venous pressure, whereas the PI, umbilical blood flow, and the calculated placental vascular resistance remained unchanged. Hypovolemia resulted in a decrease in fetal heart rate, arterial pressure, umbilical venous pressure, and umbilical blood flow. The PI increased by 42%, and the placental vascular resistance was unchanged (Fig 4–3). Thus, a

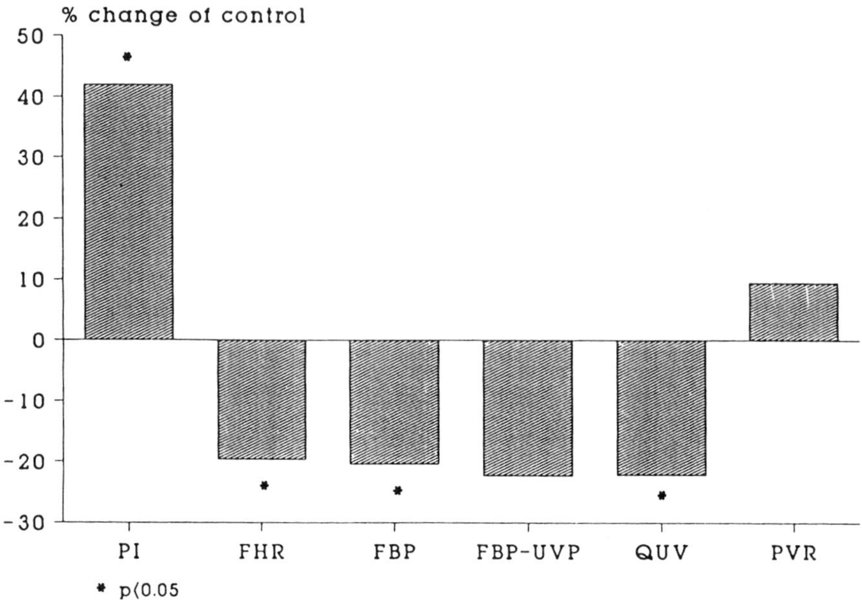

Fig 4–3.—The percent changes from control in umbilical artery pulsatility index, fetal heart rate, fetal blood pressure, umbilical blood flow, and placental vascular resistance after withdrawal of 50 mL of fetal blood. (Courtesy of van Huisseling H, Muijsers GJJM, de Haan J, et al: *Eur J Obstet Gynecol Reprod Biol* 43:149–155, 1992.)

10% to 15% increase in fetal circulating blood volume did not affect the umbilical artery PI or the placental vascular resistance, whereas an acute reduction in fetal blood volume with the same amount was associated with an increase in the umbilical artery PI without a change in placental vascular resistance.

Conclusion.—Increased umbilical artery blood velocity indices are not necessarily related to placental vascular pathology, but they may be a sign of fetal hypotension.

▶ Blood flow patterns in the fetal vessels have come under close scrutiny to determine fetal well-being. Absent or reversed end-diastolic flow velocities in the fetal umbilical artery indicate fetal jeopardy. The fetus may die or have a greater risk of requiring admission to the intensive care unit. The authors used a chronically instrumented lamb preparation to unravel the mysteries of the umbilical artery pulsatility index. The responses to hypervolemia and hypovolemia were closely monitored. Indeed, acute blood volume changes produced short-lasting changes on the cardiovascular variables. Hypervolemia increased blood pressure by almost 30%, but it was well tolerated, producing minimal change in the PI. However when the lamb is rendered hypotensive by acutely reducing the blood volume by 10% to 15%, the heart rate is almost 40 beats slower and the pulsatility index changes dramatically, triggering the "on" signal for all the statistical lights. Fetal hypoxemia did not contribute to the rise in PI, because the hematocrit and arterial oxygen content were not altered by the acute hemorrhage. The pulsatility index was noted to increase without a concomitant increase in the placental vascular resistance, leading to the not-so-profound conclusion that the increased umbilical velocity indices may be a sign of fetal hypotension (with reduced end-diastolic velocities) and do not necessarily relate to placental vascular pathology. Were these lambs sacrificed for nought?

Stick to one thing and all will come; aim at everything and all will go.—Jackson Brown, Jr.

A.A. Fanaroff, M.B.B.Ch.

Middle Cerebral Artery Flow Velocity Waveforms in Normal and Small-for-Gestational-Age Fetuses

Mari G, Deter RL (Yale Univ, New Haven, Conn; Baylor College of Medicine, Houston)

Am J Obstet Gynecol 166:1262–1270, 1992 4–8

Background.—Normal values for the velocity waveforms of different cerebral arteries in the fetus have been reported. In the first longitudinal report on the cerebral blood flow velocity waveforms early in the second trimester of pregnancy, the pulsatility index of the middle cerebral artery was compared in normal fetuses and small-for-gestational-age (SGA) fetuses.

Methods.—Study data were obtained from 16 normal fetuses (group 1), 128 normal fetuses in a cross-sectional study (group 2), and 33 SGA fetuses (group 3). No growth abnormalities or congenital anomalies were found in the first 2 groups. Doppler ultrasonography examinations of the middle cerebral artery were carried out at various intervals, starting at 15 or 20 weeks. Three consecutive waveforms were analyzed, and the results were averaged.

Results.—In group 1, the middle cerebral artery waveforms exhibited a higher diastole at 15–20 weeks and at the end of gestation. This finding was associated with a lower pulsatility index value between 15–20 weeks' gestation and a higher value at 25–30 weeks' gestation. In 9 of 16 infants studied longitudinally, no significant difference was observed in pulsatility index values at the end of gestation and 1 month after delivery. Nine of the 33 SGA fetuses had a middle cerebral artery pulsatility value below the normal range. The SGA fetuses with abnormal pulsatility index values had a significantly higher incidence of abnormal fetal heart rate and admission into the neonatal intensive care unit. The SGA fetuses with abnormal pulsatility index values also had a higher rate of mortality than did the SGA fetuses with normal values (33.3% vs. 12.5%).

Conclusion.—In the normal human fetus, the pulsatility index of the middle cerebral artery has a parabolic pattern during pregnancy. An abnormal index in the SGA fetus is associated with a worse fetal outcome. A brain-sparing effect can be present as early as 20 weeks' gestation and can indicate a high-risk fetus.

▶ The normative data for middle cerebral artery flow velocity waveforms are gradually being accumulated (1, 2). As a result, it may be possible to distinguish the patterns from appropriately growing and SGA infants. An exciting aspect of this research has been the attempt to correlate the observations on the middle cerebral artery resistance with the classic brain growth studies of Dobbing and Sands (3), who demonstrated major brain cell multiplication at 15–20 weeks gestation, and again in the third trimester. Mari and Deter have noted that these periods of maximal brain growth coincide with the lowest resistance; they also have speculated that this lower impedance accomodates the increased metabolic requirements of the brain. Extrapolating indirect measurements of middle cerebral artery blood flow with brain sparing in a growth-retarded fetus may be considered a reach. On the other hand, the proposition is conceptually sound, feasible, and plausible. Furthermore, those fetuses with abnormal pulsatility index had a greater incidence of adverse perinatal outcome. Factors accounting for changes in the pulsatility index include fetal hypoxemia, anemia, or ciculatory changes induced by changing flow through the ductus arteriosus.

The selection of the study population will raise some eyebrows, as some of these subjects had been included in other publications. However, this is stated up front, and everyone is in the business of maximizing the data. I was more concerned with the technical aspects of the study. The ultrasonic energy ouput exceeded the Food and Drug Administration's recommendation for fetal Doppler ultrasonography. The instrumentation permitted better data collection and the authors justified its use citing "no independently confirmed significant biologic effect in mammalian tissues noted with focused ultrasonographic intensities below 1W/cm2"(4). As there are no clinical decisions made from the above measurements, we need reassurance that no harm will come to the fetus as a result of these measurements.—A.A. Fanaroff, M.B.B.Ch.

References

1. 1992 YEAR BOOK OF NEONATAL AND PERINATAL MEDICINE, pp 65–66.
2. 1991 YEAR BOOK OF NEONATAL AND PERINATAL MEDICINE, pp 44–45.
3. Dobbing J, Sands J: *Nature* 226:639, 1970.
4. American Institute of Ultrasound in Medicine: *J Ultrasound Med* 9:S1, 1988.

Inferior Vena Cava Flow Velocity Waveforms in Appropriate- and Small-for-Gestational-Age Fetuses

Rizzo G, Arduini D, Romanini C (Università Cattolica S Cuore, Rome; Università di Ancona, Italy)

Am J Obstet Gynecol 166:1271–1280, 1992 4–9

Background.—Fetal pathologic conditions including anemia, nonimmune hydrops, and arrhythmias and fetal growth retardation have been associated with abnormal inferior vena cava flow velocity waveforms. There has been little research on the reference ranges of the longitudinal changes occurring in inferior vena cava blood flow patterns with the progression of normal pregnancy, or in growth-retarded fetuses with different degrees of compromise. Doppler ultrasonography was used to establish the reference ranges of velocity waveforms.

Method.—Blood flow velocity waveforms of 118 appropriate-for-gestational-age (AGA) fetuses of 18–40 weeks' gestation and 79 small-for-gestational-age (SGA) fetuses were recorded with color and pulsed Doppler equipment. The systolic-to-diastolic ratios for the peak velocities and time velocity intervals were calculated. The percentage of reverse flow with atrial contraction was quantified as the percentage of time velocity intervals during atrial contraction with respect to total forward time velocity intervals. The 79 SGA fetuses were divided into 3 groups according to umbilical artery velocity waveforms, group 1 having normal pulsatility index values, group 2 having an abnormal pulsatility index with the presence of end-diastolic velocities, and group 3 having no end-diastolic velocities (table). Some of the SGA fetuses were also studied longitudinally at weekly intervals until delivery.

Results.—In AGA fetuses, no changes were evident in peak velocity and time velocity interval ratios, whereas the percentage of reverse flow significantly decreased with gestation. Group 1 SGA fetuses had similar results, but those in groups 2 and 3 showed a significant increase in peak velocity and time velocity interval ratios and in percentage of reverse flow. Those SGA fetuses in groups 2 and 3 who had a percentage of reverse flow above the 95% confidence interval had a poorer perinatal outcome than did the fetuses of the same groups that had reverse flow values in the normal range. Among the 14 SGA fetuses followed up longitudinally, there was a significant and progressive increase in peak velocity and time velocity interval ratios and in percentage of reverse flow, despite minimal changes in pulsatility indexes from the umbilical artery and different peripheral fetal vessels.

Conclusion.—In SGA fetuses, abnormal flow patterns in the inferior vena cava appear to be a result of uteroplacental insufficiency and seem to be unrelated to the abnormalities present in Doppler-measured vascular resistances in fetal arterial vascular beds. The modified flow velocity

Characteristics of Fetuses Studied

		SGA			*Significance**			*Significance**		
	AGA (n = 118)	*Group 1 (n = 26)*	*Group 2 (n = 33)*	*Group 3 (n = 20)*	*AGA vs group 1*	*AGA vs group 2*	*AGA vs group 3*	*Group 1 vs group 2*	*Group 1 vs Group 3*	*Group 2 vs group 3*
Gestational age at Doppler recordings (wk)	29.6 ± 5.1	30.3 ± 2.6	31.0 ± 2.5	28.3 ± 5.2	NS	NS	NS	NS	NS	NS
Umbilical artery pulsatility index (Δ value)	−0.12 ± 0.99	0.33 ± 0.94	3.04 ± 1.13	4.12 ± 1.62	NS	$p \le 0.001$	$p \le 0.001$	$p \le 0.001$	$p \le 0.001$	$p \le 0.001$
Descending aorta pulsatility index	1.94 ± 0.21	1.97 ± 0.26	2.46 ± 0.41	2.64 ± 0.55	NS	$p \le 0.001$	$p \le 0.001$	$p \le 0.001$	$p \le 0.001$	NS
Renal artery pulsatility index (Δ-value)	0.03 ± 0.83	0.21 ± 0.96	2.24 ± 1.45	3.19 ± 1.84	NS	$p \le 0.001$	$p \le 0.001$	$p \le 0.001$	$p \le 0.001$	$p \le 0.05$
Internal carotid artery (Δ-value)	−0.06 ± 0.87	0.27 ± 0.75	-2.67 ± 1.44	-3.19 ± 1.46	NS	$p \le 0.001$	$p \le 0.001$	$p \le 0.001$	$p \le 0.001$	NS
Middle cerebral artery pulsatility (Δ-value)	0.12 ± 0.88	0.31 ± 0.92	-2.95 ± 1.21	-3.32 ± 1.33	NS	$p \le 0.001$	$p \le 0.001$	$p \le 0.001$	$p \le 0.001$	NS
Gestational age at birth (wk)	39.7 ± 1.9	38.4 ± 2.5	34.8 ± 3.2	32.1 ± 4.2	NS	$p \le 0.001$	$p \le 0.001$	$p \le 0.001$	$p \le 0.001$	$p \le 0.05$
Birth weight (gm)	3654 ± 412	2320 ± 316	1635 ± 521	1135 ± 363	$p \le 0.001$	$p \le 0.001$	$p \le 0.001$	$p \le 0.001$	$p \le 0.001$	$p \le 0.001$
Umbilical artery pH	—	7.251 ± 0.029	7.223 ± 0.034	7.188 ± 0.042	—	—	—	$p \le 0.001$	$p \le 0.001$	$p \le 0.005$
Antepartum late heart rate decelerations (%)	0 (0)	0 (0)	13 (39.4)	14 (70.0)	NS	$p \le 0.001$	$p \le 0.001$	$p \le 0.002$	$p \le 0.001$	$p \le 0.01$
Cesarean section (%)	9 (7.6)	3 (11.5)	28 (84.5)	20 (100)	NS	$p \le 0.001$	$p \le 0.001$	$p \le 0.001$	$p \le 0.001$	NS
5 min Apgar score <7	0 (0)	0 (0)	9 (27.2)	9 (45.0)	NS	$p \le 0.001$	$p \le 0.001$	$p \le 0.005$	$p \le 0.002$	NS
Neonatal mortality	0 (0)	0 (0)	1 (3.0)	4 (20.0)	NS	NS	$p \le 0.005$	NS	$p \le 0.05$	NS

Note: values are mean ± 1 SD or number and percentage. Because pulsatility index values obtained from umbilical, renal, internal carotid, and middle cerebral arteries change with gestation, the data are expressed as the number of standard deviations from the normal mean for gestation.

Abbreviation: NS, not significant.

* By unpaired *t* test and Fisher's exact test.

(Courtesy of Rizzo G, Arduini D, Romanini C: *Am J Obstet Gynecol* 166:1271–1280, 1992.)

patterns in the inferior vena cava seem to deteriorate progressively with advancing gestation.

▶ The database expands excruciatingly slowly as the blood flow velocity patterns are laboriously accumulated from one fetal vessel at a time. Nonetheless, a profile is emerging, and the inferior vena caval flow patterns in healthy AGA infants are distinguishable from a subset of growth-retarded infants. As usual, the SGA infants comprise a heterogenous group. In view of the diverse etiologies for growth retardation, any other findings would have been open to question. I remain puzzled that the inferior vena caval flows reflect placental pathology, but I was, nonetheless, convinced that persistence of reverse flow in distole predicts a poor perinatal outcome. The pathophysiologic sequences are all inferred, but all may express progressive cardiac deterioration and, although the significance is the same, they are independent from patterns measured in fetal arterial vascular beds. Fetal distress in labor may be predicted in fetuses with abnormal inferior vena caval flow patterns. Technology has opened the windows into the fetal vascular flow patterns. To use this information in a meaningful clinical manner, a large number of fetuses will need to be studied. See also References 1 and 2.—A.A. Fanaroff, M.B.B.Ch.

Hear the other side.—Roman Law Principle

References

1. 1992 YEAR BOOK OF NEONATAL AND PERINATAL MEDICINE, pp 65, 66.
2. 1992 YEAR BOOK OF NEONATAL AND PERINATAL MEDICINE, pp 61, 62.

The Prevalence, Aetiology and Clinical Significance of Pseudo-Sinusoidal Fetal Heart Rate Patterns in Labour

Murphy KW, Russell V, Collins A, Johnson P (John Radcliffe Hosp, Oxford, England)
Br J Obstet Gynaecol 98:1093–1101, 1991 4–10

Introduction.—The fetal heart rate (FHR) usually fluctuates during labor and delivery. The sinusoidal pattern as seen in the FHR recording may indicate a serious loss of the beat-to-beat variability; however, such a pattern does not often occur during labor. Fetal heart rate patterns were assessed to determine the prevalence of the sinusoidal and the pseudosinusoidal patterns in women monitored during labor.

Methods.—The study population included all women who underwent fetal monitoring during labor in one 6-month period. A total of 1,520 patients were identified. In some patients, intrapartum ultrasound was used to determine whether fetal sucking or mouth movements occurred during a pseudosinusoidal pattern recording. Every tenth woman moni-

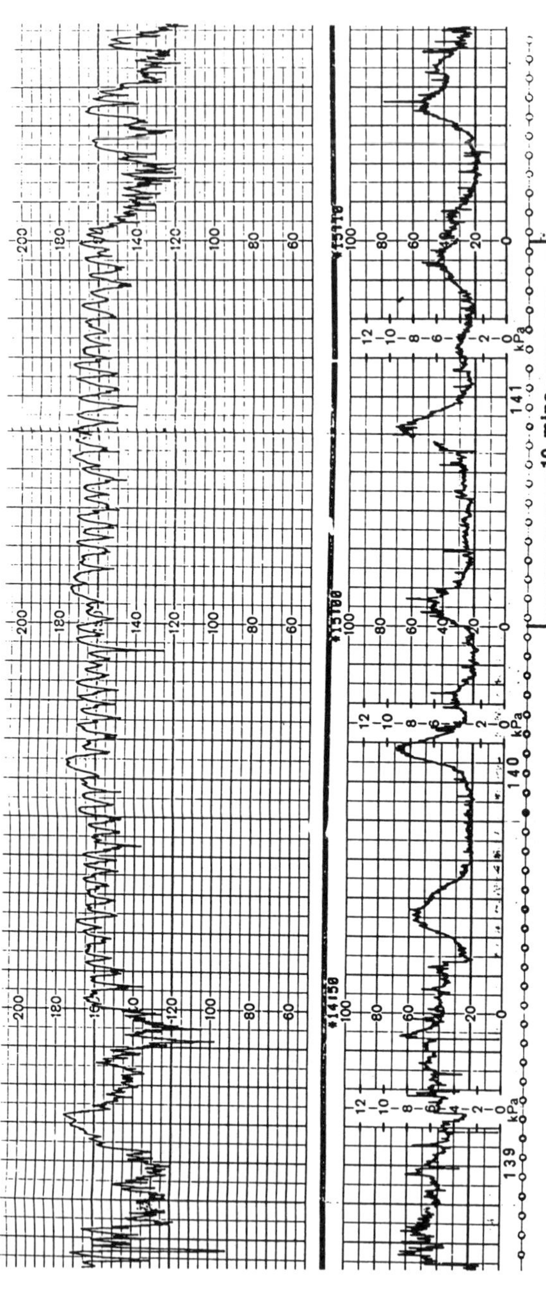

Fig 4–4.—Intermediate pseudosinusoidal FHR pattern showing oscillations with an amplitude of 15–20 beats/min and a frequency of 2–3 cycles/min. The baseline FHR increased during the oscillatory period. This pattern was caused by non-nutritive, fetal sucking. Fetal outcome was normal. (Courtesy of Murphy KW, Russell V, Collins A, et al: *Br J Obstet Gynaecol* 98:1093–1101, 1991.)

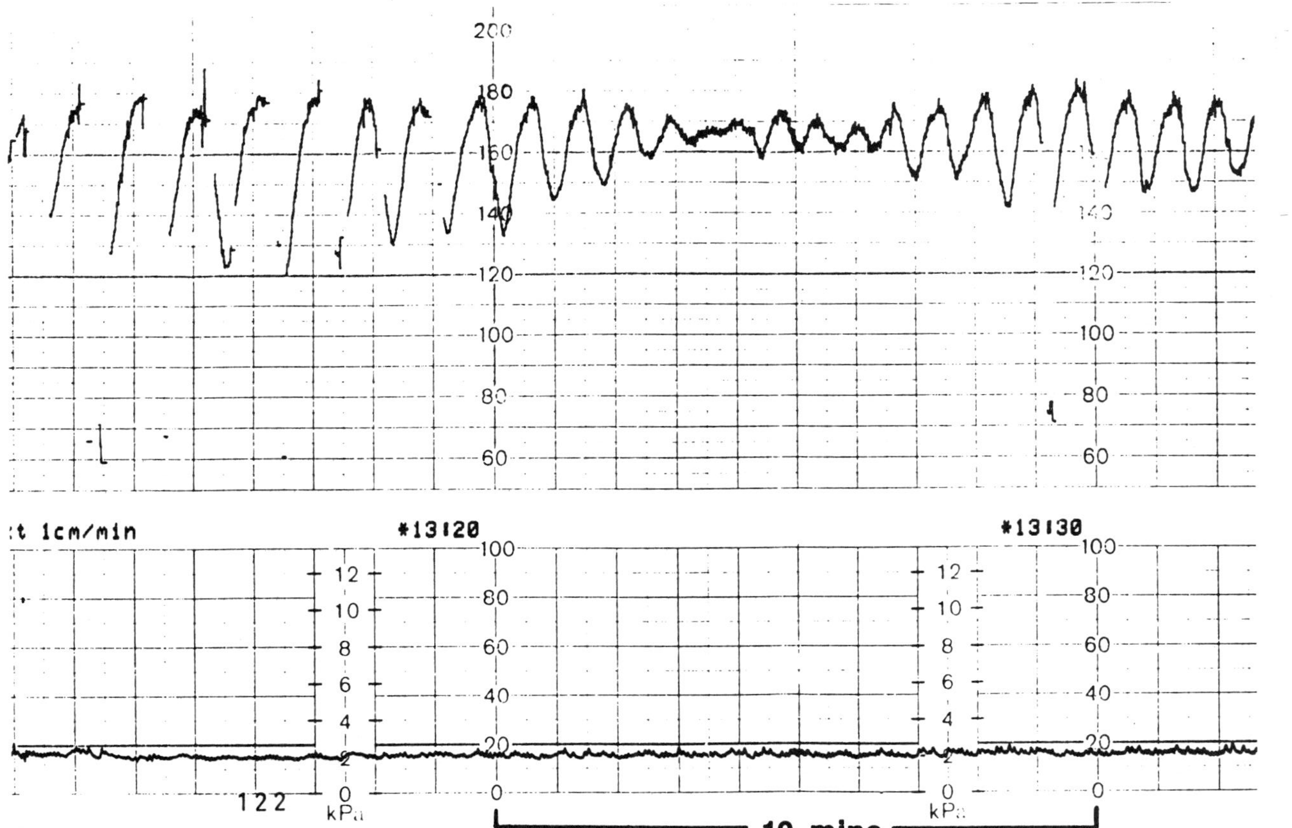

Fig 4–5.—Major pseudosinusoidal FHR pattern showing oscillations with an amplitude of 10–60 beats/min and a frequency of 1–2 cycles/min. This pattern followed an antepartum cordocentesis to measure fetal platelets. Acute cord hemorrhage occurred and a hypovolemic infant was born by emergency cesarean section. (Courtesy of Murphy KW, Russell V, Collins A, et al: *Br J Obstet Gynaecol* 98:1093–1101, 1991.)

tored who did not have a sinusoidal or pseudosinusoidal pattern served as a control.

Results.—A total of 1,520 cardiotocographs (CTGs) underwent review, resulting in not 1 case of an FHR sinusoidal pattern. A total of 230 pseudosinusoidal FHR patterns were recorded, however, for a prevalence of 15%. Of the 230 pseudosinusoidal FHR patterns, 219 were rated as minor occurrences and 11 were judged as intermediate (Fig 4–4). The mean time for this pattern was 21 minutes. Most of these pseudosinusoidal FHR patterns had occurred during the first stage of labor. Figure 4–5 illustrates a major pseudosinusoidal FHR pattern. Women with pseudosinusoidal FHR patterns differed significantly from controls in receiving 100 mg of intramuscularly administered pethidine (60% compared with 36%, respectively), in receiving an epidural analgesic (57% compared with 39%), in receiving oxytocin (65% compared with 51%), and in having a longer labor. The intermediate pseudosinusoidal FRH pattern occurred during fetal sucking in utero.

Conclusion.—Pseudosinusoidal FHR patterns may arise to compensate for the hypoxia experienced by the cardiac center in the medulla. Most fetuses will have a normal outcome even after having a recorded pseudosinusoidal FHR pattern.

▶ Lamentably, FHR monitoring has remained an inexact science. Despite extensive exposure and education over the past 2 decades and elaborate, expensive central monitoring stations in many labor suites, no clear advantage over intermittent auscultation has been established. An aspect of the problem is punctuated by this report on pseudosinusoidal patterns in labor. There remains much confusion with regard to the classification and interpretation of fetal heart rate patterns.

A sinusoidal pattern is usually regarded as ominous. Disorders associated with sinusoidal patterns include Rh isoimmunization, severe diabetes, prolonged pregnancy, amnionitis, umbilical cord compression, fetomaternal hemorrhage, administration of alphaprodine and even normal labor. A sinusoidal pattern implies baseline oscillations at a frequency of 2 to 5 per minute, varying from 5 to 15 per minute, with an absence of FHR reactivity. Central hypoxia has been inferred in the etiology of this pattern. Good reactivity just before or after the sinusoid-like pattern renders it pseudosinusoidal, which by definition means artificial or spurious. The pseudosinusoidal pattern has been attributed to fetal sucking or mouthing and maternal opiate usage.

Murphy prospectively determines that minor pseudosinusoidal patterns are relatively common in normal labor, intermediate pseudosinusoidal patterns are less common, and major pseudosinusoidal patterns are rare. No true sinusoidal patterns were observed in this study. Although there was an association between pseudosinusoidal patterns and the administration of oxytocics and analgesics to the mother, no correlation was established with fetal outcome. The authors present a number of interesting hypotheses to explain the pseudosinusoidal patterns. These include altered fetal temperature, varying fetal behavioral state, and fluctuations in uteroplacental flow. No definitive cause is established, and they point out the flaws in their arguments.

This manuscript generated some novel information. I remain confused as to the distinction between true sinusoidal and major pseudosinusoidal patterns. Because the fetus is in jeopardy with both these patterns, immediate delivery is necessary, so perhaps the distinction is not necessary. It is imperative not to misclassify the minor and moderate pseudosinusoidal patterns. These fetuses will do okay, and they don't need to be snatched surgically from the womb. See also Abstracts 4–1 and 4–3.—A.A. Fanaroff, M.B.B.Ch.

Maternal Serum α-Fetoprotein Testing: Physician Experience and Attitudes and Their Influence on Patient Acceptance

Madlon-Kay DJ, Reif C, Mersy DJ, Luxenberg MG (St Paul-Ramsey Med Ctr, St Paul, Minn)

J Fam Pract 35:395–400, 1992 4–11

Background.—Commercial kits for estimating maternal serum α-fetoprotein (MSAFP) were approved by the Food and Drug Administration in 1983. Indications other than identifying open neural tube defects have evolved. The test process requires a high level of cooperation among physicians, laboratories, genetic counselors, and prenatal diagnosis centers.

Survey.—A questionnaire was sent to 849 members of the American Academy of Family Physicians in Minnesota, and 84% responded. Approximately 80% of the 593 respondents providng prenatal care were men, and nearly as many were residency-trained. All but 3% were board-certified. The mean patient age was 40 years.

Findings.—Eighty-seven percent of family physicians offered MSAFP testing to patients receiving prenatal care before 18 weeks' gestation. Of those, 63% offered testing to all their patients, but 41% of those offering the test reported that very few patients accepted the test. Only 22% of respondents found that more than half their patients accepted testing. Thirty-seven percent of the physicians offering the test had had at least 1 abnormal result. Few physicians believed that MSAFP testing is cost effective. Fifty-seven percent expressed concern over the possibility of a malpractice lawsuit. The strongest predictor of test availability by far was a belief that the test is medicolegally necessary.

Conclusion.—Physicians appear to have many concerns about the MSAFP test and its limitations. Those in this survey are motivated more from fear of being sued than from a belief that the test is an accurate screen for neural tube defects or Down syndrome.

▶ One major question that is not easily explored but may possibly be at the root of physician attitudes is their actual knowledge of the subject. With the addition of serum estriol and choriogonadotropin, the value and importance of prenatal testing increases (as noted in this abstract and Abstract 7–18) and should encourage a greater educational effort by physicians.—M.H. Klaus, M.D.

Prenatal Screening for Down's Syndrome With Use of Maternal Serum Markers

Haddow JE, Palomaki GE, Knight GJ, Williams J, Pulkkinen A, Canick JA, Saller DN Jr, Bowers GB (Found for Blood Research, Scarborough, Me; Women and Infants Hosp, Providence, RI)

N Engl J Med 327:588–593, 1992 4–12

Background.—Approximately one third of all cases of Down syndrome in fetuses can be detected by measuring maternal serum α-fetoprotein in the second trimester. Recent case-control studies have shown that this detection rate may be doubled by measuring serum levels of unconjugated estriol and chorionic gonadotropin. In women carrying fetuses with Down syndrome, the serum level of estriol is abnormally low, and the level of chorionic gonadotropin is abnormally high. The

Comparison of Current Study With an Earlier Study in Which Screening Process Was Based on Maternal Age and Serum Levels of Alpha-Fetoprotein in Women Younger Than Age 35 Years

Variable	Earlier Study	Current Study
No. screened	77,273	23,975
Second-trimester risk cutoff used	1:270	1:190
Initial positive rate (%)	4.7	6.1
% Offered amniocentesis	2.7	3.2
% Choosing amniocentesis *	2.1	2.6
Cases of Down's syndrome identified	18	17
No. of amniocenteses per case of Down's syndrome identified	89	38
Detection rate of Down's syndrome (%)	25	58

Note: The results of the earlier study were published in 1989.

*Seventy-five percent and 82% of women or adolescents offered amniocentesis in the 2 studies, respectively, chose to have the procedure; 1,593 and 655 amniocenteses, respectively, were actually performed in 2 studies.

(Courtesy of Haddow JE, Palomaki GE, Knight GJ, et al: *N Engl J Med* 327:588–593, 1992.)

effects of adding these 2 measurements to routine prenatal screening protocols at 2 centers were investigated.

Methods.—The study population consisted of 25,207 women and adolescents in the second trimester of pregnancy. Each was assigned a risk of fetal Down syndrome by using an algorithm that took into account measurements of all 3 serum markers combined with maternal age. This formula predicted that 1,661 women and adolescents (6.6%) had a second trimester risk of Down syndrome of at least 1 in 190. After calculation of gestational age by ultrasonography, 962 (3.8%) were offered amniocentesis for chromosomal analysis.

Findings.—Seven hundred sixty women and adolescents chose to have amniocentesis. Twenty cases of fetal Down syndrome were found, along with 7 other chromosomal disorders. One additional case of Down syndrome occurred among the 202 women who chose not to have amniocentesis. Thus, the rate of detection of fetal Down syndrome was 58%, and the frequency of identifying a Down syndrome fetus in those undergoing amniocentesis was 1 per 38 amniocenteses. In the table, these results are compared with those of an earlier study.

Conclusion.—Measuring serum levels of α-fetoprotein, chorionic gonadotropin, and estriol is more effective than measuring the maternal serum level of α-fetoprotein alone in screening for Down syndrome. This expanded protocol can easily be incorporated into existing prenatal screening programs.

Free Beta Human Choriogonadotropin in Down's Syndrome Screening: A Multicentre Study of Its Role Compared With Other Biochemical Markers

Spencer K, Coombes EJ, Mallard AS, Ward AM (Oldchurch Hosp, Romford, England; Queen Alexandra Hosp, Portsmouth, England; Royal Cornwall Hosp, Truro, England; Royal Hallamshire Hosp, Sheffield, England)

Ann Clin Biochem 29:506–518, 1992 4–13

Introduction.—A number of biochemical markers have been assessed for their value in screening for Down syndrome. In a large multicenter study including the largest collection of cases of Down Syndrome ever reported, the maternal levels of serum free β-human choriogonadotropin (β-hCG), total hCG, α-fetoprotein (AFP), and unconjugated estriol (UE3) were evaluated as markers.

Methods.—The Down Syndrome study population consisted of women who were seen through neural defect screening programs. Each of 3 centers established its own normative data for free β-hCG, total hCG, AFP, and UE3. Ninety singleton pregnancies associated with Down syndrome were identified with maternal serum samples taken between 14 and 21 weeks' gestation and before amniocentesis. Also included were 2,862 controls matched for maternal and gestational age.

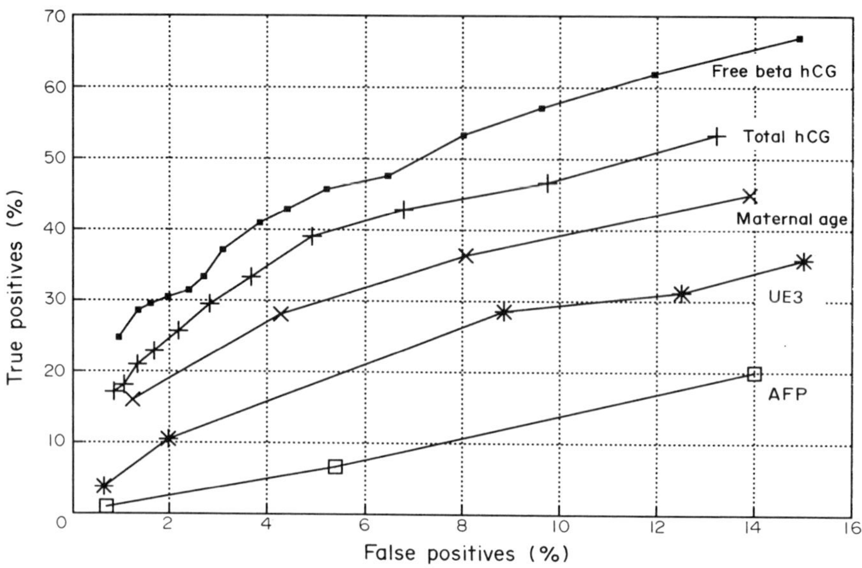

Fig 4–6.—Receiver-operator characteristic curves showing variation of false positive rate with true positive rate for markers of Down syndrome analyzed independently. *Filled squares,* free β-hCG; +, total hCG; x, maternal age; * UE3; *open squares,* AFP. (Courtesy of Spencer K, Coombes EJ, Mallard AS, et al: *Ann Clin Biochem* 29:506–518, 1992.)

The results for each center were expressed in multiples of the median for unaffected pregnancies at the same gestational age.

Results.—Free β-hCG was found to have more discriminating power alone than AFP, UE3, or total hCG (Fig 4–6). Alone, AFP and UE3 contributed relatively little to the detection of Down Syndrome. The use of UE3 alone resulted in a 1% increase in the false positive rate. When used in early gestation (14–16 weeks) in combination with AFP and maternal age, free β-hCG will enable detection of 77% of Down syndrome cases. In women younger than age 30 years, the free β-hCG combination detects 100% more cases than does the total hCG combination.

Conclusion.—Free β-hCG is a superior marker to total hCG, yielding a significant difference in detection rates. If 90% of pregnant women in the United Kingdon were screened with the free β-hCG, AFP, and age protocol, 90 more cases of Down syndrome would be detected each year than with the total hCG protocol.

Thickened Nuchal Fold in Fetuses Not at Risk for Aneuploidy

Benacerraf BR, Laboda LA, Frigoletto FD (Harvard Med School, Boston)

Radiology 184:239–242, 1992 4–14

Introduction.—Sonographic detection of a thickened nuchal fold in second-trimester fetuses is thought to be superior to advanced maternal

Findings in Fetuses With Abnormal Karyotypes

Case No.	Maternal Age (y)	Gestational Age (wk)	Indication for Sonography	Other Sonographic Findings	Karyotype	Serum AFP Level
1	23	21	Dating	Fetal hydronephrosis	Trisomy 21	Normal
2	31	18	Abnormal level 1 sonogram	None	Trisomy 21	Normal
3	32	17	Exposure to vitamin D	Heart defect	Trisomy 21	Low
4	33	19	Low maternal serum AFP level	None	Trisomy 21	Low
5	33	17	Bleeding	None	Trisomy 21	Low
6	29	16	Possible amniotic bands	None	Trisomy 21	Normal
7	32	14.7	Dating	Fetal hydronephrosis	Trisomy 21	Normal
8	32	21	Abnormal level 1 sonogram	Hydrocephalus, hydronephrosis	Trisomy 21	. . .
9	30	18	Low maternal serum AFP level	Heart defect, hydronephrosis	Trisomy 21	Low
10	34	16	Size, dating	Fetal hydronephrosis	Trisomy 21	. . .
11	28	17	Arrhythmia	None	Trisomy 21	Low
12	30	15.5	Exposure to medication	None	XYY	Normal
13	29	15.5	Dating	None	XO	Normal
14	31	15	Bleeding	None	XXX	Normal

(Courtesy of Benacerraf BR, Laboda LA, Frigoletto FD: *Radiology* 184:239–242, 1992.)

age or low serum α-fetoprotein (AFP) levels in identifying fetuses at risk for trisomy 21. This sonographic sign is also highly predictive in younger women at low risk for aneuploidy.

Methods.—Included in the study were women younger than 35 who were not planning to undergo amniocentesis but had a thickened nuchal fold at sonographic examination. The fold was considered wider than normal if it measured at least 6 mm from the outer aspect of the occiptal bone to the outer aspect of the skin edge. The patients were advised of this finding and offered cytogenetic testing.

Results.—Two of the 42 women had a low serum AFP before sonography, but the others had no indications suggesting a need for karyotyping. Fourteen of the 42 fetuses were found to have abnormal karyotypes (table). Included in this group were the patients with low serum AFP; their fetuses had Down syndrome. There had been no known indications for amniocentesis in the remaining 12 cases. Without the sonographic finding of a thickened nuchal fold, 9 fetuses (6 with trisomy 21) would not have been identified before birth. In 1 case, however, amniocentesis would have been performed because of the sonographic finding of hydrocephalus.

Conclusion.—The yield of an abnormal karyotype was high (22%) in these patients with no known risk for aneuploidy. More than half of fetuses with Down syndrome will not be identified if cytogenetic studies are limited to women 35 or older or those with serum AFP levels. Although universal screening is not recommended at this time, karyotyping should be performed when a thickened nuchal fold is found on sonograms of second-trimester fetuses, regardless of the reason for imaging.

▶ These 3 reports (Abstracts 4–12 through 4–14) on the screening for Down syndrome represent the present state of the art in the United States and England. In the table included with the Haddow report, there has been, since 1989, a marked improvement in the detection rate (from 25% to 58%) and a reduction in the number of amniocentesis required (from 89 to 38) to identify an infant with Down syndrome. A recent report by Wald et al. (1) confirms the value of the 3 markers, concluding that the cost of picking up 1 infant with Down Syndrome was 38,000£. I have included a status report on the value of the thickened nuchal fold, because I believe this will improve the detection rate.—M.H. Klaus, M.D.

Reference

1. Wald N, et al: *BMJ* 305:391, 1992.

Comparison of Dynamic Image and Pulsed Doppler Ultrasonography for the Diagnosis of the Small-for-Gestational-Age Fetus

Miller JM Jr, Gabert HA (Louisiana State Univ, New Orleans)

Am J Obstet Gynecol 166:1820–1826, 1992 4–15

Setting.—The effectiveness of real-time ultrasonography and Doppler velocimetry for the identification of small-for-gestational-age (SGA) fetuses was examined in a prospective study. Specifically, the estimated fetal weight relative to gestational age and the utility of the velocimetric systolic-diastolic ratio of the umbilical artery were compared with receiver-operator characteristic curves in 136 women who were at risk for fetal growth abnormalities. All patients were delivered within 3 weeks of ultrasonography and had liveborn, nonanomalous, singleton infants.

Findings.—There were 46 SGA infants (33.8%). Both relative estimated fetal weight and the systolic-diastolic ratio were strongly associated with SGA; however, analysis of the area under the curve indicated

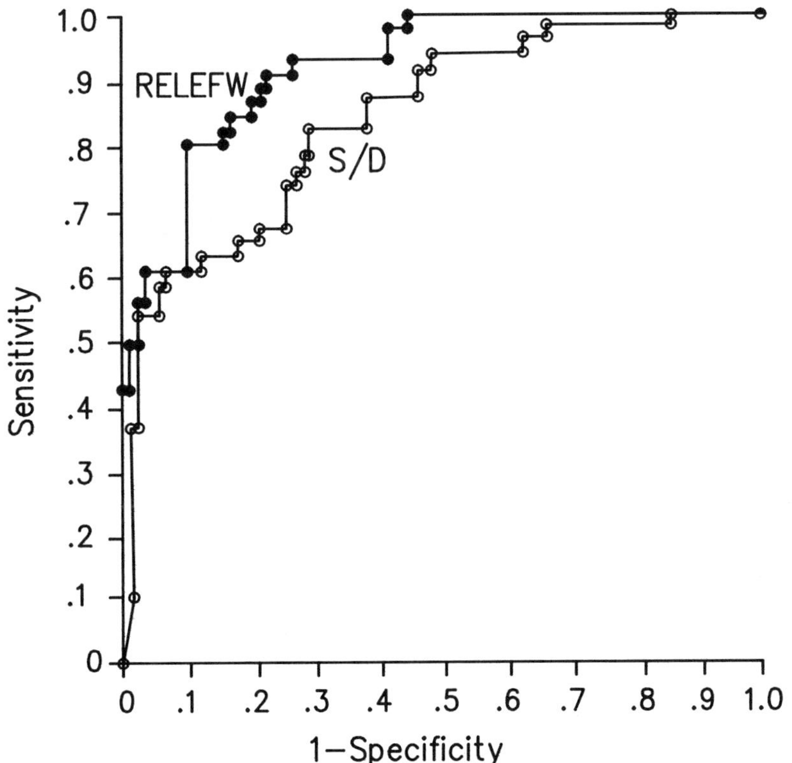

Fig 4–7.—Receiver-operator characteristic curves of ultrasonographic variables in detection of SGA fetuses. *Abbreviations: RELEFW,* relative estimated fetal weight; *S/D,* systolic-diastolic ratio. (Courtesy of Miller JM Jr, Gabert HA: *Am J Obstet Gynecol* 166:1820–1826, 1992.)

Contingency Tables for Ultrasonographic Variables vs. SGA with Preselected Boundary

Variable	*SGA*	*Non-SGA*	*Significance*	*Positive predictive value*	*Negative predictive value*	*Sensitivity*	*Specificity*
Relative estimated fetal weight							
≤0.80	38	13	$p < 0.001$	75%	91%	83%	86%
>0.80	8	77					
Systolic/diastolic ratio							
≥3.0	31	22	$p < 0.001$	59%	82%	67%	76%
<3.0	15	68					

(Courtesy of Miller JM Jr, Gabert HA: *Am J Obstet Gynecol* 166:1820–1826, 1992.)

that the curve for relative weight was significantly better than that for the systolic-diastolic ratio (Fig 4–7). The positive predictive value and specificity for relative weight was approximately 20% greater than those of the systolic-diastolic ratio (table). When an arbitrary boundary on the curve was selected for maximal sensitivity and specificity, the optimal break point for relative weight was .784, and that for systolic-diastolic value was at least 2.85.

Conclusion.—Relative estimated fetal weight, derived from ultrasonography, should be the preferred parameter for antenatal identification of an SGA fetus.

▶ It is entirely logical that a technique that predicts size from direct measurements of the fetus would more accurately predict SGA than would a physiologic measurement. Advanced logic would dictate that combining these measurements would give a broader dimension of the fetal status. That these deductions actually come to pass is reassuring—at least for the reader, if not always for the fetus.

Do not be intimidated by the receiver-operating characteristic (ROC), which is a fashionable method to evaluate the overall performance in a test in discriminating between the diseased and healthy population. In the above report, the ROC was constructed for relatively mature fetuses (36 ± 3 weeks), which cannot be extrapolated to infants less than 33 weeks.

What do we learn? First, that ultrasonography is a better way of predicting fetal size and deriving a relative weight (estimated fetal weight divided by the median birth weight for the gestational age at which the study was done) than Doppler velocimetry. Second, we are reminded that SGA infants comprise a heterogenous group. Doppler velocimetry correlates best with neonatal morbidity and mortality.

We conclude that ultrasound will assist in identifying the growth-retarded fetus, and that Doppler will help in detection when fetal status is deteriorating and intervention is indicated. Please see References 1–3.

Nothing will ever be attempted if all possible objections must be first overcome.—Samuel Johnson

A.A. Fanaroff, M.B.B.Ch.

References

1. 1992 Year Book of Neonatal and Perinatal Medicine, pp 61–62.
2. 1992 Year Book of Neonatal and Perinatal Medicine, pp 65–66.
3. 1992 Year Book of Neonatal and Perinatal Medicine, pp 66–67.

Serial Thoracic Versus Abdominal Circumference Ratios for the Prediction of Pulmonary Hypoplasia in Premature Rupture of the Membranes Remote From Term

D'Alton M, Mercer B, Riddick E, Dudley D (Tufts Med Univ, Boston; Univ of Tennessee, Memphis; Univ of Ottawa, Ont)

Am J Obstet Gynecol 166:658–663, 1992 4–16

Background.—Premature rupture of the membranes before 26 weeks' gestation is associated with a high rate of perinatal mortality. Pulmonary hypoplasia is a major cause of death in these infants. The fetal thoracic vs. abdominal circumference ratio in the prediction of pulmonary hypoplasia after preterm premature rupture of the membranes was evaluated.

Methods.—To obtain normal values, ultrasonographic measurements of fetal thoracic and abdominal circumferences were performed in 120 uncomplicated pregnancies. Seventeen patients with premature rupture of fetal membranes that occurred before 26 weeks' gestation were then assessed serially with ultrasonography to obtain thoracic vs. abdominal circumference ratios and amniotic fluid estimations. The results were correlated to fetal outcome and autopsy data.

Results.—Sixteen of the 17 women who elected to continue their pregnancies were delivered of 13 infants after 26 weeks' gestation. The 3 infants delivered before 26 weeks' gestation, and 5 of the 13 delivered after this date died. The mean time from premature rupture of fetal membranes to delivery was 61.8 days. All 6 infants whose abnormally low thoracic vs. abdominal circumference ratio predicted pulmonary hypoplasia died of this condition. Two infants with normal ratios died in the early neonatal period; 1 was found to have pulmonary dysplasia.

Conclusion.—As a predictor of neonatal death from pulmonary disease, the thoracic vs. abdominal circumference ratio had a sensitivity of 75%, a specificity of 100%, a positive predictive value of 100%, and a negative predictive value of 80%. Serial ultrasonographic evaluation is

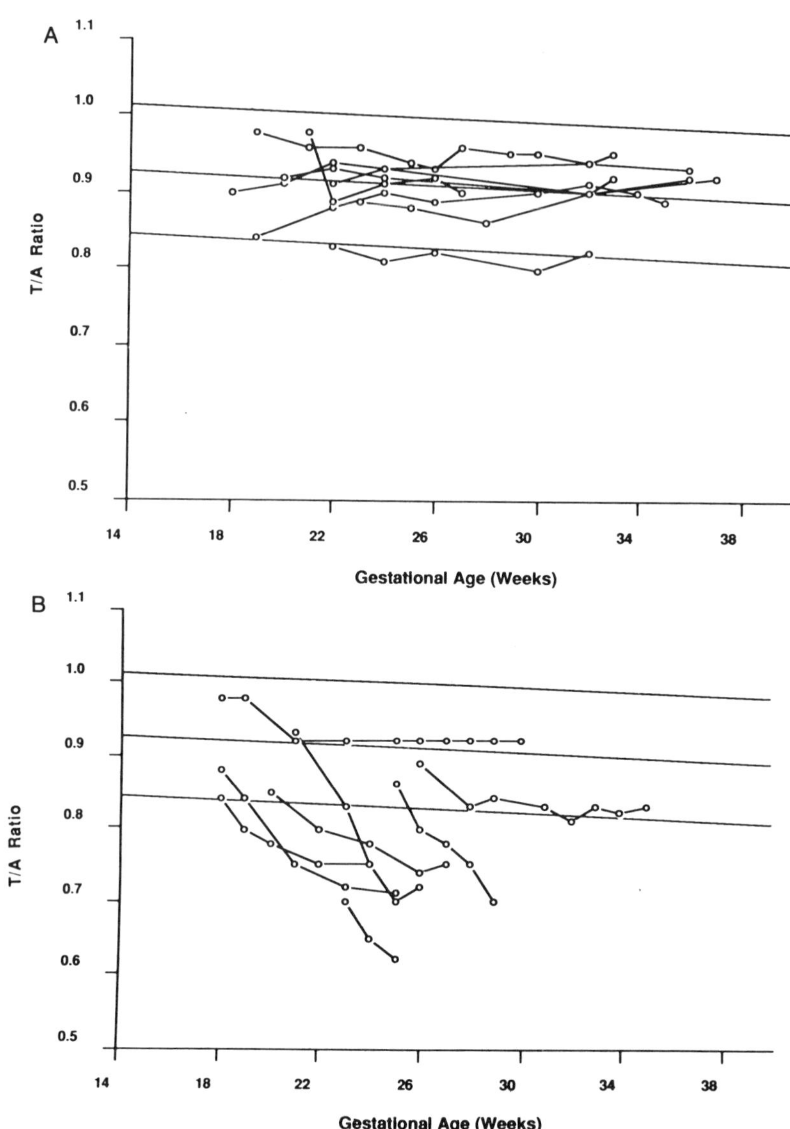

Fig 4–8.—A, serial thoracic vs. abdominal circumference ratios vs. gestational age for surviving infants. **B,** serial thoracic vs. abdominal circumference ratios vs. gestational age for nonsurviving infants. (Courtesy of D'Alton M, Mercer B, Riddick E, et al: *Am J Obstet Gynecol* 166:658–663, 1992.)

helpful, for progressive growth failure occurs in infants destined to have pulmonary hypoplasia (Fig 4–8).

▶ Respiratory disorders continue to lead the lethal disorders encountered in the neonatal period. Surfactant therapy has helped salvage many immature infants with respiratory failure, hoisting pulmonary hypoplasia into the limelight. The relationship between premature rupture of the membranes, oligohydramnios, and pulmonary hypoplasia retain central stage. It has been established beyond reasonable doubt that rupture of the membranes before 26 weeks' gestation is a potentially lethal event. Moretti reported a mortality of 87% with rupture before 23 weeks (1).

In this report, the fetal thoracic vs. abdominal circumference ratio is presented as a predictor of pulmonary hypoplasia. The addition of the abdominal circumference serves as an internal "control" correcting for variation in fetal size and refines the report by Nimrod (2). In the series outlined in this report, chest circumference alone would have missed pulmonary hypoplasia.

The crux of all these investigations hinges on the diagnosis of pulmonary hypoplasia. In D'Alton et al.'s series, the criteria established by Wigglesworth (3) and based on lung weight were used. This does not distinguish the various lung elements. Detailed morphometric studies, including counts of alveoli and the number of generations of branches of the bronchi and bronchioles, are laborious, costly, and impractical. However, using cruder parameters introduces an element of subjectivity regarding the diagnosis of pulmonary hypoplasia. Pediatric pathologists, in moments of weakness, will reveal that recognizing pulmonary hypoplasia sometimes requires the same definition that the Supreme Court uses for pornography: "You recognize it when you see it." Nonetheless, the profile of pulmonary hypoplasia is becoming clearer, and interventions to stimulate and facilitate lung development are on the horizon. See also Abstract 4–18 and References 4 and 5.—A.A. Fanaroff, M.B.B.Ch.

References

1. Moretti M, Sibai B: *Am J Obstet Gynecol* 159:390, 1988.
2. Nimrod C, et al: *Am J Obstet Gynecol* 148:540, 1984.
3. Wigglesworth J, Desai R: *Arch Dis Child* 56:601, 1981.
4. Songster GS, et al: *Obstet Gynecol* 73:261, 1989.
5. Vintzileos AM, et al: *Am J Obstet Gynecol* 161:606, 1989.

Extended Fetal Echocardiographic Examination for Detecting Cardiac Malformations in Low Risk Pregnancies

Achiron R, Glaser J, Gelernter I, Hegesh J, Yagel S (Chaim Sheba Medical Centre, Tel Hashomer, Israel; Shaare Zedek Medical Centre, Jerusalem; Tel Aviv Univ, Israel; et al)

BMJ 304:671–674, 1992 4–17

Objective.—Because most neonates with congential heart disease are born to women who lack known risk factors, prenatal selection of women for detailed fetal echocardiographic assessment would seem to be inadequate. Extended examination of a low-risk population was done to increase the detection rate of congenital heart disease.

Diagnostic Accuracy of Abnormal Results on Four-Chamber View and Extended Echocardiography

	Sensitivity	Specificity	Positive predictive value	Negative predictive value
Abnormal four chamber view (n=11)	11/23 (48%)	5323/5324 (99·9%)	11/12 (92%)	5323/5335 (99·8%)
95% Confidence interval	(38% to 58%)		(88% to 96%)	
Abnormal extended examination (n=18)	18/23 (78%)*	5323/5324 (99·9%)	18/19 (95%)	5323/5328 (99·9%)
95% Confidence interval	(71% to 85%)		(93% to 97%)	

*P = .0078 compared with 4-chamber view by correlated chi-square test.
(Courtesy of Achiron R, Glaser J, Gelernter I, et al: *BMJ* 304:671–674, 1992.)

Methods.—A toal of 5,400 fetuses in low-risk pregnancies at 18–24 weeks' gestation underwent echographic screening using sector scanners. In addition to routine 4-chamber views, and left and right ventricular outflow tracts and the main pulmonary artery and its branches were visualized. Doppler, M-mode, and color flow mapping methods were used in cases with abnormal findings.

Findings.—Eighteen of 21 infants with major structural and functional heart disorders had heart disease diagnosed prenatally, 11 by the 4-chamber view alone, which was 48% sensitive. Extended echocardiographic examination was 78% sensitive (table). There was a single false positive finding.

Conclusion.—Extended echocardiography detected 86% of the major cardiac abnormalities in this low-risk population. Extended echocardiography should be part of the routine prenatal ultrasonographic assessment.

▶ The incidence of cardiac structural abnormalities in the newborn approaches 8–10 per 100 live births (1). However, the midtrimester incidence is probably higher, because complex cardiac anomalies, in isolation or as part of chromosomal abnormalities or malformation syndromes, may result in fetal losses. In the absence of uniform screening, detailed fetal cardiac evaluation should be undertaken if major extracardiac anomalies are detected or if the mother has congenital heart disease, diabetes, a history of exposure to cardiac teratogens (e.g., alcohol, lithium, or phenytoins), a hydropic fetus, or polyhydramnios. Rare disorders such as tuberous sclerosis would also warrant a fetal cardiac examination.

During the past 2 decades, the ultrasound examination of the heart has increased in scope. The standard views for fetal echocardiography include the 4-chamber view, the left ventricular long-axis view with visualization of the aortic outflow tract, the short-axis view with visualization of the pulmonary outflow tract, and ductus arteriosus and longitudinal views of the aortic arch. Fetal echocardiography has advanced to the point whereby perinatologists are provided with detailed and accurate assessment of cardiovascular anatomy. The combination of 2-dimensional imaging, M-mode scanning, pulsed and continuous-wave Doppler measurements, and color flow mapping provide exquisite detail of the cardiac abnormalities and the associated hemodynamic changes. Furthermore, the elucidation and treatment of fetal arrythmias is much more reliable (2, 3).

Many families have been reassured by the confirmation of normal anatomy and rhythm. On the other hand, when an abnormality is detected in utero, the management team has the opportunity to comprehensively evaluate the fetus for other anomalies and, when appropriate, determine the fetal karyotype. Decisions can also be made regarding the optimal site for delivery and management of the cardiac lesion before and after delivery.

Although there has been tremendous technologic progress, I do not believe that we can justify an extended echocardiographic examination in all pregnancies, as suggested by Achiron and co-workers. I *do* support routine ultrasound evaluations in pregnancies, and that (together with other features pointing to an increased prevalence of cardiac problems) would be the basis for the extended cardiac evaluation of the fetus.

If you think you can do a thing or think you can't do a thing, you're right.—Henry Ford

A.A. Fanaroff, M.B.B.Ch.

References

1. Hoffman JI, Christianson R: *Am J Cardiol* 42:641, 1978.
2. Copel JA, et al: *Obstet Gynecol* 78:1, 1991.
3. Kleinman C, et al: *Ultrasound Obstet Gynecol* 1:286, 1991.

Decreased Amniotic Fluid Index in Term Pregnancy: Clinical Significance

Jeng C-J, Lee J-F, Wang K-G, Yang Y-C, Lan C-C (Mackay Mem Hosp, Taipei, Taiwan)

J Reprod Med 37:789–792, 1992 4–18

Objective.—Phelan's amniotic fluid index (AFI), reflecting estimates from 4 quadrants, has been modified, and an index that represents a normal distribution of amniotic fluid has been developed. The clinical importance of the AFI was investigated, and results of the index were compared with the single largest pocket measurement.

Study Plan.—A 4-quadrant method was used to obtain AFI measurements in 331 term pregnancies. All were singleton pregnancies at gestational ages of 37–42 weeks. All deliveries occurred within a week of measurement. The single largest vertical diameter of fluid in each quadrant was measured in centimeters, and the sum of 4 diameters taken as the AFI.

Results.—Application of the 2-cm rule led to only 4 patients (2%) being classified as oligohydramnios. Only 2 patients had a single largest

Comparison Between AFI and Single Largest Pocket Measurement for Predicting Fetal Outcome

	Sensitivity *	Specificity	Positive predictive value	Negative predictive value
AFI	31.2%	98.0%	89.5%	72.5%
Single largest pocket (2 cm)	1.9%	99.0%	50.0%	66.1%

Note: Patients with any 2 or more poor fetal outcome parameters were counted only once.
*$P < .05$.
(Courtesy of Jeng C-J, Lee J-F, Wang K-G, et al: *J Reprod Med* 37:789–792, 1992.)

pocket less than 1 cm. An AFI of 8 cm or less was significantly more sensitive in predicting a poor fetal outcome (table) than the single pocket measurement. No significant reduction in specificity or predictive value was noted using AFI measurements. Three of 4 women with intrauterine growth retardation had a normal AFI.

Conclusion.—Measuring the AFI is a superior means of predicting poor fetal outcomes. An index of less than 8 cm signals the need for close attention.

▶ The fetus may be compromised in the presence of disorders of amniotic fluid volume. Refinements of ultrasonographic techniques have made recognition of these disorders more precise in addition to often providing evidence of the underlying etiology of the disorder. Amnioinfusion is emerging as a form of interventional therapy for these disorders both before or during labor.

Determination of amniotic fluid volume has shifted from subjective to very objective measurements. The amniotic fluid index (AFI), first suggested by Phelan, is emerging as the gold standard. Jeng and colleagues have modified the technique a smidgen and have redefined the standards of "normality." From a clinical standpoint, no substantive change occurs. The ultrasonographer is directed to measure the single largest vertical diameter of amniotic fluid in each quadrant, irrespective of gestational age, and then sum the results. (Phelan had not used 4 quadrants before 20 weeks' gestation.) Jeng determined that 8 and 24 cm defined the 5th and 95th percentiles, respectively (1). In this report, he notes that meconium staining, abnormal fetal heart rate monitoring, cesarean section deliveries, and lower Apgar scores are prevalent if the AFI is below 8 cm, with no distinction between the group with an index of less than 5 cm and the 5.1- to 8-cm group, the group Phelan previously designated severe oligohydramnios. The AFI was more sensitive than the single pocket (< 2 cm) in predicting poor fetal outcome. Any AFI less than 8 cm near term merits close monitoring and attention.

The total uterine volume increases linearly with gestational age; however, the amniotic fluid shows a steady increase until 25 weeks and then increases gradually until 30 weeks' gestation; it peaks at a volume of 900–1,000 mL. Near term there is a normal decline in amniotic fluid volume. Trimmer and associates, after carefully measuring urine production ultrasonographically, concluded that the decreased urine production in the post-term infant with oligohydramnios was the result (not the cause) of the oligohydramnios. Structural changes in the amniotic epithelial layer have been documented with oligohydramnios. The abnormal membranes thus become part of the vicious cycle, because the amniotic fluid volume will not be reconstituted. As we expand our knowledge and understanding of the relationship between the fetus and the amniotic fluid, it can be translated into better pregnancy management and improved perinatal outcomes. For more information on this topic please see References 2–6.—A.A. Fanaroff, M.B.B.Ch.

References

1. Jeng CJ, et al: *J Reprod Med* 35:674, 1990.
2. 1991 Year Book of Neonatal and Perinatal Medicine, pp 67–69, 104–108.
3. 1992 Year Book of Neonatal and Perinatal Medicine, pp 49–50.
4. 1992 Year Book of Neonatal and Perinatal Medicine, pp 51–52.
5. 1992 Year Book of Neonatal and Perinatal Medicine, pp 53–54.
6. 1991 Year Book of Neonatal and Perinatal Medicine, pp 67–69.

5 Labor and Delivery

Erythromycin Therapy in Preterm Premature Rupture of the Membranes: A Prospective, Randomized Trial of 220 Patients

Mercer BM, Moretti ML, Prevost RR, Sibai BM (Univ of Tennessee, Memphis)

Am J Obstet Gynecol 166:794–802, 1992 5–1

Introduction.—Most studies on the use of antibiotics in preterm premature rupture of the membranes, a major cause of maternal, fetal, and neonatal morbidity, have been poorly designed. Although 2 recent articles report mezlocillin and ampicillin to be beneficial, no randomized studies have investigated the use of erythromycin. The efficacy of oral erythromycin therapy in increasing the latency period and reducing the incidence of maternal and neonatal infectious morbidity in patients with premature rupture of the membranes was investigated.

Methods.—Eligible women who consented to take part in the study were between 20 weeks and 34 weeks plus 6 days of gestation. They were randomized in a double-blind fashion to receive erythromycin, 333 mg (106 women), or placebo (114 women) every 8 hours until delivery. The women and neonates received whatever additional treatment and procedures that were standard for their condition.

Results.—Both groups had a surprisingly high incidence of clinical abruptio placentae. No differences in the incidences of clinical chorioamnionitis or endometritis were observed. Amniotic fluid cultures were positive in 17.9% of the placebo group and in 18.4% of the erythromycin group. Erythromycin therapy was associated with a significant prolongation of latency from randomization to delivery, particularly in those who would have chorioamnionitis and those with oligohydramnios. Subsequent to the first week after randomization, no differences in latency were seen. Infant morbidity and mortality and maternal morbidity were not significantly reduced by erythromycin therapy.

Conclusion.—Prophylactic oral erythromycin therapy significantly prolonged the latency period in patients with preterm premature rupture of the membranes. The combination of this drug with broader spectrum agents might be more effective in treating the organisms identified in the amniotic fluid.

▶ Preterm premature rupture of the membranes (PROM) is a major cause of perinatal morbidity. The issue of antibiotic therapy after PROM has been addressed by several studies using heterologous populations and a variety of agents not appropriate for use in pregnancy. More recent prospective studies have indicated that parenteral Mezlocillin or ampicillin, followed by oral ampicillin, prolonged latency and reduced infections in the mother and newborn (1, 2).

The above represents a prospective blinded study designed to evaluate erythromycin in women with PROM. The protocol was strictly enforced with active monitoring of chorio amnionitis, fetal well-being, and maturity. It was encouraging to observe the appropriate use of steroid therapy for those with immature pulmonary indices. Although erythromycin prolonged the latency period, during the first week it did not affect the incidence of positive amniotic fluid cultures or the morbidity of the mothers or infants. Therefore, the authors are forced to conclude that erythromycin alone is not the answer for this particular problem. We concur. (See also References 3 and 4.)

Passion you see can be destroyed by a doctor. It cannot be created.—Peter Schaffer

References

1. Johnson MM, et al: *Am J Obstet Gynecol* 163:743, 1990.
2. Amon E, et al: *Am J Obstet Gynecol* 159:539, 1988.
3. 1990 Year Book of Neonatal and Perinatal Medicine, pp 82–83.
4. 1990 Year Book of Neonatal and Perinatal Medicine, pp 81–82.

A.A. Fanaroff, M.B.B.Ch.

Treatment of Preterm Labor With the Beta-Adrenergic Agonist Ritodrine

Moutquin J-M, for the Canadian Preterm Labor Investigators Group (Quebec City, Canada)

N Engl J Med 327:308–312, 1992 5–2

Introduction.—Even though β-adrenergic agonists have been widely used for 2 decades to arrest premature labor, few studies have assessed the potential risks and benefits of these drugs to the mother and infant. In a randomized, controlled, multicenter trial, researchers compared the use of the β-adrenergic agonist ritodrine with placebo.

Methods.—The study group included 708 women with preterm labor, 352 of whom were assigned to ritodrine and 356 to placebo. Assignment was made with stratification according to 4 categories of gestational age. Two hundred forty-six of the surviving infants were followed up at the age of 18 months. The women received intravenous drug or placebo upon presentation with threatened preterm delivery, followed by oral medication for 5 days if uterine contractions stopped.

Results.—The mean length of time from randomization to delivery did not differ significantly for the 2 groups: 27.8 days for the ritodrine group and 24.5 days for the placebo group. The incidence of delivery before 37 weeks' gestation and the proportion of infants weighing less than 2,500 g were also similar for the 2 groups. There were 23 deaths (6.1%) in the ritodrine group and 25 (6.4%) in the placebo group. Maternal morbidity tended to be higher in the ritodrine group, but neonatal morbidity was similar in both groups. One infant in the ritodrine group and 5 in the placebo group were found to have cerebral palsy at 18-month evaluation. Ritodrine treatment was associated with a slightly improved score on the Bayley Psychomotor Development Index, but it is not significant.

Conclusion.—The use of ritodrine to arrest premature labor yields no significant beneficial effects on perinatal mortality, delay of delivery, or birth weight. Use of the drug is not recommended for gestational ages greater than 28 weeks.

▶ This large randomized trial agrees with the meta-analyses of a large number of previous trials. It is a pity that all of the patients in both groups did not also receive glucocorticoids, because they are known to decrease the incidence of respiratory distress, necrotizing enterocolitis, and neonatal mortality. This study possibly would have supported the combination of ritodrine and betamethasone, because a significant reduction in the number of mothers who delivered within the first 48 hours after treatment occurred among those who received ritodrine. Is it time to standardize some procedures, such as administering glucocorticoids to every mother in early labor?—M.H. Klaus, M.D.

Outcome of Breech Delivery at Term

Thorpe-Beeston JG, Banfield PJ, Saunders NJStG (St Mary's Hosp, London)
BMJ 305:746–747, 1992 5–3

Introduction.—The optimal management of breech presentation at term remains controversial, and most data on this entity are derived from retrospective studies. Data obtained prospectively from the St.

Numbers of Low Apgar Scores (< 7) at 5 Minutes, Neonatal Intubations, and Admissions to Special Care Infant Unit According to Method of Breech Delivery

	Vaginal Delivery (n = 961)	Emergency lower segment cesarean section (n = 1029)	Elective lower segment cesarean section (n = 1457)	Relative risk* (95% confidence interval)
Low Apgar score	44 (4.6)	44 (4.3)	32 (2.2)	2.0 (1.3 to 2.9)
Intubation	86 (8.9)	98 (9.5)	61 (4.2)	2.2 (1.6 to 2.9)
Special care baby unit	54 (5.6)	72 (7.0)	75 (5.1)	1.2 (0.9 to 1.6)

Note: Numbers in parentheses are percentages.
* Relative risk for vaginal delivery and emergency vs. elective cesarean section.
(Courtesy of Thorpe-Beeston JG, Banfield PJ, Saunders NJStG: *BMJ* 305:746–747, 1992.)

Mary's maternity information system were used for a population-based study to define neonatal morbidity and early morbidity in term breech infants delivered vaginally or by cesarean section.

Setting.—Intrapartum and neonatal mortality, low Apgar scores, intubation at birth, and admission to special infant-care units were analyzed in 3,447 singleton fetuses presenting by the breech at ≥ 37 weeks' gestation.

Outcome.—After exclusion of infants with congenital anomalies, the incidence of intrapartum and neonatal death with vaginal delivery was .83% (8/961) compared with .03% with cesarean section (relative risk, 20; 95% confidence interval, 2.5–163). Furthermore, the frequency of low Apgar scores and neonatal intubation doubled in infants delivered vaginally or by emergency cesarean section compared with those delivered by elective cesarean section (table).

Conclusion.—The risk of intrapartum and neonatal loss in vaginal delivery of a term breech fetus approaches 1%. The authors believe that most mothers would opt for elective cesarean section if informed of this disturbing statistic before delivery.

▶ The level of tension and anxiety tends to rise meteorically in those moments before an infant in the breech position is finally delivered. It is a feeling similar to that experienced by passengers when the yellow plastic cups fall from their compartments into their airplane seats. Will the fetus (turned newborn) survive this traumatic transition turned upside down? How extensive a resuscitation will be needed? The equipment is checked for the umpteenth time! How sweet is the sound when the infant, in the firm grasp of the obstetrician, starts to cry and is obviously moving all extremities.

The above analysis once again demonstrates the advantages of cesarean section for the fetus still in the breech position at term (1). There were fewer deaths and fewer infants that required active resuscitation or a stay in the neonatal intensive care unit.

Furthermore, as the obstetric trainee has less and less experience with vaginal breech deliveries, the "wholesale elective section" will become the only option. However, to place this in the proper perspective, only about 3% of infants are in the breech position at term, and vaginal birth after a section will be an option for these women in subsequent pregnancies (see Reference 2.)

Life is not meant to be easy, my child; but take courage: it can be delightful.—George Bernard Shaw

A.A.Fanaroff, M.B.B.Ch.

Reference

1. Bingham P, Lilford RJ: *Obstet Gynecol* 69:965, 1987.

The Safety of Home Birth: The Farm Study

Durand AM (Commonwealth of the Northern Mariana Islands, Rota Health Ctr, Rota, MP)

Am J Public Health 82:450–452, 1992 5–4

Objective.—The safety of home delivery has not been established. The results of the largest comparative study of planned lay midwife-attended home births have now been reported.

Setting.—The outcome of 1,701 relatively low-risk pregnancies delivered between 1971 and 1989 through a home birth service run by lay midwives in rural Tennessee was compared retrospectively to that of 14,033 physician-attended hospital deliveries derived from the 1980 US National Natality Survey-National Fetal Mortality Survey (NNS-NFMS).

Results.—There were no significant differences between the 2 groups regarding fetal and neonatal death, low 5-minute Apgar scores, and composite index of labor complications (table). The rate of assisted delivery, particularly cesarean section, was significantly lower in lay midwife-attended home births than in the physician-attended hospital deliveries (16.46 vs. 1.46). The most common causes of the 17 perinatal deaths that occurred during the home births were lethal congenital anomalies and complications related to prematurity.

Implications.—For relatively low-risk pregnancies, lay midwife-attended home births can be accomplished as safely as, and with less intervention than, physician-attended hospital deliveries.

▶ Although the present paradigm of Western medicine dictates that hospital birth is safer than home delivery, there are not satisfactory data to support

Association Between Intended Site of Delivery and Selected Pregnancy Outcomes

Outcome	% Farm group	% NNS/ NFMS	Crude RR	Adjusted OR *	(95% CI)	*P* value
Perinatal death	1.00	1.33	0.75	0.69	(0.38–1.26)	.23
Labor-related complications	6.27	7.29	0.86	0.81	(0.63–1.04)	.09
Bleeding	1.93	1.02	—	—	—	—
labor >24 hours	2.87	2.76	—	—	—	—
Birth injury	0.23	3.34	—	—	—	—
RDS	1.41	3.65	—	—	—	—
Assisted delivery †	2.11	26.60	0.08	0.04	(0.03–0.05)	.00
Cesarean section	1.46	16.46	0.09	0.09	(0.08–0.10)	.00
5-minute Apgar<7	1.62	2.40	0.68	0.69	(0.40–1.19)	.18

Abbreviations: RR and OR, risk and odds ratios; *CI*, confidence interval; *RDS*, respiratory distress syndrome.

* Adjusted odds ratios were obtained by logistic regression and controlled for maternal age, parity, education, marital status, birth weight, smoking, and number of prenatal visits.

† Assisted delivery is use of any of following: cesarean section, forceps, or vacuum extractor.

(Courtesy of Durand AM: *Am J Public Health* 82:450–452, 1992.)

this dictum. In fact, studies suggest that, with the proper precautions, home delivery is associated with a reduced maternal morbidity without an increased infant mortality. This study is especially valuable, because the authors used many methods to select and evaluate a comparable control group. I have always hoped for a randomized study of mothers who wanted to deliver at home. One step removed from the study is a comparison of low-risk pregnant women booked for delivery in 2 systems of care (consultant or an integrated family practice unit) in the same hospital (1). In this study, there were fewer interventions by family practice physicians compared with obstetricians, and there were no significant differences in morbidity. Further trials are necessary to answer these important questions (1).—M.H. Klaus, M.D.

Reference

1. Klein M, et al: *Br J Obstet Gynaecol* 90:118, 1983.

Brachial Plexus Palsy: An Old Problem Revisited

Jennett RJ, Tarby TJ, Kreinick CJ (St Joseph's Hosp and Med Ctr, Phoenix, Ariz)

Am J Obstet Gynecol 166:1673–1677, 1992 5–5

Background.—It is generally accepted that brachial plexus palsy is caused by extreme lateral traction on the head during delivery of the shoulders. Reports in the neurologic literature of brachial plexus impairments that were almost certainly of intrauterine onset prompted a review of a perinatal database involving 57,597 births from 1977 through 1990. Separate searches were conducted for all cases of shoulder dystocia and all diagnoses of brachial plexus impairment.

Findings.—Seventeen of the 39 brachial plexus impairments diagnosed (43.5%) were associated with shoulder dystocia, but the other 22 (56%) had no such association. Maternal age of less than 20 years was 5 times greater in the non–shoulder-dystocia group (32%) than in the shoulder-dystocia group (6%), and nulliparity was more than twice as common (64% versus 29.4%). In addition, a birth weight of less than 3,500 g was significantly more frequent in the non–shoulder-dystocia group (60%) compared with the shoulder-dystocia group (6%).

Implications.—It appears that factors other than force during delivery of the fetal shoulders may account for brachial plexus impairment. Intrauterine maladaptation may play a role in brachial plexus impairment. Uterine maladaptation associated with young maternal age and nulliparity may be associated with a higher incidence of intrauterine pressures that result in nerve impairment. Brachial plexus impairment should not be considered prima facie evidence of shoulder dystocia.

▶ Brachial plexus injuries render the obstetrician vulnerable to medicolegal action (1). The plaintiff's attorneys imply that the injuries are preventable, as shoulder dystocia is predictable. Fuel was added to the fire by the report of excessive and prolonged force, as measured by force sensing devices applied to the fetus in deliveries complicated by shoulder dystocia (2). The revisitation of brachial plexus injuries by dredging the Arizona database produces striking findings. A significant number of injuries to the brachial plexus result from intrauterine forces and posture, totally unrelated to the delivery process. The profile of the pregnancy wherein the fetus may have been injured before labor and delivery is very different from traditional shoulder dystocia (3). The mothers are more likely to be young prima gravidas and the infants are smaller, lighter, and less mature. Other nerve involvement is also more likely in the non–shoulder-dystocia group. The plea for the use of the term "brachial plexus impairment" appears reasonable, and the evidence presented in this study speaks to the unpredictability of such impairment.

The report speaks to the value of a regional database; however, the limitations of retrospective reviews must be acknowledged. The fact that the medical record does not reflect shoulder dystocia or other traction problems does not preclude extreme lateral traction on the fetal head, particularly in those infants delivered in the breech position. Further prospective studies with similar findings will stem the tide of litigation after brachial plexus impairment.

Everyone is ignorant, only on different subjects.—Will Rogers

A.A. Fanaroff, M.B.B.Ch.

References

1. Gross TL, et al: *Am J Obstet Gynecol* 156:1408, 1987.
2. 1990 Year Book of Neonatal and Perinatal Medicine, pp 84–86.
3. Gonik B, et al: *Am J Perinatol* 8:31, 1991.

A Randomized Trial of Psychosocial Support During High-Risk Pregnancies

Villar J, for The Latin American Network for Perinatal and Reproductive Research (World Health Org, Geneva, Switzerland)

N Engl J Med 327:1266–1271, 1992 5–6

Background.—Psychological and social support and health education for women at high risk of delivering low-birth-weight infants is often advocated as a way to improve pregnancy outcomes. However, the evidence is inconclusive. In prospective trial, a program of home visits designed to provide psychosocial support during pregnancy was assessed.

Methods.—Four centers in Latin America participated in the study. A total of 2,235 women at higher-than-average risk for delivering a low-birth-weight infant were recruited before 20 weeks' gestation. They were randomly assigned to an intervention or control group. The former received 4–6 home visits from a nurse or social worker in addition to routine prenatal care. The control group received only routine prenatal care.

Findings.—The women in the intervention group did not have significantly different outcomes from those in the control group. The 2 groups had similar risks of low birth weight, preterm delivery, and intrauterine growth retardation. The intervention did not appear to affect type of delivery, length of hospitalization, perinatal mortality, or neonatal morbidity significantly in the first 40 days. The psychosocial support program did not appear to have any protective effect, even among the mothers at greatest risk.

Conclusion.—Interventions aimed at providing psychosocial support and health education during high-risk pregnancies are not likely to improve maternal health or the incidence of low-birth-weight among the infants. Clinics and hospitals should focus on consistently providing the prenatal care that has been proved effective.

▶ It seems such a logical and reasonable intervention, yet it joins 10 other similar studies of social support that revealed no difference between the control and experiment groups (1). In closely reading the details of the intervention, the support women were trained social workers who were encouraged to increase the mothers' social network and to discuss any worries. However, a large part of the interaction involved health education. Several nonrandomized pilot studies suggest a different approach. Intensive psychotherapy that uses hypnosis at the beginning of the actual premature labor to probe for the inciting cause has shown interesting results. These early studies note that each mother had a different and specific cause for her labor. Thus, a standardized intervention may not be appropriate.—M.H. Klaus, M.D.

Reference

1. Chalmers I, et al (eds): *Effective Care in Pregnancy and Childbirth, Vol I.* Oxford, England, Oxford Univ Press, 1989, pp 221–236.

Prevention of Excess Neonatal Morbidity Associated With Group B Streptococci by Vaginal Chlorhexidine Disinfection During Labor

Burman LG, Christensen P, Christensen K, Fryklund B, Helgesson A-M, Svenningsen NW, Tullus K, and the Swedish Chlorhexidine Study Group (Natl Bacteriological Lab, Stockholm; Central Hosp, Kristianstad, Sweden; Univ Hosp, Lund, Sweden, et al)

Lancet 340:65–69, 1992 5–7

Introduction.—Group B hemolytic *Streptococcus* is associated with a high rate of mortality in neonates infected from the vagina during birth. Antibiotic prophylaxis has not been entirely effective in preventing transmission of group B streptococci. The results of a new approach, the sup-

Rate of Admission of Infants to Special-Care Neonatal Unit by the Group B Streptococci Carrier State of Mothers and by Treatment Group

	No *(%)* infants admitted who were born to:			
Treatment group	Mother with vaginal group B streptococci	Mother without vaginal group B streptococci	RR (95% CI)	p (chi-square test)
Placebo (n = 2203)	22 *(5·4)*	43 *(2·4)*	2·31 (1·39–3·86)	0·002
Chlorhexidine (n = 2181)	11 *(2·8)*	34 *(1·9)*	1·51 (0·76–2·99)	0·24
Both treatment groups (n = 4384)	33 *(4·1)*	77 *(2·1)*	1·97 (1·31–2·96)	0·002

(Courtesy of Burman LG, Christensen P, Christensen K, et al: *Lancet* 340:65–69, 1992.)

pression of *Streptococcus agalactiae* during labor by intravaginal applications of chlorhexidine, have been reported.

Methods.—The double-blind, randomized, placebo-controlled trial took place at 10 Swedish hospitals. Data were available on 4,483 mothers and their full-term infants. Swabs were taken for culture when the women arrived in the delivery room. Vaginal flushing was performed with either 60 mL of chlorhexidine diacetate (2 g/L) or saline placebo. This procedure was repeated every 6 hours until delivery. The study end points were the rate of admission of infants to special-care neonatal units within 48 hours of delivery and the morbidity diagnoses of these infants.

Results.—The rate of vaginal carriers of *S. agalactiae* in this group was 18.4%. A total of 111 (2.5%) infants were admitted to special-care neonatal units within 48 hours of delivery. Infants whose mothers were carriers of group B streptococci and who received placebo flushings had a 2.3-fold increased risk of admission to special-care units. Overall, vaginal colonization of the mother with *S. agalactiae* was strongly associated with subsequent admission of the infant to special units (table). Disinfection with chlorhexidine of colonized mothers also reduced the overall risk of early respiratory disorder and diagnosed or probable infection. The prophylaxis caused no adverse effects in infants.

Conclusion.—Antepartum disinfection of the vagina with chlorhexidine reduced early morbidity by 31% in all infants and by 48% in infants born to mothers who were carriers of group B streptococci. This method of prophylaxis is inexpensive, safe, and effective.

▶ Commenting on this article is Julie Kulhenjian, M.D., Associate, Infectious Disease, Children's Hospital, Oakland, California:

▶ During the past 2 years, committees of the American College of Obstetricians and Gynecologists and the American Academy of Pediatrics have reviewed strategies for the prevention of perinatal transmission of group B *Streptococcus* (GBS). There is concurrence that intrapartum antibiotic chemoprophylaxis is effective in interrupting the transmission of GBS from colonized mothers to their infants during delivery. It is believed that this approach will prevent substantial numbers of early-onset neonatal infection and will also decrease the incidence of maternal postpartum amnionitis.

Selection of patients for intrapartum chemoprophylaxis remains the most controversial issue regarding prevention of GBS transmission. There continues to be no consensus as to the appropriate timing of antenatal screening for predicting carriage of GBS at delivery. Currently available rapid diagnostic techniques continue to be imperfect. Choosing women for intrapartum chemoprophylaxis based solely on the presence of risk factors at the time of hospitalization would be efficacious. However, this approach would result in unnecessary antibiotic exposure for women who are not carriers.

This study is important because it describes an alternative to parenteral antibiotics as a treatment regimen for prevention of GBS transmission in situations where the mother's carrier status is unknown. It has been demonstrated that GBS may be suppressed during labor by introvaginal applications of the disinfectant chlorhexadine (1). In the study, the rate of admission for infants born to chlorhexidine-treated GBS carrier mothers was significantly less than that for infants of colonized, placebo-treated mothers. Intravaginal administration of chlorhexadine was not associated with any serious adverse effects in the treated women. Unfortunately, this study was not able to address the issue of potential toxicity of chlorhexadine to premature infants. It is also not clear that using readmission as an end point, irrespective of probable or proven GBS invasive disease, is valid.—J. Kulhenjian, M.D.

Reference

1. Dykes AK, et al: *Eur J Obstet Reprod Biol* 16:167, 1983.

Maternal Death Due to Rupture of a Low Transverse Cesarean Section Incision During Labor at Home

Catanzarite VA, Foster E, Robinette P, Cousins LM, Schneider JM (Sharp Mem Hosp Women's Ctr, San Diego, Calif)

West J Med 157:454–455, 1992 5–8

Introduction.—Several studies have supported the selection of vaginal birth by women who have had a cesarean section delivery. Women with normal pregnancies who have had only 1 low-transverse cesarean section and who have no obstetric contraindication for vaginal delivery are frequently offered a trial of labor. About 1% of these women will have life-threatening emergencies. One woman who had a previous cesarean section selected to have a vaginal delivery, but a rupture of the surgical incision led to her death.

Case Report.—A woman in her eighth pregnancy, after 3 live births and 4 abortions, decided to have a vaginal delivery after a prior cesarean delivery. She did not have regular medical care and had changed physicians 3 times during the pregnancy. She wanted to have early labor at home with a birth coach, although she was warned of the dangers of this action. At 41 weeks' gestation the large 4,424-g fetus was in breech presentation; a cesarean section was recommended and the patient agreed. However, she left the hospital 30 minutes before the scheduled procedure; when contacted the next day, the procedure was rescheduled. However, she did not return to the hospital, and, when contacted, she expressed a desire for a second opinion. She called later in the day to say that another doctor had found the fetus to be in a vertex presentation, so she would remain home and await onset of labor. Three days later the patient was found at home, alone and dead as a result of a maternal hemorrhage that resulted from uterine rupture.

Discussion.—This patient had considered vaginal delivery safe and cesarean section dangerous. Although she had received detailed information about the great danger of remaining at home during labor, she did not accept this medical advice.

Conclusion.—Women who choose a vaginal delivery after a cesarean section should be evaluated during early labor and monitored appropriately in a hospital capable of rapidly mobilizing for obstetric emergencies.

▶ As we now categorize each pregnancy, it is important that parents fully understand why some pregnancies are truly high risk.—M.H. Klaus, M.D.

6 Infectious Diseases and Developmental Immunology

Defective Production of Interleukin-6 in Very Small Premature Infants in Response to Bacterial Pathogens

Yachie A, Takano N, Ohta K, Uehara T, Fujita S, Miyawaki T, Taniguchi N (Kanazawa Univ, Japan)

Infect Immun 60:749–753, 1992 6–1

Objective.—Dysfunction of mononuclear phagocytes is 1 major factor that predisposes newborns to bacterial infections. Interleukin-6 (IL-6) is a monocyte-derived product mediating the host defense against infectious agents. The ability of preterm and term newborn infants to produce IL-6 in response to major bacterial pathogens was examined using a unique whole-blood culture system, apparently mimicking neonatal bacteremia.

Methods.—Cord blood samples were obtained from 19 preterm ($<$ 38 weeks' gestation) and 7 term ($\geq$ 38 weeks' gestation) infants who were free of obvious bacterial infection at birth. The levels of IL-6 production induced by 4 major bacterial pathogens, group B streptococci, *Escherichia coli, Listeria monocytogenes,* and *Streptococcus pneumoniae* were examined in the whole-blood culture.

Results.—Cord blood from term infants induced IL-6 production at levels comparable to those of adult peripheral blood. In contrast, the levels of IL-6 production were significantly lower in preterm infants, particularly those born before 30 weeks' gestation, for each pathogen. In addition, the IL-6 response to lipopolysaccharide, a potent stimulant of monocyte cytokine production, was reduced in preterm infants, significantly so in newborns with gestation less than 30 weeks.

Conclusion.—These findings suggest an inherent defect in monocyte functions in preterm newborn infants. The reduced IL-6 production may partly account for the susceptibility of preterm newborns to bacterial infections.

▶ The interplay between the cells and the cytokines is the key to keeping unwanted organisms out of the neonate. However, the problem is debated much like the question regarding the chicken and the egg. Which comes first, and what is ultimately responsible for the increased susceptibility of the neonate to infection? Volumes have been filled describing the disorders of the white cells: their reduced number, impaired chemotaxis and phagocytosis, deficiencies in immunoglobulin and complement and, more recently, the inadequate production of cytokines in response to appropriate stimuli. Abstract 12–3 outline some of the T-cell production problems.

Interleukin-6 has surfaced as an important monocyte-derived product that helps to protect against infectious agents by mediating acute-phase responses and regulating immune reactions (1–3). Interleukin-6 revs up the T cells, stimulating proliferation and preparation for killing, and it also promotes B-cell multiplication and differentiation in addition to stimulating thrombopoiesis. Furthermore, IL-6 induces acute-phase protein production by the hepatocytes.

Using a unique whole-blood culture system, the authors unequivocally demonstrated that monocytes from full-term newborns are stimulated to produce amounts of IL-6 equal to those in adults when exposed to a variety of pathogens commonly encountered in the neonatal period. As might have been suspected (and certainly the oddsmakers refused to take bets otherwise), the preterm infants did not generate the same responses to any of the pathogens. The diminished amount of IL-6 could be incriminated in the susceptibility of the preterm infants to infection. More likely, it is the cumulative constellation of defects in the host defenses that opens the flood gates for the bacteria. However, I am of the opinion that as the broader picture of the immune problems in the immature infant emerges, it will facilitate finding the strategies and solutions to protect them.—A.A. Fanaroff, M.B.B.Ch.

References

1. Gauldie J, et al: *Proc Natl Acad Sci USA* 84:7251, 1987.
2. May LT, et al: *J Biol Chem* 263:7760, 1988.
3. Tosato G, et al: *Science* 239:502, 1988.

Diminished *Clostridium difficile* Toxin A Sensitivity in Newborn Rabbit Ileum Is Associated With Decreased Toxin A Receptor

Eglow R, Pothoulakis C, Itzkowitz S, Israel EJ, O'Keane CJ, Gong D, Gao N, Xu YL, Walker WA, LaMont JT (Univ Hosp, Boston; Mount Sinai Med Ctr, Boston; Massachusetts Gen Hosp, Boston; et al)

J Clin Invest 90:822–829, 1992 6–2

Background.—*Clostridium difficile* is the most common cause of antibiotic-associated diarrhea and colitis in animals and humans. However, human newborns and infants are relatively resistant to C. *difficile* infection compared with adults. Because toxin A is the major cause of intestinal damage with this organism, toxin A receptor binding and biological effects were compared in newborn and adult rabbit ileum.

Methods.—Purified toxin A was labeled with tritium or biotin with full retention of biological activity. The binding of biotinylated toxin A to rabbit ileal brush border from different ages was examined by using immunohistochemical techniques. The biological response to toxin A was studied by inhibition of in vitro protein synthesis and light microscopy.

Findings.—There was an age-related increase in C. *difficile* toxin A-receptor binding to rabbit ileal brush border. There was minimal [^{3}H] toxin A-specific binding in rabbit ileal brush border aged 2 and 5 days, with a gradual increase to adult levels in rabbits aged 90 days. This was confirmed further by immunohistochemical studies, being absent in newborn and present in adult rabbits. Toxin A, in doses ranging from 50 ng to 20 μg/mL, significantly inhibited protein synthesis in adult ileal loops in a dose-dependent fashion. In contrast, inhibition of protein synthesis in ileum aged 5 days occurred only at the highest toxin A doses. At all doses tested, the inhibitory effect of toxin A on protein synthesis was significantly less in newborn ileum than in adult ileum. Furthermore, adult ileum exposed to 5 μg of toxin A exhibited marked mucosal damage, whereas ileal explants aged 5 days exposed to the same concentration of toxin A remained normal.

Discussion.—There is a relative absence of specific intestinal binding sites for C. *difficile* toxin A in newborn rabbits. This may explain the lack of biologic responsiveness to purified toxin and the absence of disease in human infants with this pathogen.

▶ The strong correlation between the age-related expression of membrane receptors for bacterial toxins and the sensitivity to enterotoxins noted in this report also probably relates to the low incidence of shigellosis in neonates, because in rabbits, the intestinal receptors for shigella toxin are absent at birth but develop by 3 weeks of life. Using the same logic, the increased susceptibility to the heat stable toxin of *Eschericheria coli* in infants and children up to 2 years of age be explained by the greater number of *E. coli* heat stable enterotoxin receptors in the human neonate (1).—M.H. Klaus, M.D.

Reference

1. Cohen MB, et al: *Gastroenterology* 94:367, 1988.

The K1 Capsule Is the Critical Determinant in the Development of *Escherichia coli* Meningitis in the Rat

Kim KS, Itabashi H, Gemski P, Sadoff J, Warren RL, Cross AS (Univ of Southern California, Los Angeles; Harbor-UCLA Med Ctr, Torrance, Calif; Walter Reed Army Inst of Research, Washington, DC)

J Clin Invest 90:897–905, 1992 6–3

Background.—*Escherichia coli* strains possessing the K1 capsule are predominant among isolates from neonatal *E. coli* meningitis. Most of

Development of Meningitis (Defined as Positive CSF Culture) in Newborn Rats With Varying Degrees of Bacteremia

Bacteremia CFU/ml of blood	Number of animals with positive CSF culture/number of animals with positive blood culture			
	Strain C5 (018+K1+)	C5 mutant (018+K1−)	Strain XYL (018−K1+)	Strain 2513 (018−K1+::Tn 10)
$< 10^4$	0/9	0/8	0/11	0/5
10^4 to $< 10^5$	2/20 (10%)	0/22	0/8	1/7 (14%)
10^5 to $< 10^6$	10/25 (40%)	0/19	5/16 (31%)	3/15 (20%)
10^6 to $< 10^7$	4/10 (40%)	0/10	7/15 (46%)	5/18 (28%)
$> 10^7$	19/23 (83%)	0/9	5/6 (83%)	8/13 (62%)

(Courtesy of Kim KS, Itabashi H, Gemski P, et al: *J Clin Invest* 90:897–905, 1992.)

these K1 isolates are also associated with a limited number of 0 polysaccharide (LPS) types. However, the basis of this association of the K1 capsule and certain 0 antigens with neonatal *E. coli* meningitis has not been clearly defined.

Study Design.—The role of the K1 capsule or 0-LPS antigen, or both, in the development of *E. coli* meningitis was studied by using a model of experimental *E. coli* bacteremia and meningitis in newborn and adult rats. The animals subcutaneously received a K1 *E. coli* strain (018+K1+) or mutants lacking either the K1 capsule (018+K1−) or 0 side chain (018−K1+). Quantitative cultures of blood and specimens of CSF were obtained 12–24 hours later.

Results.—*Escherichia coli* organisms were isolated from CSF in both newborn and adult rats infected with K1+ strains, regardless of LPS phenotype, and they also had a high degree of bacteremia (10^4 colony-forming units/mL of blood) (table). In contrast, none of the animals that were infected with the unencapsulated mutant 018+K1− and that developed a similar level of bacteremia had positive cultures of CSF. Histopathologic studies of the brains of selective animals with positive cultures of CSF showed gram-negative rods in the subarachnoid space, without concomitant inflammatory cells.

Implications.—The presence of the K1 capsule and a high degree of bacteremia are key determinants in the development of *E. coli* meningitis. It appears that the prevention of bacteria multiplication in the blood may be a feasible approach to the prevention of meningitis. The 0 serogroups that are associated with the K1 encapsulated *E. coli* strains may be relevant to the pathogenesis of the bacteremic stage of the disease. Further studies are warranted to define the role of immunotherapy (e.g., hyperimmune globulin) in controlling neonatal *E. coli* sepsis and meningitis.

▶ Commenting on this article is Julie Kulhenjian, M.D., Associate, Infectious Disease, Children's Hospital, Oakland, California:

▶ Human neonates are predisposed to bacterial sepsis and meningitis caused by *Escherichia coli* (*E. coli*). In the United States, *E. coli* is the second most common bacterial pathogen isolated from the blood stream of neonates. The development of effective adjunctive passive or active immunotherapy for the treatment of neonatal gram-negative bacteremia and meningitis is dependant upon an adequate understanding of the host response to this infection.

The *E. coli* strains possessing the K-1 capsule are predominant among isolates from neonatal cases of *E. coli* meningitis. Based on these authors' findings, a critical number of bacteria-1 *E. coli* and the presence of K1 capsular antigen are key to CNS infection in young rats. They propose that the addition of hyperimmunogobulin containing opsonic antibodies theoretically has a role in decreasing the level of bacteremia.

Other authors have tried to assess the mechanisms responsible for the increased susceptibility of the neonate to gram-negative infections (1). The 2 most important deficits associated with neonatal sepsis are quantitative and qualitative changes in the phagocytic system and defects in antibody-mediated humoral immunity. Specifically passive, bacteriolysis of pathogenic *E. coli* mediated by the classical complement pathway has been shown to be inefficient in the serum of healthy full-term human neonates. In addition, neonatal serum may deposit IgG onto *E. coli* inefficiently. The potential benefits of adjunctive therapies such as granulocyte transfusions, intravenous immunoglobulin, and granulocyte–colony-stimulating factor are currently being investigated.—J. Kulhanjian, M.D.

Reference

1. Lassiter HA, et al: *Infect Dis J* 165:290, 1992.

Receiver Operating Characteristic Curves for Comparison of Serial Neutrophil Band Forms and C Reactive Protein in Neonates at Risk of Infection

Russell GAB, Smyth A, Cooke RWI (Liverpool Maternity Hosp, Liverpool, England)

Arch Dis Child 67:808–812, 1992 6–4

Background.—There is a wide variation in the performance of indirect tests of infection in the newborn because of differences in techniques, including diagnostic cutoff levels. The receiver operating characteristic

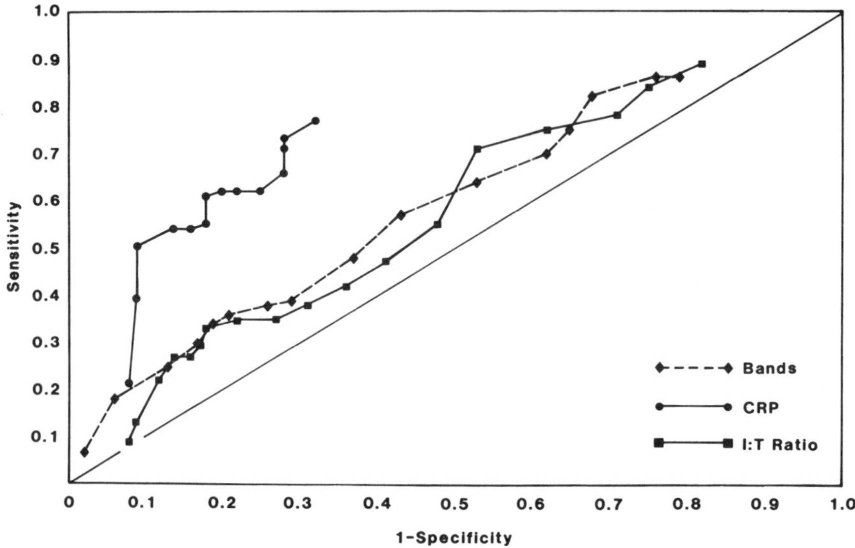

Fig 6–1.—Receiver operating characteristics curves of infection indices. 1-Specificity is equal to the false positive rate. (Courtesy of Russell GAB, Smyth A, Cooke RWI: *Arch Dis Child* 67:808–812, 1992.)

(ROC) curve permits direct comparison of tests regardless of diagnostic cutoff levels.

Study Design.—The ROC was used to compare the performance of serial neutrophil band forms and C reactive protein measured by rate nephelometry in neonates with suspected infection. The "gold standard" was a positive culture. The operational diagnostic cutoff values for the tests were: C reactive protein > 8 mg/L; immature: total neutrophil ratio (I:T ratio) > .2; and neutrophil band count > 5%.

Results.—For the 172 septic screens on 56 patients, the overall positive culture rate was 32.5%. The sensitivity of C reactive protein was 71.4%, which was similar to the sensitivity of the band count (69.6%) but significantly better than the I:T ratio (34%). The specificity of C reactive protein (72.4%) was significantly better than the band count (38.8%) but no better than the I:T ratio (73%). The ROC curves were constructed for all cutoff values, and the C reactive protein showed superior performance, compared with band count and I:T ratio, at any given diagnostic level (Fig 6–1). When the ROC curve was used, a diagnostic cutoff level of 7 mg/mL for C reactive protein achieved a sensitivity of 75%, a specificity of 71%, and a positive predictive accuracy of 55%.

Conclusion.—In neonates, serial C reactive protein is a useful indicator of early infection. A more rapid and sensitive detection method should be developed to exploit the potential of C reactive protein as an early marker of infection. The ROC curve permits comprehensive and graphic comparison between tests and the calculation of optimal diagnostic cutoff values.

▶ Judging from the steady stream of publications related to infections in the neonatal period, this line of investigation will continue to support a number of academicians. By constructing ROC curves, Russell et al. have offered a novel approach to distinguishing between the tests used to separate infected from noninfected newborns. Early signs of infection in the newborn are not specific, and laboratory indicators are necessary to assist the clinician. In selecting the laboratory tests and their interpretation, the clinician may follow many options. The glass-is-half-full group searches for sensitivity (the proportion of positive cultures detected by the test), and the glass-is-half-empty supporters seek specificity (the proportion of negative cultures correctly identified by the test). The majority no doubt yearn for efficiency (the proportion of all culture results correctly determined by the test, i.e., the sum of sensitivity and specificity).

The blood culture is, of course, referred to as the "gold standard." This too can be challenged. In the above series, the majority of infections, including one seen on the first day of life, were caused by *Staphylococcus epidermidis.* Should these not have been verified with repeat blood cultures?

I look forward to other reports using ROC curves and, for the present, I can accept the idea that throughout the neonatal period, the C reactive protein is the best indicator. Repeating the test improves the performance, and the availability of a rapid kit for C reactive protein would be welcome in most nurseries. Through this report, I became aware that the I:T ratio performs well only during the first week of life, and I noted (for future reference) that, unlike the CBC, the CRP was not invalidated by the use of steroids (in the few patients studied). This study reaffirmed that the adjunctive determination of infection has a low specificity. See Abstracts 6–6, 6–7, and 6–14.—A.A. Fanaroff, M.B.B.Ch.

Development of Cutaneous Microflora in Premature Neonates

Keyworth N, Millar MR, Holland KT (Royal Hampshire County Hosp, Winchester, England; Univ of Leeds, England)

Arch Dis Child 67:797–801, 1992 6–5

Background.—Coagulase-negative staphylococci (C-NS) are frequently isolated from the blood of premature infants. Bacteremia usually is associated with the presence of an intravascular catheter, and it seems likely that the strains of C-NS that cause bacterial sepsis originate on the skin surface.

Objective.—A swab wash method was used to sample the cutaneous microflora of 9 premature neonates admitted to an intensive care unit with respiratory distress syndrome. Gestational ages ranged from 25 to 32 weeks.

Findings.—Bacteria were identified on the skin surface within 6 hours after birth. The most common bacterial isolates were C-NS. The number of staphylococci at skin sites increased rapidly in the first week of postnatal life (Fig 6–2). *Staphylococcus epidermidis* was the predominant

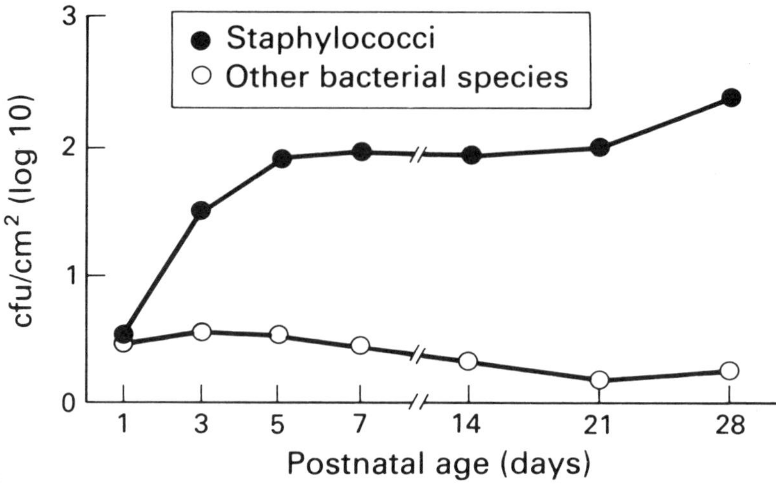

Fig 6–2.—Quantitative changes in cutaneous microflora with postnatal age. Measurements are logarithmically transformed and taken at 8 sites in 9 neonates. (Courtesy of Keyworth N, Millar MR, Holland KT: *Arch Dis Child* 67:797-801, 1992.)

species. All infants had antibiotic-resistant C-NS by the end of the first week of life. Changes in cutaneous staphylococci and in the proportion resistant to antibiotics in 1 infant are shown in Figure 6–3.

Implications.—The finding that C-NS on the skin surface increase rapidly in the first week of postnatal life suggests the need for good skin preparation — using an efficient disinfectant — before insertion of an intravenous catheter. Ongoing care of the insertion site is necessary because the skin repopulates within 18 hours.

▶ A mother lode of data is accumulated from this longitudinal study of 9 preterm infants. This represents the maiden attempt to quantitate and classify the bacteria colonizing the skin. It was a little surprising that coagulase-negative staphylococci were already prevalent by 6 hours of life, with scant representation by the infamous vaginal flora. The patterns of acquisition were similar in infants passing through the birth canal and those delivered by cesarean section. It was not surprising that staphyloccoci predominated beyond 6 hours, and that resistance to antibiotics was rampant. Resistance to antibiotics that are not used in the neonatal intensive care unit, such as chloramphenicol, suggested "linkage of genes coding for resistance to antimicrobials on the same plasmid." During the study, more than 2,500 staphylococci were identified, and *Staphylococcus epidermidis* reigned supreme, accounting for 82% of the total colonial counts of staphylococci. The rest of the list reads like a "Who's Who in Staphylococci."

The tale is one of good news/bad news. The good news is that the skin of the immature infant is not supportive of a stable microbial system. The bad news is that there is a constant change of organisms in the skin. The prema-

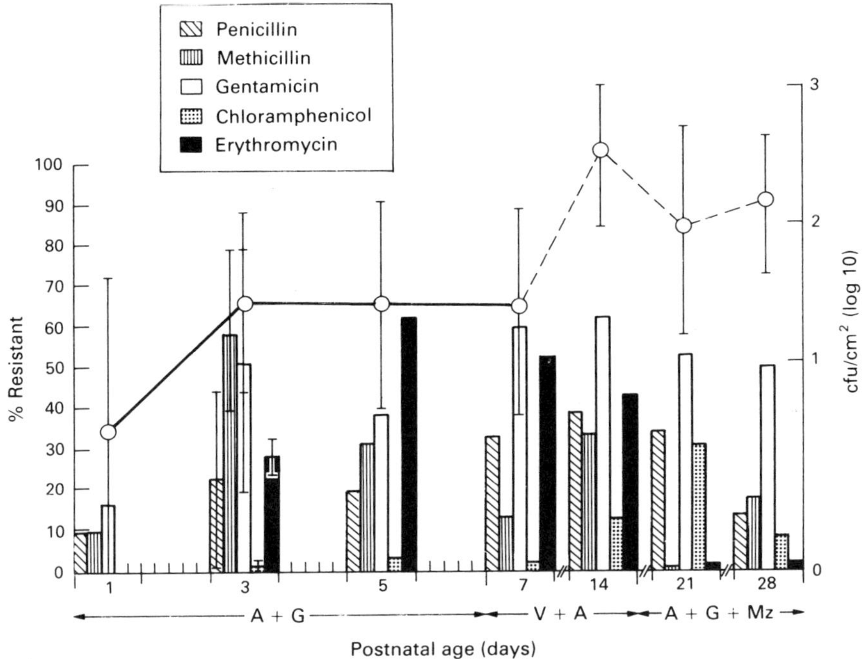

Fig 6–3.—Quantitative changes in cutaneous staphylococci and percentage resistant to antibiotics with postnatal age. Resistance is shown in relation to treatment: ampicillin (A) and gentamicin (G) given to day 6, the vancomycin (V) and ampicillin, followed by ampicillin, gentamicin, and metronidazole (Mz). (Courtesy of Keyworth N, Millar MR, Holland KT: *Arch Dis Child* 67:797–801, 1992.)

ture skin is capable of sustaining staphylococci, but it is not as supportive for other microorganisms. The skin is fragile, and every effort should be made to maintain its integrity. Careful skin preparation before inserting intravenous lines is a prerequisite to diminish the risk of infection. Continued antisepsis around the catheter is wise and, of course, the old standby, good handwashing, is a must.—A.A. Fanaroff, M.B.B.Ch.

Relatedness of Strains of Methicillin-Resistant Coagulase-Negative *Staphylococcus* Colonizing Hospital Personnel and Producing Bacteremias in a Neonatal Intensive Care Unit

Patrick CH, John JF, Levkoff AH, Atkins LM (Med Univ of South Carolina, Charleston)

Pediatr Infect Dis J 11:935–940, 1992 6–6

Introduction.—Recently, the methicillin-resistant coagulase-negative *Staphylococcus* species has emerged as a major bacterial pathogen in neonatal intensive care units (NICUs). It was hypothesized that health-care personnel in NICUs constitute a reservoir of resistant strains that colonize and/or infect high-risk neonates.

Methods.—During a 12-month period, methicillin-resistant coagulase-negative *Staphylococcus* strains isolated from blood cultures of NICU patients were characterized using newer molecular methods including plasmid profiles, genomic DNA restriction endonuclease digestion patterns, and restriction fragment length polymorphisms with the use of ribosomal RNA probe (ribotype). The results were compared with bacterial strains isolated from surveillance nasal cultures of the nursing, physician, and respiratory therapy staff.

Results.—Sixty-two percent of the nurses carried methicillin-resistant coagulase-negative *Staphylococcus,* and the species were similar to those found in bacteremia isolates from NICU infants. Plasmid profiles showed a moderate degree of similarity between neonatal and personnel strains, but genomic DNA restriction patterns showed more diversity. Ninety percent of the strains from nares of personnel and 50% of the neonatal bacteremic strains had similar ribotype patterns, whereas the remainder had distinctly different appearances.

Implications.—The NICU health-care workers displayed a high rate of colonization with strains of methicillin-resistant coagulase-negative *Staphylococcus* that shares some biomolecular traits with the strains recovered from bacteremia isolates in neonatal patients. This observation does not establish the cause of colonization or infection in infants, but it is hypothesized that related methicillin-resistant strains may be transferred among personnel and neonates in the NICU.

▶ Jill E. Baley, M.D., Associate Professor of Pediatrics at Case Western Reserve University, made the following observations:

▶ This study is an example of the complexity of the issues regarding methicillin-resistant coagulase-negative *Staphylococcus* species colonization and infection among very-low-birth-weight infants. The authors performed a sophisticated study analyzing any relationship of the strains among bacteremic infants and nasally-colonized personnel. After consultation with local experts, it became evident that the riboprobe patterns did not perform as expected in that the infant and personnel strains had patterns very similar to the control strains. In addition, although there was a high degree of similarity in plasmid profiles, speciation did not always correspond to these profiles. Thus, the differentiation fell to genomic DNA restriction patterns, and these patterns showed more diversity. All the appropriate studies were performed to compare the relatedness of the strains, but the data generated were not terribly illuminating, other than to direct attention to the high degree of colonization with methicillin-resistant coagulase-negative *Staphylococcus* species among nursing personnel, who had the highest degree of physical contact with the patients.—J.E. Baley, M.D.

Comparison of Blood Cultures With Corresponding Venipuncture Site Cultures of Specimens From Hospitalized Premature Neonates

Hammerberg O, Bialkowska-Hobrzanska H, Gregson D, Potters H, Gopaul D, Reid D (St Joseph's Health Ctr, London, Ont, Canada)

J Pediatr 120:120–124, 1992 6–7

Introduction.—Coagulase-negative staphylococci are the most common cause of nosocomial bacteremia in neonatal intensive care units. Because coagulase-negative staphylococci also make up commensal skin flora, it is possible that blood cultures are contaminated with skin flora in these children, especially because their blood culture collection is technically difficult.

Methods.—Blood culture isolates were compared with residual commensal skin flora after cleaning the venipuncture site in 677 blood culture specimens and corresponding venipuncture site swabs obtained from 488 premature infants. Coagulase-negative staphylococcal species were identified with standard commercial methods; restriction-endonuclease fingerprinting of chromosomal DNA and plasmid-profile analysis were performed for the molecular typing of staphylococcal strains.

Results.—Organisms grew in 58 blood cultures; in 9, the corresponding venipuncture site cultures also yielded organisms. Of these blood cultures, 42 (73%) yielded coagulase-negative staphylococci; in 5, the corresponding venipuncture site cultures also yielded coagulase-negative staphylococci. Analysis by restriction-endonuclease fingerprinting of chromosomal DNA and plasmid content showed that growth was caused by identical strains in 3 of these 5 specimens.

Conclusion.—Overall, only 3 (7%) of 42 of coagulase-negative staphylococcal blood culture isolates from hospitalized premature neonates were associated with identical skin isolates. The contamination rate resulting from the skin flora of blood cultures of these neonates in this setting seems very low, and the growth of blood cultures seems to be caused by bacteremia in most infants.

▶ Jill E. Baley, M.D., Associate Professor of Pediatrics at Case Western Reserve University, critiqued this study in the following manner, with appropriate help from other consultants who, however, shall remain nameless:

▶ Previously written off as a contaminant or a very indolent infection causing minimal or no symptoms, *S. epidermidis* has risen to the forefront, both as the most common cause of nosocomial infections in the neonatal intensive care unit and as an infection associated with an increasing array of symptomatology. Certainly, *S. epidermidis* has developed an impressive pattern of antibiotic resistance. Despite this, physicians are still troubled by the possibility that blood and other sterile body-fluid cultures yielding *S. epidermidis* might be contaminants, resulting in unnecessary, potentially toxic therapy prolonging the hospitalization. This report adds to several prior reports attempting to address this issue. Analysis of the data is complicated by the lack of an adequate means to determine the presence of sepsis when not using a definition dependent on a positive blood culture. This problem is experienced by investigators who use quantitation of blood cultures as a means of validation. How do you validate the validation?

These investigators take a different approach, determining skin colonization after cleansing of the venipuncture site. Only 3 of 42 (7%) blood cultures of *S. epidermidis* had an identical isolate from the skin. The authors appropriately acknowledge that their culture mechanism might miss organisms in the stratum corneum. A more pressing issue is whether the presence of identical isolates from both sites is truly an indication of contamination. It has been shown with other organisms, such as group B *Streptococcus,* that the more heavily the skin is colonized, the more likely the infant is to become septic. Thus, with cleansing of the skin, blood culture contamination appears to be an infrequent problem.

Another factor that lends some confusion to the data is the means of skin cleansing. The skin often will not dry completely by 30 seconds after the application of 10% iodine. It may not result in the most optimum skin cleansing, but it is probably fairly reflective of the usual skin cleansing administered in nurseries.—J.E. Baley, M.D.

Intravenous Immune Globulin for the Prevention of Nosocomial Infection in Low-Birth-Weight Neonates

Baker CJ, for the Multicenter Group for the Study of Immune Globulin in Neonates (Baylor College of Medicine, Houston)

N Engl J Med 327:213–219, 1992 6–8

Introduction.—Premature infants now survive longer but often only to succumb to nosocomial infection, particularly those neonates weighing less than 1,500 g at birth. Because little maternal IgG is transmitted to the fetus before 32 weeks' gestation, the efficacy of intravenous administration of immunoglobulin low-birth-weight infants during the first 2 months of life was examined in a randomized, multicenter, double-blind trial.

Methods.—The study population included premature infants weighing between 500 and 1,750 g at birth, who had an expected survival of greater than 48 hours at 6 United States hospitals. The infants were given either immunoglobulin, 500 mg/kg, or placebo at enrollment, 1 week afterward, and every 14 days thereafter, until they had received a total of 5 infusions or were discharged.

Results.—Two hundred ninety-seven premature infants received 1,163 infusions of placebo, and 287 received 1,125 infusions of immunoglobulin. There were 5 adverse reactions in each group, including mild alterations in blood pressure, heart rate, or temperature. At the beginning of the study the mean level of IgG of the placebo group was 520 mg/dL, and that of the immunoglobulin group was 536 mg/dL. The mean level of IgG in the placebo group decreased immediately, but that of the immunoglobulin group remained above birth level, a significant difference. Infants who received immunoglobulin had a significantly lower risk of a first infection than did the infants in the placebo group. Most of the bacterial infections were severe and were seen as septicemia without other identified foci of infection.

Conclusion.—For premature infants weighing between 500 and 1,750 g at birth, treatment with intravenous infusions of immunoglobulin is safe and reduces the risk of nosocomial infection. This treatment also reduced the average hospital stay for the immunoglobulin-treated group by about 6 days, compared with the placebo group.

▶ Melvin Berger, M.D., Ph.D., Director of Immunology at Rainbow Babies and Children's Hospital, and Associate Professor of Pediatrics at Case Western Reserve University, offers the following:

▶ The use of intravenous immunoglobulin (IVIG) continues to be controversial in low- and very-low-birth-weight infants who are deprived of the maternal IgG that is normally transported across the placenta in the last trimester of pregnancy. Although the rationale for IgG supplementation is clear and several small studies suggest beneficial effects, confirmation in large multicenter trials has been considered a necessary prerequisite to large-scale recommendation of IVIG prophylaxis. In this well-designed study of 588 infants at 6 centers, bacteria were responsible for 85% of all nosocomial infections, and more than half of these were caused by coagulase-negative *Staphylococcus* species and *Staphylococcus aureus*. Interestingly, group B *Streptococcus* accounted for less than 1% of infections. As in most other studies, IVIG was remarkably free from side effects. The IVIG-treated infants had a significantly lower incidence of infection. The mortality rate was so low in both groups that no significant effect could be attributed to the IVIG. Perhaps more importantly, the IVIG-treated group had fewer days of hospitalization than the placebo group. Although the large doses of IVIG used for Kawasaki Syndrome and idiopathic thrombocytopenic puerpera can be quite expensive, the cost of the dose of IVIG used in these small infants (500 mg/kg x 5 doses x $30 per g of IVIG) is less than $100 each, which pales compared with current hospital charges of more than $1,000 per day at most centers. It should be noted that not all studies of IVIG in neonates have had equally favorable outcomes; therefore, it may still be too soon to advocate the widespread use of IVIG prophylaxis in all low- and very-low-birth-weight infants.—M. Berger, M.D., Ph.D.

Intravenous Immune Globulin Therapy for Early-Onset Sepsis in Premature Neonates

Weisman LE, Stoll BJ, Kueser TJ, Rubio TT, Frank CG, Heiman HS, Subramanian KNS, Hankins CT, Anthony BF, Cruess DF, Hemming VG, Fischer GW (Walter Reed Army Med Ctr, Washington, DC; Emory Univ, Atlanta, Ga; Tripler Army Med Ctr, Honolulu, Hawaii; et al)

J Pediatr 121:434–443, 1992 6–9

Rationale.—Infants who are born before term may have both quantitative and qualitative deficiencies of IgG and, as a result, may be at risk of infection by encapsulated bacteria. Intravenously administered immunoglobulin contains opsonic antibody for many relevant pathogens, but previous studies have failed to give definite evidence of benefit.

Study Design.—A prospective double-blind trial of intravenously administered immunoglobulin (IVIG) therapy enrolled 753 newborn infants with a gestational age of 34 weeks and less. The infants were assigned to receive either 500 mg of IVIG per kg or 5 mg of albumin per kg. The medications were given over 2 hours before age 12 hours of life.

Results.—Early-onset sepsis developed in 4.2% of the infants. The most frequent isolates were group B streptococci and *Escherichia coli.* Seven of the infected infants (23%) died. During the 7 days for which serum IgG levels were higher in actively treated infants, there were 5 deaths among control infants and none in the IVIG-treated group. Survival at age 8 weeks did not differ significantly. Adverse reactions to the infusion were less frequent in the IVIG group than in infants given albumin.

Conclusion.—When added to appropriate antibiotic therapy, intravenously administered immunoglobulin is quite safe and may lessen early mortality in high-risk neonates with early-onset sepsis. The overall survival, however, is not significantly reduced. Specific hyperimmune or monoclonal antibody preparations might prove more effective.

▶ Melvin Berger, M.D., Ph.D., Director of Immunology at Rainbow Babies and Children's Hospital, and Associate Professor of Pediatrics at Case Western Reserve University, supplemented his editorial comments in the *Journal of Pediatrics* on this manuscript with the following thoughts:

▶ It is important to note that the use of IVIG for the *treatment* of established infections raises questions that differ considerably from those involved in its prophylactic use. The potential for blockade of the reticuloendothelial system (RES) and more rapid generation of the immune complexes that can induce inflammatory mediators, as well as the detrimental results in some animal models of neonatal infection, have caused most investigators to focus on prophylaxis and to exclude infants that may already be infected. Nevertheless, several small clinical studies (1) have shown decreased morbidity and/or mortality in infants treated with IVIG plus antibiotics as compared to those treated with antibiotics alone. This paper by Weisman et al. reports part of a larger study in which IVIG was administered within 12 hours of birth, regardless of the infant's status. Those infants found to have positive cultures at the time of randomization and treatment were then analyzed separately from uninfected infants. The IVIG resulted in a significant decrease in mortality at 7 days, but the effect was not sustained, and the mortality rate was equal at 56 days. The latter result is not surprising, because only a single dose of IVIG was given, and the treated group did not maintain an increase in IgG levels. The use of IVIG cannot yet be routinely recommended as adjunctive therapy for neonatal sepsis; however, the safety and efficacy reported in this study are encouraging and should lead to additional, larger trials.—M. Berger, M.D., Ph.D.

Reference

1. Schreiber, Berger: *J Pediatr* 121:401, 1992.

Randomized Trial of Granulocyte Transfusions Versus Intravenous Immune Globulin Therapy for Neonatal Neutropenia and Sepsis

Cairo MS, Worcester CC, Rucker RW, Hanten S, Amilie RN, Sender L, Hicks DA (Children's Hosp, Orange, Calif; Children's Hosp, Los Angeles)

J Pediatr 120:281–285, 1992 6–10

Introduction.—Neonatal sepsis occurs in about 10% of live births and is more common in premature infants. To improve the high mortality rate, treatment with adjuvant granulocyte transfusions was compared with intravenous immunoglobulin (IVIG) infusions in addition to standard supportive care in 35 neonates with sepsis and neutropenia.

Methods.—Half of the infants were premature, and the average postnatal age was 5 days. There were no significant differences between the groups with regard to serum immunoglobulins, total hemolytic complement values, hypoxia, acidosis, or hypotension.

Results.—The most commonly identified infection was group B *Streptococcus,* which accounted for nearly 33% of all bacterial isolates. The survival rate was 100% in the group receiving polymorphonuclear leukocyte transfusions and 64% in the group receiving IVIG transfusions. This difference was significant. No significant complications were associated with both treatment regimens.

Conclusion.—Granulocyte transfusions may be more beneficial than IVIG in the treatment of neonates with sepsis and neutropenia. Larger, randomized, prospective multicenter trials should be conducted to determine the efficacy and safety of this procedure in the treatment of neonates with sepsis.

▶ After reviewing and re-reviewing this manuscript, I concluded that the definitive study on the use of granulocyte transfusions for neonatal neutropenia and sepsis has not yet hit the launchpad. With all the difficulties inherent in conducting such a trial, my hunch is that it will get no further than the drawing board. A priori, it is necessary to separate the infants with neutropenia alone from those with neutropenia and sepsis. Then it would be ideal to match the infants with bone marrow neutrophil storage pool depletion in the various treatment groups. These are tasks easily accomplished in laboratory models but not in the clinical arena. Furthermore, granulocyte-macrophage colony-stimulating factors will imminently be available for clinical trials.

The above randomized trial included only 1 infant with neutrophil storage pool depletion. How many truly needed granulocyte transfusions? Furthermore, were the multiple transfusions indicated? The trial intermingles infants with bacterial-proven sepsis and those manifesting a clinical sepsis syndrome. This confounds the picture. In addition, the size of the trial minimizes its power. To their credit, the authors summarize by indicating that this single-center trial should serve as the springboard for a multicenter effort with granulocytes or the testing of other adjuvants. As I have had the opportunity to review all the prior trails involving the clinical use of granulocytes (1), my investment would be in cytokines or other means of boosting the neonatal host defense.—A.A. Fanaroff, M.B.B.Ch.

Reference

1. Baley JE, Fanaroff AA: Neonatal infections, part 2, in Sinclair JC, Bracken MB (eds): *Effective Care of the Newborn Infant.* Oxford University Press, 1992, pp 477–506.

Group B Streptococcal Sepsis in Piglets: Effect of Combined Pentoxifylline and Indomethacin Pretreatment

Gibson RL, Truog WE, Henderson WR Jr, Redding GJ (Univ of Washington, Seattle)

Pediatr Res 31:222–227, 1992 6–11

Background.—Group B *Streptococcus* (GBS) is a common neonatal gram-positive pathogen causing similar pathophysiology in human newborns and animal neonates. Animal models of GBS sepsis have revealed a 2-phase response. In the acute phase, increased pulmonary artery pressure (P_{pa}) and reduced arterial oxygen pressure (PaO_2) are associated with increased serum thromboxane B_2 (TxB_2); in the late phase, persistently increased P_{pa} and reduced PaO_2, reduced systemic arterial pressure, and progressive decline in cardiac output are associated with increased serum TxB_2, 6-keto-prostaglandin $F_{1\alpha}$ (6-keto-$PGF_{1\alpha}$), and tumor necrosis factor-α ($TNF\alpha$). It was hypothesized that pretreatment of piglets with pentoxifylline (PTF) and indomethacin would inhibit GBS-induced TxB_2, 6-keto-$PGF_{1\alpha}$, and $TNF\alpha$ and also prevent the acute- and late-phase physiologic responses to GBS sepsis.

Methods and Results.—Combined PTF and indomethacin pretreatment of anesthetized, mechanically ventilated piglets infused with GBS for 4 hours prevented GBS-induced increases in P_{pa} at 1 hour. It also markedly attenuated increases in P_{pa} at 4 hours. Pentoxifylline plus indomethacin prevented GBS-induced decreases in mixed and venous oxygen pressure and PaO_2 at 1, 2, and 4 hours and attenuated GBS-induced drops in cardiac output. This combination also significantly attenuated GBS-induced serum TNF**α** polypeptide levels at 4 hours and blocked GBS-induced increases in serum TxB_2 and 6-keto-$PGF_{1\alpha}$. Alone, indomethacin pretreatment prevented GBS-induced increases in serum TxB_2 and 6-keto-$PGF_{1\alpha}$ levels, but it did not significantly inhibit GBS-induced TNF**α** production. In addition, it did not attenuate GBS-induced P_{pa} increases at 4 hours, nor did it prevent latephase decreases in PaO_2 and mixed venous oxygen pressure.

Conclusion.—Treatment of GBS sepsis with PTF plus indomethacin is better than treatment with either agent alone in piglets. Inhibition of blood eicosanoid and TNF**α** production may constitute an adjunctive treatment for human newborns with sepsis and pulmonary hypertension.

▶ In the 1992 edition of the YEAR BOOK, we abstracted the data on the modulation of neutrophil function by pentoxifylline (1). To provide an update for those few readers with short memories (like myself), a brief review of pentoxifylline follows. Pentoxifylline is a xanthine derivative related to caffeine and theophylline; it was introduced into the clinical arena to treat vasoocclusive disease. It increases red blood cell and polymorphonuclear flexibility, enhances polymorphonuclear motility, stimulates chemotaxis, and reduces blood viscosity. Other actions it provokes include inhibition of TNF and reduction of pulmonary vascular permeability and pulmonary sequestration.

The above series of experiments was designed to use the property of inhibition of TNF. In combination with indomethacin, which inhibits eiconosanoids, PTF reduced pulmonary hypertension induced by GBS in a piglet model. The pathophysiology of bacterial-induced pulmonary hypertension is progressively emerging. Modulation of the inflammatory response can reduce the pulmonary vascular pressure. However, these are short-term experiments, and the ramnifications of altering so many factors in the newborn are uncertain. I am concerned that some of the fail-safe mechanisms will be blocked, and that although the pulmonary hypertension will resolve, we will lose the patient. Testing these new therapeutic approaches in the neonate will require great caution and courage. Skepticism is allegedly the chastity of academia. I retain a healthy dose of the same and will need much more convincing laboratory data before trying this therapeutic approach.—A.A. Fanaroff, M.B.B.Ch.

Reference

1. 1992 YEAR BOOK OF NEONATAL AND PERINATAL MEDICINE, pp 258–260.

Bone and Joint Infections Caused by Multiply Resistant *Staphylococcus aureus* in a Neonatal Intensive Care Unit

Ish-Horowicz MR, McIntyre P, Nade S (Westmead Hosp, Westmead, New South Wales, Australia)

Pediatr Infect Dis J 11:82–87, 1992 6–12

Introduction.—In 1981–1987, 20 patients were treated for osteomyelitis and/or septic arthritis caused by multiply resistant *Staphylococcus aureus* in an Australian tertiary neonatal unit. Eighteen cases occurred in a 3-year period (1985–1987), for an incidence in that time of 9.6 per 1,000 admissions.

Clinical Aspects.—All cases of osteomyelitis and/or septic arthritis involved ill premature infants who required intensive support; 11 weighed less than 1,500 g at birth. In 70% of the patients, an intravascular device served as the portal of entry. Initially, systemic symptoms predominated, and local signs developed within a week. Nearly all patients had radiologic abnormalities within 10 days, but bone scans were uninformative. In 11 infants, multiple osteomyelitis was diagnosed; involvement of the large joints was infrequent.

Treatment and Course.—Infants received vancomycin intravenously for a mean of 1 month. There was 1 septicemic death. No surgical drainage was necessary. One third of the patients had residual signs in the affected extremity at follow-up. Most of the infants with residual deficit had had associated arthritis. In no patient was limb function significantly impaired.

Conclusion.—This experience supports the empirical use of vancomycin in neonates suspected of having sepsis in an area where multiply resistant *S. aureus* is prevalent.

▶ After reading this report from Down Under, there can be no Doubting Thomases regarding the devastation that can be brought about by the virulent multiply resistant *Staphylococcus aureus*. The mighty *S. aureus* was the scourge of the nurseries in the '50s, but it has been more recently replaced in eminence by its cousins—the coagulase-negative staphylococci and group B streptococci. Thirteen percent of colonized infants had significant infection, and 6% had bacteremia; this is "the largest series of MRSA skeletal infection in any age group." Osteomyelitis/septic arthritis was diagnosed by clinical and radiologic features. All sites of osteomyelitis should be apparent after 10–14 days of therapy. Technetium scanning detected only 1 additional site of osteomyelitis and was not otherwise useful in early diagnosis.

Vancomycin remains the treatment of choice for MRSA; however, in many respects, the duration of therapy is arbitrary (1, 2). The authors concluded that a minimum of 3 weeks of parenteral vancomycin was prudent; others have recommended 3–4 weeks after defervescence (3). Surgical intervention is mandatory for septic arthritis, but it is rarely indicated for osteomyelitis. Those infants manifesting residual problems had joint involvement. A pleasant surprise for the authors was the lack of residual problems in even the most severe cases of osteomyelitis. However, their joy may be short lived as the potential for abnormalities in growth persists.

Osteomyelitis and septic arthritis are serious conditions in the neonatal period. Clinicians must be alerted to these entities, especially in the presence of MRSA outbreaks. Vancomycin therapy must be commenced promptly, and surgical drainage must be performed to preserve the large joints if there is septic arthritis.—A.A. Fanaroff, M.B.B.Ch.

References

1. Kline MW, Mason EO: *Paediatr Clin North Am* 35:613–624, 1988.
2. James A, et al: *Antimicrob Agents Chemother* 32:1320–1322, 1987.
3. Marcy SM: Bacterial infections of the bone and joints. In Remington JS, Klein JO (eds): *Infectious Diseases of the Foetus and Newborn Infant.* Philadelphia, WB Saunders, 1983, pp 755–770.

Lack of Evidence of Efficacy of Cohorting Nursing Personnel in a Neonatal Intensive Care Unit to Prevent Contact Spread of Bacteria: An Experimental Study

Ehrenkranz NJ, Sanders CC, Eckert-Schollenberger D, Hufcut RM, Macdonald N, Stone J, Sanders WE Jr (Florida Consortium for Infection Control, South Miami; Creighton Univ, Omaha, Neb; Broward Gen Med Ctr, Ft Lauderdale, Fla)

Pediatr Infect Dis J 11:105–113, 1992 6–13

Background.—In some hospitals with large nurseries, cohorting of newborn infants is routine to minimize transmission of infectious agents. Cohorting often is the ultimate measure used to contain nursery outbreaks of infection. It requires that nursing personnel strictly limit care to specified patients. The practice imposes increased demands on the number of skilled nursing personnel.

Objective and Methods.—Nurse cohorting was investigated during 99 days in a modern neonatal intensive care unit, where 100 infants were assigned to cohort or noncohorted care. Colonizing isolates were identified by plasmid profile analyses and biotyping. Surveillance cultures were acquired at weekly intervals.

Results.—In the first week, 3 infections occurred in the cohorted infants and none occurred in the noncohorted group. No secondary spread occurred, and no definitive cluster of colonization was evident. The rate of initial colonization at any site was .53 per patient-week in the noncohorted group and .3–.4 per patient-week in the cohorted units. Respiratory colonization with species other than usual skin bacteria was more frequent in cohorted infants, as was rectal colonization by species other than *Escherichia coli.*

Implications.—Strict cohorting is a costly and burdensome practice of unproved value. It may lower nursing morale and result in understaffing elsewhere. Modern infection control measures, including hand antisepsis with alcohol, should preclude the need for cohorting.

▶ The initial gratification for a clinical investigator is precipitated by a letter from an editor accepting a manuscript for publication. Continued satisfaction denotes that the research findings have an impact on care. This report has such potential, as it lays to rest the case for routine cohorting in the neonatal intensive care unit.

This well-performed epidemiologic study was carried out in a spacious, well-equipped nursery with a predominantly inborn population. The severity of the condition of the subjects admitted to the unit was difficult to read. Hence, some doubt lingers as to whether the data can be extrapolated to all neonatal intensive care units, as cohorting is more expensive, is bad for morale, and may place the infants at risk as a result of inadequate nursing coverage. The benefit of doubt would be to avoid cohorting in the absence of an epidemic (an aspect not evaluated in this data set). Nursing administrators will, no doubt, applaud this recommendation. A thorny issue that is conspicuously absent from this discussion is the routine practice of gowning, which was done in the unit under surveillance. That concept, which falls into neither the "art" nor the "science" of medicine, remains part of the mystique of the neonatal intensive care unit. Is it effective or necessary? Baley (1), in reviewing this topic, concluded that it was not.

The abiding message and theme reiterated throughout the manuscript concerns the importance of washing one's hands. The use of hand antisepsis with ethyl alcohol or isopropanol is superior to a bland soap hand wash (2). The appropriate use of gloves is also acceptable. Nobody will query these recommendations. Nosocomial infections remain a major cause of morbidity in the neonatal intensive care unit, and hand washing remains our most potent weapon.

Epidemiologic studies are often given biblical weight but they don't constitute proof. I don't see any glaring faults in this study but it's just an association — It doesn't prove it.—Dr. William Connell

A.A. Fanaroff, M.B.B.Ch.

References

1. Baley J, et al: *Effective Care of the Newborn Infant.* Oxford, England, Oxford Univ Press, 1992, p 461.
2. Ehrenkrantz NJ, Alphonso BC: *Infect Control Hosp Epidemiol* 12:654, 1991.

Outbreak of *Candida* Bloodstream Infections Associated With Retrograde Medication Administration in a Neonatal Intensive Care Unit
Sherertz RJ, Gledhill KS, Hampton KD, Pfaller MA, Givner LB, Abramson JS,

Dillard RG (North Carolina Baptist Hosp, Winston-Salem; Wake Forest Univ, Winston-Salem, NC; Univ of Iowa, Iowa City)
J Pediatr 120:455–461, 1992 6–14

Background.—The incidence of nosocomial *Candida* outbreaks has been increasing. Investigation and successful intervention in an outbreak of candidemia involving 5 infants receiving total parenteral nutrition (TPN) in a neonatal intensive care unit were examined.

Methods.—The outbreak occurred in January of 1990. All infants were receiving antibiotics before and during *Candida* infection. The infants' mean weight was 1,400 g, and their mean duration of hospitalization at the time of infection was 35 days. When the outbreak was first recognized, a search was initiated for a *Candida albicans* reservoir in lotions or soaps, barrier syringe solutions, and in-line fluids at the time that intravenous tubing was changed. Two months before the outbreak, the frequency of intravenous line changes was decreased from every 24 hours to every 72 hours.

Results.—The fluids from barrier syringes and waste syringes used for retrograde medication administration were more likely to grow *Candida* (4.1%) than were the other fluids sampled (.3%). An in vitro simulation revealed that catheter lumina were significantly less likely to be contaminated with C. *albicans* if intravenous tubing was changed every 24 hours than if it was changed every 48 or 72 hours. There was a significant association between candidemia and both TPN and retrograde medication administration.

Conclusion.—The outbreak apparently developed after the frequency of changing the intravenous tubing was decreased. Investigators also discovered a number of nursing practices that may have led to line contamination and cross infection. When syringes were used only once and intravenous tubing was changed every 24 hours, the outbreak was terminated. The authors advise neonatal intensive care units to carefully examine their TPN administration practices.

▶ Jill E. Baley, M.D., Associate Professor of Pediatrics at Case Western Reserve University, had the following thoughts:

▶ This report is a superb illustration of the kinds of detailed and discriminating analyses needed regarding every aspect of neonatal intensive care. The authors were able to track the mechanism of the *Candida* outbreak in the neonatal intensive care unit to contaminated retrograde medication syringes, exacerbated by a reduction in the frequency of intravenous tubing changes from 24 to 72 hours. The problem was remedied by adherence to stricter techniques that resulted in less contamination of the intravenous fluid apparatus. Of note were their experiments regarding the selective growth advantage for *Candida* from TPN solution. This is reminiscent of the study by Weese-Mayer and colleagues, in which the duration of central catheter use was not longer among *Candida*-infected infants, but the duration of use of hyperalimentation fluids was significantly longer. Once again, we note the importance of evaluating the benefits vs. the risks of TPN in each individual infant.—J.E. Baley, M.D.

Reference

1. Weese-Mayer DE, et al: *Pediatr Infant Dis J* 6:190, 1987.

Resurgence of Congenital Rubella Syndrome in the 1990s: Report on Missed Opportunities and Failed Prevention Policies Among Women of Childbearing Age

Lee SH, Ewert DP, Frederick PD, Mascola L (Ctrs for Disease Control, Los Angeles; Los Angeles County Dept of Health Services)

JAMA 267:2616–2620, 1992 6–15

Introduction.—In 1990, 189 cases of rubella were reported in 4 southern California counties, more than double the number reported the previous year (Fig 6–4). It is likely that a large part of the epidemic went unnoticed and unreported because of a large measles epidemic in the same area.

Methods.—Data were reviewed on 21 women who recently delivered infants with congenital rubella syndrome.

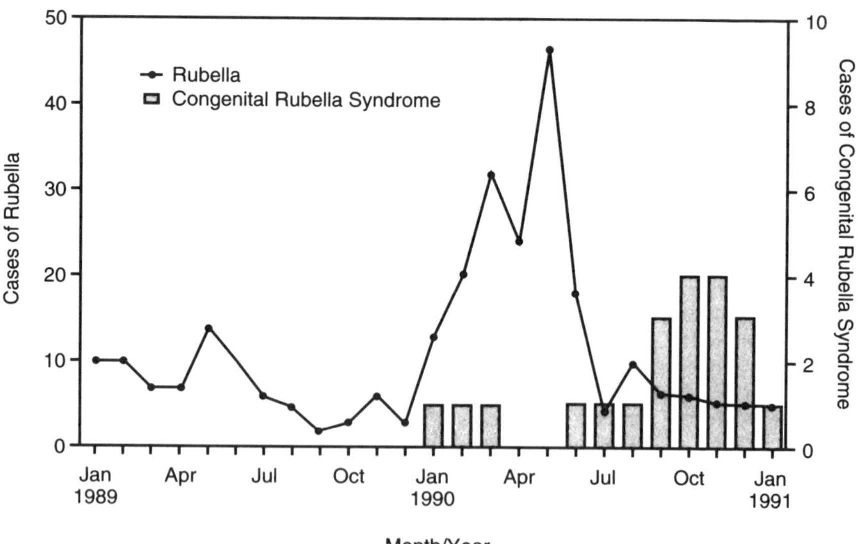

Fig 6–4.—Reported cases of rubella and congenital rubella syndrome in southern California (January 1989 through January 1991). (Courtesy of Lee SH, Ewert DP, Frederick PD, et al: *JAMA* 267:2616-2620, 1992.)

Criteria for Classification of Cases of Congenital Rubella Syndrome (CRS)

CRS Confirmed: Defects present and one or more of the following:
- (*a*) Rubella virus isolated
- (*b*) Rubella-specific IgM present
- (*c*) Rubella hemagglutination-inhibition titer, or equivalent rubella antibody test result in the infant persisting above and beyond that expected from passive transfer of maternal antibody (ie, rubella hemagglutination-inhibition titer in the infant that does not fall off at the expected rate of one twofold dilution per month)

CRS Compatible: Laboratory data insufficient for confirmation and any two complications listed below in *a*, or one from *a* and one from *b:*
- (*a*) Cataracts or congenital glaucoma (either or both count as one), congenital heart disease, loss of hearing, pigmentary retinopathy
- (*b*) Purpura, splenomegaly, jaundice, microcephaly, mental retardation, meningoencephalitis, radiolucent bone disease

CRS Possible: Some compatible clinical findings that do not fulfill the criteria for a compatible case

Congenital Rubella Infection Only: No defects present but laboratory evidence of infection

(Courtesy of Lee SH, Ewert DP, Frederick PD, et al: *JAMA* 267:2616–2620, 1992.)

Results.—Of the 21 women, 12 had 22 known missed opportunities for rubella screening or vaccination; 3 women failed to be screened when they married, 2 during previous pregnancies, and 5 during induced abortion. Twelve women missed a chance to be vaccinated after induced abortion or delivery. Only 4 of 12 women educated in California were subject to the 1982 California school rubella immunization requirement. Criteria for the classification of congenital rubella syndrome are provided in the table.

Conclusion.—Concerted efforts are needed to counsel and vaccinate susceptible women wherever they come into contact with the health-care system. Rubella screening and vaccination should be routine at university student health centers, family planning clinics, and facilities for abortion, treatment of sexually transmitted diseases, and during rehabilitation.

▶ This report reads a bit like an Agatha Christie mystery as it tracks down how congenital rubella could have been prevented. As we enter the new era of disease prevention, the whole society will have to participate, and the health record of each individual should be in his or her possession. Every woman should carry a copy of her own unified health record and, at the same time, care givers should be able to recover in a few moments each patient's record on a computer. When a physician treats an acute disease, he has quick feedback on his actions; however, disease prevention is usually inexpensive, less dramatic, and the rewards are rarely observed. As we move into the era of disease prevention, our system of health care will have to change.—M.H. Klaus, M.D.

The Outcome of Congenital Cytomegalovirus Infection in Relation to Maternal Antibody Status

Fowler KB, Stagno S, Pass RF, Britt WJ, Boll TJ, Alford CA (Univ of Alabama, Birmingham)

N Engl J Med 326:663–667, 1992 6–16

Introduction.—Congenital infection with cytomegalovirus (CMV) is often asymptomatic at birth, but sensorineural hearing loss, chorioretinitis, mental retardation, and neurologic deficits develop in 5% to 17% of

TABLE 1.—Clinical Findings in the First Month of Life in 24 Newborns With Symptomatic CMV Infection After a Primary Maternal Infection

Finding	No. (%)
Jaundice	15 (62)
Petechiae	14 (58)
Hepatosplenomegaly	12 (50)
IUGR*	8 (33)
Preterm birth†	6 (25)
Microcephaly	5 (21)
Hydranencephaly	1 (4)
Death	1 (4)

* IUGR denotes intrauterine growth retardation, defined as a birth weight less than the tenth percentile of gestational age.
† Any birth before 37 completed weeks of gestation.
(Courtesy of Fowler KB, Stagno S, Pass RF, et al :N *Engl J Med* 326:663–667, 1992.)

TABLE 2.—Sequelae in Children With Congenital CMV Infection According to Type of Maternal Infection

Sequela	Primary	Recurrent	P Value
	% (no. with sequela/ total no. evaluated)		
Sensorineural hearing loss	15 (18/120)	5 (3/56)	0.05
Bilateral hearing loss	8 (10/120)	0 (0/56)	0.02
Speech threshold ≥60 dB*	8 (9/120)	0 (0/56)	0.03
IQ ≤70	13 (9/68)	0 (0/32)	0.03
Chorioretinitis†	6 (7/112)	2 (1/54)	0.20
Other neurologic sequelae‡	6 (8/125)	2 (1/64)	0.13
Microcephaly	5 (6/125)	2 (1/64)	0.25
Seizures	5 (6/125)	0 (0/64)	0.08
Paresis or paralysis	1 (1/125)	0 (0/64)	0.66
Death§	2 (3/125)	0 (0/64)	0.29
Any sequela	25 (31/125)	8 (5/64)	0.003

* For the ear with better hearing.
† Of the 7 children with chorioretinitis, 3 (43%) in the primary-infection group had visual impairment.
‡ Of the 8 childrren, 4 (50%) had more than 1 abnormality.
§ After the newborn period.
(Courtesy of Fowler KB, Stagno S, Pass RF, et al: *N Engl J Med* 326:663–667, 1992.)

affected infants. Symptomatic CMV infection results in much more frequent and more severe sequelae. Transmission of CMV infection can occur from mother to fetus when maternal infection occurs during pregnancy or when the maternal infection occurred years before conception.

Method.—The degree of protection afforded an infected infant by the presence of antibody in the mother before infection was investigated in 197 children with congenital CMV infection. The children were classified as those whose mothers had primary and those whose mothers had recurrent CMV infections during pregnancy, based on seroconversion determined from stored maternal serum samples. Sequelae were assessed in 125 infants from the primary infection group and 64 from the recurrent-infection group.

Results.—Of the children born to mothers with primary CMV infections during pregnancy, 18% had symptoms as neonates, most commonly jaundice, petechiae, and hepatosplenomegaly (Table 1). No children born to mothers with recurrent infections had neonatal symptoms. After a mean follow-up of 4.7 years, 25% of the children in the primary-infection group had sequelae, significantly more than 8% in the recurrent infection group. The most common sequelae were sensorineural hearing loss, bilateral hearing loss, and an IQ of 70 or less (Table 2). These sequelae were significantly more frequent in children in the primary-infection group, and multiple sequelae occurred only among children in the primary infection group. The sequelae among children in the primary-infection group were most commonly seen during the first year of life.

Conclusion.—Pre-existing maternal antibody to CMV is associated with fetal protection and reduces the severity of the sequelae of congenital CMV infection. It is possible that vaccination of seronegative women of childbearing age could prevent up to 6,000 damaging congenital CMV infections annually.

► Mary-Lou Kumar, M.D., Professor of Pediatrics at Case Western Reserve University, and Director of Infectious Disease at Metrohealth-St Luke, our local expert on cytomegalovirus infections, had the following remarks to add to these abstracts:

► The Alabama team responsible for this excellent long-term study of children with congenital CMV infection again reminds us of the importance of maternal immunity in predicting the severity of neurobehavioral sequelae. Such sequelae developed in 25% of congenitally infected children if the child's mother experienced a *primary* CMV infection in pregnancy, whereas sequelae (usually milder) occurred in only 8% of those children in whom the maternal infection was classified as *recurrent.* The criterion used to identify primary infection was the presence of CMV-specific IgM antibody. As pointed out by the authors, this is a less-than-perfect test. Some mothers with primary infection but a negative IgM test (an estimated 25% of primary infections are IgM-negative) were probably misclassified as having recurrent infection, and the true risk of sequelae in congenitally-infected infants born to mothers with recurrent infection is less than 8%. The demonstrated protective effect of maternal immunity argues FOR further efforts to develop a vaccine that could be given to CMV-seronegative women to prevent CMV infection in pregnancy. Such a vaccine would probably be a recombinant "sub-unit" vaccine consisting of an immunogenic CMV envelope glycoprotein. As stressed by Drs. Gail Demmler and Martha Yow (1), congenital CMV is a *now* problem, and we need to work toward a solution to the problem—M. Kumar, M.D.

Reference

1. Demmler GJ, Yow M: N *Engl J Med* 326:702, 1992.

Lethal Cytomegalovirus Infection in Preterm Infants: Clinical, Radiological, and Neuropathological Findings

Perlman JM, Argyle C (Univ of Texas, Dallas)

Ann Neurol 31:64–68, 1992 6–17

Background.—Cytomegalovirus (CMV) infection is associated with a variety of neurologic manifestations. Abnormalities in term infants have received considerable attention, but there are limited data on preterm infants with symptomatic congenital CMV infection. The medical records of 21 affected preterm infants seen at Parkland Memorial Hospital in Dallas between 1975 and 1989 were examined.

Methods.—The records, including autopsy reports and histologic slides, were studied to determine the clinical, neuroradiologic, and neuropathologic characteristics of CMV infection in preterm infants. Diagnosis was based on isolation of the virus from urine during the first week of life and also from the appearance of typical intranuclear inclusion bodies in greatly enlarged cells from at least 2 systemic organs at autopsy.

Results.—Sufficient data were available for analysis in 15 cases. Six of these infants were stillborn; 9 were live-born but died at a mean postnatal age of 18 days. Intrauterine growth retardation was apparent in 10 infants. The common clinical findings in live-born infants included microcephaly (77%), seizures (55%), hypotonia (33%), and multiple contractures (18%). The eyes of 4 live-born infants were examined; all had abnormal findings. Two of 6 infants who underwent an antenatal sonogram had ventriculomegaly. Meningoencephalitis was observed in 12 of 15 infants. Cerebellar hypoplasia occurred in 5 cases, and diffuse calcification frequently involving the convexity of the gyri was seen in 6. In the 21 original infants, the organs most commonly involved were the kidney (95%), the lung (90%), and the liver (38%).

Conclusion.—Preterm infants with lethal CMV infection have several atypical features rarely found in term infants. Hypotonia, multiple contractures, periventricular leukomalacia, and optic atrophy are among these features.

▶ Mary-Lou Kumar, M.D., Professor of Pediatrics at Case Western Reserve University, and Director of Infectious Disease at Metrohealth-St Luke, our local expert on cytomegalovirus infections, had the following remarks to add to this abstract:

▶ This article serves as a reminder of the remarkable spectrum of congenital CMV infections, ranging from totally asymptomatic infection to severe systemic disease, with the potential for remarkable neuropathology as described in this study. Of the estimated 40,000 CMV-infected infants born each year in the United States (1% of 4,000,000 births), approximately 7% have symptomatic disease; approximately 12% of these symptomatic infections are fatal.

Antiviral therapy for several life-threatening CMV infections (pneumonia in bone marrow transplant patients and CMV retinitis in patients with AIDS) has now become the standard of care. It is not surprising that the NIH-sponsored Collaborative Antiviral Study Group (CASG), under the direction of Dr. Richard Whitley, has undertaken an evaluation of ganciclovir in infants with symptomatic congenital CMV infections.

Congenital CMV infection presents unique treatment challenges and, clearly, no one anticipates that antiviral therapy will ameliorate all the adverse consequences of a devastating intrauterine infection. However, milder cases of symptomatic congenital infection may be helped. Recruitment for the meticulously-conducted CASG studies is never easy, particularly for this study, which requires 6 weeks of intravenous treatment. With licensure of ganciclovir, the drug becomes available off-protocol, and I know from personal experience that it is being used for congenitally infected infants. We must remember that there are no data yet regarding the drug's efficacy in this situation. Rather than jumping in with a potentially toxic treatment of unproven efficacy, we should be making every effort to assist the CASG in completion of the phase III ganciclovir trial. If you have questions about the trial, Dr. Richard Whitley would be happy to hear from you (205-934-5316)!—M.-L. Kumar, M.D.

Presence of Non-Maternal Antibodies in Newborns of Mothers With Antibody Deficiencies

Hahn-Zoric M, Carlsson B, Björkander J, Osterhaus ADME, Mellander L, Hanson LÅ (Univ of Göteborg, Sweden; Rijksinstitut voor Volksgezondheid en Milieuhygiene, Bilthoven, Holland)

Pediatr Res 32:150–154, 1992 6–18

Background.—Previous research has shown that antibodies can be found at birth in the newborn without previous known exposure to the antigen. The mechanism for the induction and production of such antibodies was investigated in a model that excluded the possibility of specific antibodies transferred from mother to fetus.

Methods.—Specific IgG, IgA, and IgM antibodies against *Escherichia coli* and poliovirus antigens were examined with enzyme-linked immunoabsorbent assay in serum, saliva, and amniotic fluid from hypogammaglobulinemic and IgA-deficient mothers and also in the cord serum, saliva, and meconium from the infants.

Findings.—Although all the mothers lacked IgA and some lacked IgM antibodies, those antibodies were found in their healthy newborns. The amniotic fluid from 1 hypogammaglobulinemic woman lacking IgA had small amounts of IgA antibodies, also present in the neonate, which suggested a fetal origin. In cord sera, there was evidence of anti-idiotypic antibodies to poliovirus.

Conclusion.—Idiotypic and/or anti-idiotypic IgG antibodies transferred through the placenta from mother to fetus may initiate specific immune responses seen in the infant. Thus, it is possible that transplacental IgG not only passively protects the newborn but also actively primes the fetus through its content of idiotypic and/or anti-idiotypic antibodies.

▶ Commenting on this article is Brian L. Hamilton, M.D., Ph.D., Director, Division of Immunology, Children's Hospital, Oakland, California:

▶ This study was performed to determine whether antibodies to environmental antigens that are present in newborn infants are derived from the mother or from the fetus/newborn. The authors measured the concentration of IgG, IgM, and IgA in the serum and saliva of mother/newborn pairs. The mothers included in the study had either selective IgA deficiency or panhypogammaglobulinemia with IgA deficiency. The mothers with panhypogammaglobulinemia were routinely given replacement therapy with intramuscular gammaglobulin. Antibodies to poliovirus type 1 and to *Escherichia coli* O antigen were measured in serum, saliva, amniotic fluid, and meconium. The antibodies were measured using an ELISA assay designed to discriminate between IgG, IgA, and IgM antibodies.

None of the mothers had detectable IgA antibodies to either the poliovirus or *E. coli* O antigen in either serum or saliva. In contrast, all 7 infants studied had IgA antibodies to both antigens in saliva, although none had IgA antibodies to either antigen in the serum. Likewise, all 4 infants of the panhypogammaglobulinemic mothers had IgM antibodies to both antigens in the saliva (but not in the serum), whereas none of the mothers had IgM antibodies to either antigen. All mothers and all infants had IgG antibodies to both antigens in the serum. These data suggest that the IgA and IgM antibodies found in the newborns were produced by the newborns and not by the mothers, because the mothers were unable to make IgM and/or IgA antibodies. The IgG antibodies were probably from the gamma globulin replacement therapy given to the mothers.

A second question addressed in this paper was the source of the antigens that stimulated IgM and/or IgA antibody production in the fetus/newborn. The authors state that it is unlikely that the fetuses would be exposed to poliovirus, because the population is routinely vaccinated with inactivated polio vaccine, which does not replicate in the vaccinated host (as does the attenuated live polio vaccine). The authors go on to demonstrate the presence of antipolio idiotypic and anti-idiotypic antibodies in both the mothers and newborns. The authors suggest that the anti-idiotypic antibodies serve as the immunogen to stimulate the antipolio antibodies found in the newborns.

It has been known for several decades that IgG crosses the placenta from mother to fetus during the third trimester. The transplacental transfer of IgG is an active process that involves Fc receptors specific for IgG that are present on the placental cells. The IgG concentration in the term infant may be greater than the serum concentration of IgG in the mother. All 4 subclasses of IgG cross the placenta in this fashion. It is also known that IgG given to the mother in the form of intramuscular gamma globulin or intravenous gammaglobulin crosses the placenta to the fetus. In contrast, neither IgM nor IgA crosses the placenta. A variety of studies have also shown that the fetus can respond to intrauterine infections with the production of IgM and IgG antibodies. Because it is difficult to separate maternal from fetal IgG antibodies, clinicians routinely measure IgM antibodies to various infectious agents in the serum of newborns to diagnose intrauterine infection. Thus, these authors' observation that newborn infants of antibody-deficient mothers could make IgM and IgA antibodies simply confirms previous observations.

The second question addressed is, perhaps, more interesting. It is generally true that the fetus could not be exposed to many antigens because maternal antibodies should bind to any antigens present in the mother, and the antigen-antibody complexes should be removed before they could reach the fetal circulation.

Antibodies are made by B cells in response to stimulation by a foreign antigen. The antibody specificity of a given B cell is determined by a stochastic rearrangement of the immunoglobulin genes that encode the structure of the heavy and light chains. It is estimated that more than 1 billion antibody specificities can be made, including antibodies to self-antigens. The production of antibody depends on a complex process that results in the selection and clonal expansion of only a small fraction of the B cells made each day in the bone marrow. The antigen-combining site of the immunoglobulins produced has a unique 3-dimensional structure that is referred to as an "idiotype." The idiotype is a unique structure that, in turn, can be recognized by the body as a "foreign" antigen. Antibodies produced against the antigen combining site of an immunoglobulin molecule are thus referred to as "anti-antibodies." The cycle then repeats, because the anti-idiotype is also unique, and it therefore can stimulate a third antibody, referred to as "anti-anti-idiotypic" antibody. Several studies have shown that the 3-dimensional structure of the "anti-idiotype" is similar to the 3-dimensional structure of the original antigen. As a result, an anti-idiotype antibody can be used to stimulate antibodies that react with the nominal antigen. For example, an anti-idiotypic antibody raised against an antipolio antibody can be used to immunize a naive subject against polio.

In this paper, the authors demonstrate the presence of idiotypic and anti-idiotypic antibodies to polio in the serum of the mothers and in cord blood. These antibodies are presumably present in the gamma globulin preparations used to treat the mothers. The authors argue that it is the anti-idiotypic antibodies that stimulate the antipolio antibody responses detected in the newborns studies.

This is an interesting hypothesis, and it may well explain the presence of the antipolio antibodies detected in this study. The phenomenon is probably of little biological importance, because the antibodies to polio were only found in the saliva and not in the serum, and also because newborns do not maintain detectable levels of antibodies to most antigens once maternal antibody had disappeared during the first 6–8 months of life. Thus, newborns must be immunized with a series of vaccine antigens to produce protective levels of antibodies. It should be noted that considerable work is in progress to develop anti-idiotypic antibodies that can be used to effectively immunize humans against a variety of infectious agents. It is hoped that these immunogens would have fewer side effects than some of the current vaccines, such as pertussis, measles, and typhoid.—B.L. Hamilton, M.D., Ph.D.

Risk Factors for Mother-To-Child Transmission of HIV-1

Peckham CS, for the European Collaborative Study (Inst of Child Health, London)

Lancet 339:1007–1012, 1992 6–19

Background.—The reported rates of transmission of HIV type 1 infection from mother to child have ranged from 7% to 39%. Some reports have indicated that the stage of maternal infection and breast-feeding pose risks of increased transmission. With data from the European Col-

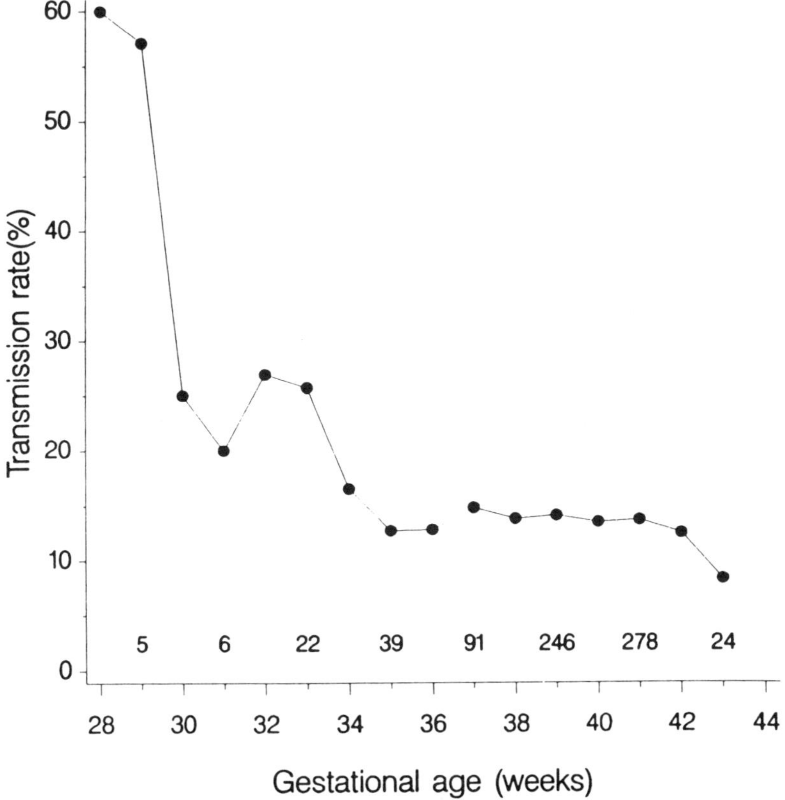

Fig 6–5.—Transmission rate by gestational age. The figure has been smoothed by plotting 3-point averages, e.g., the value at 36 weeks is the observed transmission rate for 35–37 weeks. The numbers born by gestational age are shown in 2-week intervals. (Courtesy of Peckham CS, for the European Collaborative Study *Lancet* 339:1007–1012, 1992.)

laborative Study, the role of these and other factors that may be associated with vertical transmission of HIV-1 were investigated.

Method.—From 1984 to 1991, 1,005 children from 19 centers were enrolled in the study. The HIV-infection status was determined in 721 children of 701 mothers. The associations between clinical and immunologic status of the mother during pregnancy; the maternal characteristics of age, parity, and race; length of gestation; mode of delivery; breast-feeding; and HIV-1 transmission were analyzed.

Findings.—The rate of vertical transmission of HIV-1 was 14.4%. Vertical transmission was not significantly associated with parity, race, maternal age at delivery, or intravenous drug use. The risk of infection was greatest for infants born to 13 women with AIDS. The odds ratio was 3.80 (1.62–8.91) in children born before 34 weeks' gestation. The duration of breast-feeding did not affect risk. The mechanism for the higher risk of infection found in children born before 34 weeks was unclear (Fig 6–5). Transmission was associated with maternal p24-antigenemia and a CD4 count of less than 700/μL. Transmission was also higher in vaginal deliveries in which episiotomy, scalp electrodes, or instruments were used, but only in centers where these procedures were not routine.

Conclusion.—Apparently, HIV-infected women with p24-antigenemia or a low CD4 count have an increased risk of vertical transmission of HIV-1. The mechanism for the higher rate of infection found in children born before 34 weeks' gestation is unclear. Possibly, the HIV infection in utero may affect fetal development and lead to premature delivery. Alternatively, women with AIDS or antigenemia may be more likely to deliver before 34 weeks or concurrent infections may increase both the risk of premature delivery and the risk of transmission of HIV infection.

► Until a satisfactory vaccine or viral therapy is available, we will have to be satisfied with simple methods of prevention. Because recent studies of twin deliveries reveal an increased incidence of HIV in the first-born twin, implicating transmission in the birth canal (1), an easy first step would be to stop using scalp electrodes for fetal monitoring (because they certainly have not been shown to be valuable in routine deliveries) as well as episiotomies, which in a significant number of cases result in greater tears and bleeding. Recent studies have not shown a significant reduction in HIV transmission with cesarean section.—M.H. Klaus, M.D.

Reference

1. Goedert JJ, et al: *Lancet* 338:1471, 1991.

HIV Replication During the First Weeks of Life

Krivine A, Firtion G, Cao L, Francoual C, Henrion R, Lebon P (Hôpital Saint-

Vincent-de-Paul, Paris; Clinique Universitaire Port-Royal, Paris)
Lancet 339:1187–1189, 1992 6–20

Background.—Human immunodeficiency virus (HIV) infection can be diagnosed in children born to HIV-positive mothers in the first 12 months. However, few studies have examined HIV status during the first weeks of life.

Methods.—Fifty infants born to HIV-1 seropositive women were enrolled in a prospective, longitudinal study. Blood samples were taken at birth and at 4–9 weeks and 5–9 months of age. Testing for HIV-1 consisted of polymerase chain reaction (PCR), viral culture, and p24 antigen measures.

Findings.—Sixteen children had a diagnosis of HIV infection by 4–9 weeks of age, according to PCR and culture. Infection could be detected in only 5 children at birth. No change in HIV status occurred between 4–9 weeks and 5–9 months in the 44 children available for retesting.

Conclusion.—With the use of PCR or viral culture, perinatal HIV-1 infection can be diagnosed in the first 2 months of life. In nearly 70% of the infants who were subsequently infected, HIV-1 infection could not be detected at birth, suggesting an active replication of HIV in the first weeks of life. These findings may favor the hypothesis that HIV-1 transmission occurs at the end of pregnancy or at delivery.

▶ Commenting on Abstracts 6–19 and 6–20 is Parvin Azimi, M.D., Director of Infectious Disease, Childrens Hospital, Oakland, California:

▶ The study by Krivine et al. (Abstract 6–20), was designed to determine the youngest age at which infection in infants born to HIV-infected women could be reliably identified. This was done through longitudinal evaluation of PCR, p24 antigenemia, and HIV cultures starting in the first week of life in 50 children born to HIV-infected women. The PCR finding was positive in all infected infants (16 of 50) before 2 months of age. The authors conclude that a positive PCR finding is the most reliable early indicator of infection. None of the tests could reliably identify all infected infants in the first week of life. The authors attribute the lack of detection of HIV during the first week of life to insufficient viral load. They postulate that active replication of HIV takes place in the first few weeks of life, resulting in positive markers in later months. The authors further suggest that this replication in the first weeks of life may reflect transmission of HIV to the offspring either late in pregnancy or perinatally, although they did not rule out the possibility of early transmission during pregnancy, followed by latency and reactivation.

In another report by the European Collaborative Study (Abstract 6–19), the HIV-infection status of 721 infants born to HIV-infected women between December 1984 and August 1991 was determined. Among the perceived risk factors studied, intravenous drug use (IVDU), maternal age, parity, and mode of delivery (vaginal vs. cesarean section) did not influence the risk of transmission. The maternal risk factors predictive of vertical transmission included low maternal CD4 count (less than 700 μL), presence of p24 antigenemia, and breast-feeding. The most significant factor influencing transmission, however, was gestational age, with transmission occurring in infants with gestational age less than 34 weeks at much higher frequencies than in those with a gestation of more than 34 weeks, as shown in Figure 6–5. The pathogenesis of this risk factor remains unclear. Among a number of possible explanations provided by the authors, the following are most plausible: (1) lack of protective effect as a result of the absence of passively transferred maternal antibodies in the premature infant; and (2) alternatively, women who have advanced disease can give birth to preterm infants who are exposed to heavy titers of virus and become infected either during pregnancy or perinatally.

Both of these reports underscore the frequency of intrapartum transmission. Although this may account for the majority of cases, transmission during pregnancy has been demonstrated by the presence of virus in fetal tissues (1). Postpartum transmission via breast milk has also been demonstrated (2).

The stage of maternal infection may influence the rate of vertical transmission. It is known that the viral burden is much greater during primary infection, as well as in late stages of the disease, which can adversely affect the rate of transmission. Conversely, transplacentally transferred antibodies may provide protection from transmission.

Our understanding of the exact timing and mechanism of transmission is critical in developing strategies for the intervention and prevention of infection in the newborn. These might include antiretrovirals, vaccines, HIV-immunoglobulin or other modalities. Even though the majority of children born to HIV-infected women are unaffected (transmission rate, 14% to 30%), vertical transmission contributes significantly to the pool of HIV infection globally. This is because of the high rate of infection in women of childbearing age in endemic countries, such as Central Africa and Haiti.

References

1. Sprecher S, et al: *Lancet* 2:288, 1986.
2. van de Perre P, et al: N *Engl J Med* 325:593, 1991.

Risk of Human Immunodeficiency Virus Type 1 Transmission Through Breastfeeding

Dunn DT, Newell ML, Ades AE, Peckham CS (Inst of Child Health, London)
Lancet 340:585–588, 1992 6–21

Introduction.—The detection of HIV-1 in breast milk by culture and polymerase chain reaction does not preclude transmission through breast-feeding. The risk of HIV-1 transmission through breast-feeding after prenatal or postnatal maternal infection was assessed through a systematic review of previously published studies.

Results.—In 4 epidemiologic studies in which all mothers were seronegative at delivery and were infected through blood transfusion after delivery, the estimated risk of transmission from breast-feeding mothers infected postnatally was 29%, with a 95% confidence interval of 16% to 42%. In 5 studies in which the mother was infected prenatally, the additional risk of transmission through breast-feeding was 14%, with a 95% confidence interval of 7% to 22%. This risk was over and above that in children infected in utero or during delivery.

Implications.—Mothers who acquire HIV-1 postnatally can transmit the infection through breast-feeding, and those with established infection have a substantial risk of transmission as well. In areas where safe alternatives to breast-feeding are available, universal named testing of pregnant women provides an opportunity to advise infected women not to breast-feed and, thus, may reduce the frequency of vertical transmission. Because breast-feeding protects against infant deaths from infectious disease, breast-feeding is still recommended in areas where infectious disease and malnutrition remain common causes of childhood deaths, despite the additional risk of transmission of HIV.

► When mothers acquire HIV-1 after birth, the summary analysis indicates a 29% risk of transmission. Infants breast-fed after birth may be at high risk of acquiring infection, especially during the viremia of the primary infection. The dilemma for those writing the WHO/UNICEF policy statements relates to the strong protection from other infectious diseases that breast-feeding conveys on infants, especially those in the developing world. The value of this study is that these collected results from a number of small studies give what is the current best estimate of the risk of breast-feeding.—M.H. Klaus, M.D.

Lack of Evidence of Vertical Transmission of Human Immunodeficiency Virus Type 2 in a Sample of the General Population in Bissau

Poulsen A-G, Kvinesdal BB, Aaby P, Lisse IM, Gottschau A, Mølbak K, Dias F, Lauritzen E (Univ of Copenhagen; Hvidovre Hosp, Copenhagen; Laboratório Nacional de Saúde Publica, Bissau, Guinea-Bissau)

AIDS 5:25–30, 1992 6–22

Background.—Human immunodeficiency virus type 2 (HIV-2), which is found primarily in West Africa, is assumed to be transmitted like HIV-1, by sexual contact, blood contact, and from mother to child during pregnancy or delivery. A previous study (begun in 1987) of the epidemiology of HIV in Guinea-Bissau was unable to document vertical transmission of HIV-2, despite a high prevalence among the adult population and positive findings for heterosexual transmission and transmission by blood tranfusion. Investigation into the issue of vertical transmission of HIV-2 in this population has continued.

Methods.—Twenty-nine HIV-2 seropositive women in Bissau were each matched for age and marital status with 2 HIV-2 seronegative women. Their clinical and pregnancy histories were compared. Western blot and enzyme-linked immunosorbent assays for HIV-1 and HIV-2 antibodies were performed on serum samples. Lymphocytes were assessed for the presence of CD4 and CD8 by immunocytochemical labeling.

Results.—Seropositive women had a mean age of 39.7 years; seronegative women had a mean age of 40.2 years. The 2 groups were similar as to the total number of pregnancies, live children, dead children, and abortions. Both groups had the same risk of having had at least 1 abortion or 1 dead child. Children from HIV-2 seropositive and seronegative mothers had no significant differences in mortality. Significantly more HIV-2 seropositive women had lower T-helper cell number and H/S ratios than HIV-2 seronegative women, but none was severely immunodeficient. Seven children born to seropositive women were not born with detectable HIV-2 infection. Based in part on retrospectively identified children of HIV-2 infected mothers, a rough estimate of the rate of vertical transmission was 0% to 4%.

Conclusion.—Among a group of Guinean women, little evidence of vertical transmission of HIV-2 was found. That finding may be attributable to specific biological properties of HIV-2, or to the absence of disease and immunodeficiency in this population.

▶ It has been rare to come across data regarding HIV that are not extremely negative. It has been observed that HIV-2 would emulate HIV and be transmitted by sexual contact, blood, or vertically. This small series suggests that the vertical transmission is insignificant (0% to 4%), and that the latency of HIV-2 is far greater than that of HIV-1. A golden nugget to be gleaned from this manuscript is the custom whereby women in Guinea abstain from sex for the duration of breast-feeding, often up to 24 months; 80% of the population complies with this custom.

The epidemic of HIV-1 infection continues unabated, with nary a glimmer of light at the end of the tunnel. In New York City, HIV infection affects approximately 1 of 150 indigent patients. It has been estimated that 25% to 50% of their offspring will eventually have the disease, becoming symptomatic by 3–6 months of life. The obituary columns of the major tabloids bear testimony to the wealth of talent, in many walks of lives, whose careers have been terminated prematurely by AIDS.

Health-care workers must strictly adhere to the universal precautions to minimize acquiring the virus in the line of duty. The risk of HIV is approximately 1–2 per 1,000 cases of parenteral or mucus membrane exposure. (This contrasts with 12% to 17% seroconversion after similar exposure to hepatitis B.)

Strictly adhering to universal precautions minimizes the risk, and perinatal health-care providers are well advised to follow these guidelines. Mechanical devices have become standard for resuscitation, and avoiding needlestick injuries is self-evident. There is less compliance with the use of gloves, gowns, caps, masks, and eye coverings that are cumbersome and inconvenient but reduce the risk of exposure to contaminated blood or body fluids. Health-care workers should also cover any exudative skin lesions.

He who has never hoped can never despair.—George Bernard Shaw

A.A. Fanaroff, M.B.B.Ch.

Chlamydia trachomatis in Neonatal Respiratory Distress of Very Preterm Babies: Biphasic Clinical Picture

Sollecito D, Midulla M, Bavastrelli M, Panero A, Marzetti G, Rossi D, Salzano M, Roggini M, Bucci G (Institute of Pediatrics "La Sapienza" Univ, Rome; Fatebenefratelli Hosp, Rome, Italy)

Acta Pediatr 81:788–791, 1992 6–23

Background.—In term infants, interstitial pneumonia attributable to *Chlamydia trachomatis* is usually mild, with tachypnea and cough. The roentgenographic findings include interstitial infiltrate and hyperexpansion. Infection with *C. trachomatis* in very preterm infants has aspecific features.

Patients.—Twelve very preterm infants were observed with a very peculiar respiratory syndrome characterized by an early onset after birth and a biphasic course. Gestational ages ranged from 24 weeks to 31 weeks, and birth weight ranged from 660 g to 1,910 g.

Findings.—The severe first phase was characterized by respiratory distress, requiring mechanical ventilation in 8 patients for a mean of 11 days. Chest radiography findings mimicked hyaline membrane disease. Gradually, the respiratory symptoms decreased. In the second phase, the infants showed significant worsening of respiratory signs. Eight infants had apneic spells, and 5 had feeding problems and abdominal distention. Chest radiographs showed lung hypoexpansion and a fine reticular pattern; only 1 patient showed pulmonary hyperinflation. *Chlamydia trachomatis* was isolated in conjunctival and pharyngeal swabs and/or tracheal aspirates obtained during the second phase. Most patients responded promptly to specific antimicrobial therapy. Three infants had persistent positive cultures for *C. trachomatis* after a short course of antibiotics, and another 2 showed no improvement. One patient had persistent wheezing, and 7 had chronic lung disease.

Summary.—Very preterm infants with chlamydial infection show clinical and laboratory features that are very different from the chlamydial pneumonia seen in term infants. *Chlamydia trachomatis* infection should be suspected in very preterm infants with apneic spells and peculiar roentgenographic findings such as lung hypoexpansion and fine reticular pattern. Other aspecific features include feeding problems and abdominal distention.

▶ Chlamydia trachomatis has been isolated from the genital tract of 2% to 12% of pregnant women, but there have been no reports of in utero transmission and congenital infection. Investigators from the Johns Hopkins Study of cervicitis and adverse pregnancy outcome reported an association between *Chlamydia trachomatis* and *Mycoplasma hominis* and intrauterine growth retardation and preterm delivery (1). A total of 60% to 70% of infants whose mothers harbor *C. trachomatis* acquire the pathogen during passage through the birth canal. Among these, as many as 50% may have conjunctivitis develop, and up to 20% may have pneumonia develop. Hammerschlag reported that cervical cultures were positive for 8% of 4,357 women screened in New York during a 2-year period. Among the 230 infants evaluated for chlamydial conjunctivitis, the incidence was 20% with silver nitrate prophylaxis, 14% with erythromycin, and 11% with tetracycline ointment (2).

Term and preterm infants have vast differences in the manner of presentation when the lung is the target organ of *C. trachomatis*. These differences are highlighted by the clinical descriptions of the 12 patients assembled by Sollecito and colleagues. Demonstrating their universal call for distress, the preterm infants become apneic rather than expending energy and signaling for help with a characteristic cough.

Finally, a word of caution when using erythomycin intravenously. It may induce quinidine-like effects on the heart. These infants thus need careful cardiac monitoring.—A.A. Fanaroff, M.B.B.Ch.

References

1. 1991 Year Book of Neonatal and Perinatal Medicine, pp 129–130.
2. 1991 Year Book of Neonatal and Perinatal Medicine, pp 128–129.

7 The Nervous System

The Brain

The Clinical Diagnosis of Asphyxia Responsible for Brain Damage in the Human Fetus

Low JA, Simpson LL, Ramsey DA (Queen's Univ, Kingston, Ont, Canada)

Am J Obstet Gynecol 167:11–15, 1992 7–1

Background.—There is debate over how much neurologic handicap results from perinatal asphyxia in the community. Although risk scoring, assessment of fetal behavior, and blood-gas and acid-base assessment have improved diagnosis of fetal asphyxia, there is no evidence that they have decreased the incidence of cerebral palsy. The clinical findings of 208 infants who died in the perinatal period and had brain damage attributable to asphyxia were studied retrospectively.

Patients.—The 208 perinatal deaths occurred in a 13-year period. Evidence of neuronal or white matter necrosis attributable to asphyxia was found in 30 cases, or 14% of the total. Pathologic criteria in the CNS were used to estimate the time of the asphyxial insult. The clinical courses of the pregnancy for 22 cases in which brain damage was attributable to fetal asphyxia were analyzed.

Findings.—The asphyxial insult occurred in the antepartum period in 17 cases, in the intrapartum period in 5, and in the newborn period in 8. In 8 cases in the antepartum asphyxia group, the insult seemed to have occurred in a clinically normal pregnancy. It occurred more than 3 days before labor in 3 term pregnancies with no risk factors. In the other 9 cases of antepartum insult, the fetuses were preterm and the pregnancies were clinically complicated. This was so despite periodic surveillance measures. In the intrapartum cases, indicators of asphyxia were not seen until after CNS injury had occurred.

Conclusion.—It is difficult to diagnose fetal asphyxia at a stage in which interventions could be made to prevent brain damage. Asphyxia can occur at any time in the latter half of the pregnancy, and half of antepartum asphyxial insults occur in low-risk pregnancies. Even when clinical fetal distress is seen during labor and blood gas abnormalities are seen at delivery, the sublethal insult causing brain damage probably began earlier.

▶ The timing of an asphyxial insult to the fetus may distinguish whether an adverse outcome could have been avoided. The prevailing consensus is that the bulk of asphyxia precedes the intrapartum period and can neither be predicted or prevented in the majority of cases. This line of thought is supported by the findings in this clinicopathologic correlation. Most of the asphyxia occurred before labor, and in half the cases there were no recognizable risk factors. Even in patients in whom fetal well-being was closely monitored, the indicators of fetal distress only appeared after brain injury had occurred.

The goal of the study was to determine how much of the burden of neurologic handicap could be attributed to perinatal asphyxia. The sequence of asphyxial changes in the brain depicted in Table 1 in the original article must be accepted by the reader, otherwise none of the findings will be accepted. It is not a perfect methodology, because no evidence of asphyxia may be apparent if the infant dies within 18 hours of the asphyxial insult. Hindsight is always perfect vision; however, it would have been nice to have more comprehensive neonatal assessments of the brain, including electroencephalography and the various scanning modalities. Nonetheless, the take-home message (that asphyxia often antedates labor in low-risk patients and is not preventable) came through loud and clear. Whether it will be audible in the courts is a matter for the future. For more information on this topic, see References 1–3 and Abstract 7–3.

I find the great thing in this world is not so much where we stand, as in what direction we are moving.—Oliver Wendell Holmes, Jr.

A.A. Fanaroff, M.B.B.Ch.

References

1. 1992 YEAR BOOK OF NEONATAL AND PERINATAL MEDICINE, pp 140–141.
2. 1992 YEAR BOOK OF NEONATAL AND PERINATAL MEDICINE, pp 143–144.
3. 1992 YEAR BOOK OF NEONATAL AND PERINATAL MEDICINE, pp 142–143.

CSF Ascorbic Acid and Lactate Levels After Neonatal Asphyxia: Preliminary Results

Oriot D, Bétrémieux P, Baumann N, Lefrançois C, Le Marec B (Univ Hosp of Poitiers, France; Univ Hosp of Rennes, France; Hôpital de la Salpétrière, Paris, France)

Acta Paediatr 81:845–846, 1992 7–2

Hypothesis.—The concentration of ascorbic acid in CSF might be modified by neonatal asphyxia because of the high neuronal concentration of ascorbic acid and the existence of a concentration gradient of ascorbic acid between neurons and CSF. Whether CSF levels of ascorbic acid were correlated with the early neurologic status of neonates with severe cerebral ischemia was investigated.

Patients.—Ten full-term neonates with a history of prenatal bradycardia and a 1-minute Apgar score below 3 were studied. The mean time of mechanical ventilation was 4 days. Four patients with stage III hypoxic-

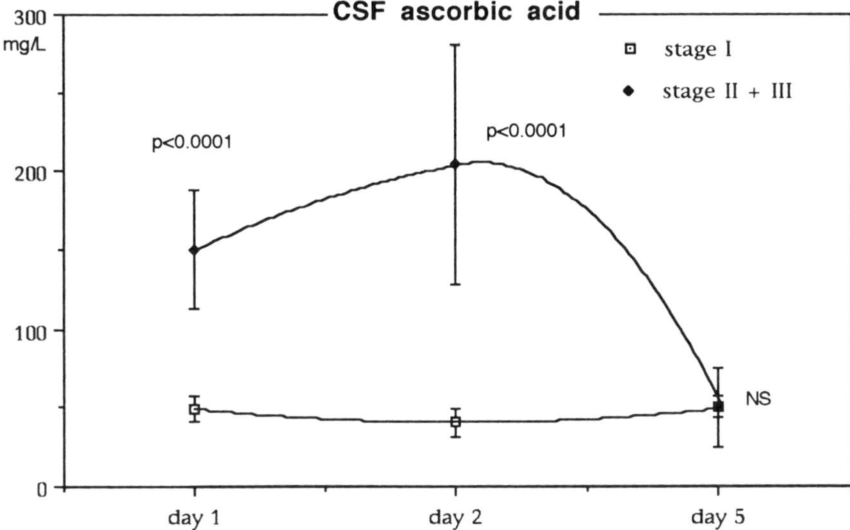

Fig 7–1.—Evolution of CSF ascorbic acid in stage I and stage II + III hypoxic-ischemic encephalopathy. *Abbreviation:* NS, not significant. (Courtesy of Oriot D, Bétrémieux P, Baumann N, et al: *Acta Paediatr* 81:845–846, 1992.)

ischemic encephalopathy died of massive cerebral edema. One with stage II encephalopathy lived with persistent electroencepalographic abnormality, whereas 5 infants with stage I encephalopathy recovered rapidly.

Methods.—Reduced ascorbic acid in CSF samples taken at 1–7 hours of life was measured using ascorbate oxidase. Lactate also was measured enzymatically.

Results.—The ascorbic acid levels in the CSF samples were significantly higher in more advanced cases of hypoxic-ischemic encephalopathy (Fig 7–1). Lactate levels also were higher in asphyxiated infants than in controls, but the group difference was not significant. Arterial pH was lower in those with stage II/III encephalopathy than in infants with stage I involvement.

Conclusion.—Reduced ascorbic acid in the CSF is increased in infants having advanced hypoxic-ischemic encephalopathy. Reduced ascorbic acid may possibly be released into the CSF after neuronal damage takes place.

▶ This short communication containing preliminary results adds a little further insight into the extraordinary changes in the CNS after an asphyxial insult. The data support the hypothesis that, with injury, ascorbic acid (which is present in high concentrations in the neurons) would leak into the CSF. As noted in Figure 7–1, the ascorbic acid is elevated in the CSF during the first 2 days of life only. This may serve as a marker of severe neuronal injury, although the clinical picture, blood gas status, electroencephalography, and imaging studies would provide the same information. It remains to be seen whether this information can be used as a springboard to gain further insight into the problem of hypoxic ischemic encephalopathy or whether it will merely serve as another roadside marker signifying cerebral injury.—A.A. Fanaroff, M.B.B.Ch.

Relation Between Cerebral Oxidative Metabolism Following Birth Asphyxia, and Neurodevelopmental Outcome and Brain Growth at One Year

Roth SC, Azzopardi D, Edwards AD, Baudin J, Cady EB, Townsend J, Delpy DT, Stewart AL, Wyatt JS, Reynolds EOR (Univ College and Middlesex School of Medicine, London; Univ College Hosp, London)

Dev Med Child Neurol 34:285–295, 1992 7–3

Objective.—Phosphorous MR spectroscopy (^{31}P MRS) was performed during the first week of life in 52 infants with clinical or biochemical evidence (or both) of birth asphyxia to determine the relationship between impaired cerebral oxidative metabolism and neurodevelopmental outcome and brain growth at age 1 year.

Setting.—The initial ^{31}P MRS was performed at a median of 34 hours (range, 3–127 hours) after birth. The minimum recorded values for cerebral phosphocreatine-inorganic phosphate concentration ratio (PCr-Pi), an index of oxidative metabolism, were correlated with neurodevelopmental outcome and brain growth at age 1 year.

Findings.—Thirty-seven infants survived at age 1 year. Twenty had neurodevelopmental impairments, including 14 with multiple major impairments and 3 with minor impairments (table). The extent of the impairment of cerebral oxidative metabolism was directly related to the severity of adverse outcome, including death, neurodevelopmental impairment, and reduced head growth, i.e., the outcome became worse as values for the PCr-Pi ratio decreased (Fig 7–2). The mean birth weight and gestational age did not affect this relationship.

Conclusion.—In a group of infants with birth asphyxia, the extent of impairment of the cerebral oxidative metabolism detected in the first days of life is directly related to the severity of adverse outcome at age 1 year.

▶ Measuring energy metabolism in the brains of asphyxiated newborns is available in a select few units worldwide. In a study of infants with increased cerebral echodensities, Hamilton noted that measurement of the PCr-Pi ratio was highly predictive of outcome (1). Infants with very low levels either died or had cerebral atrophy. Azzopardi (2) arrived at the same conclusions, as 19 of 28 infants with PCr-Pi ratios below the 95% confidence limit died, and 7 of 9 survivors had serious multiple impairments. This abstract further sup-

Birth Weight, Gestational Age, and Impairments in Surviving Infants According to Outcome at 1 Year

Outcome group	*N*	*Birthweight (g)*	*Gestational age (wk)*	*Neuromotor impairments*			*Abnormal axial tone*	*Sensory-neural hearing loss*	*Cortical blindness*	*GQ <80*
				Tetraplegia	*Hemiplegia*	*Diplegia*				
Normal	17	2946 (1633-3900)	39 (33-42)	0	0	0	0	0	0	0
Impaired										
minor	3	3618 (3460-4450)	40 (38-40)	0	0	2	2(1)*	0	0	0
major	3	3358 (2667-3420)	40 (40-41)	2	0	0	3(1)*	0	0	0
multiple	14	3005 (730-3800)	40 (29-43)	6	1	5	12(2)*	2	7	11
Died	15	2860 (1116-4190)	39 (33-44)	-	-	-	-	-	-	-

* *Numbers in brackets* indicate the number of infants with abnormal axial tone as isolated neuromotor impairment.
(Courtesy of Roth SC, Azzopardi D, Edwards AD, et al: *Dev Med Child Neurol* 34:285–295, 1992.)

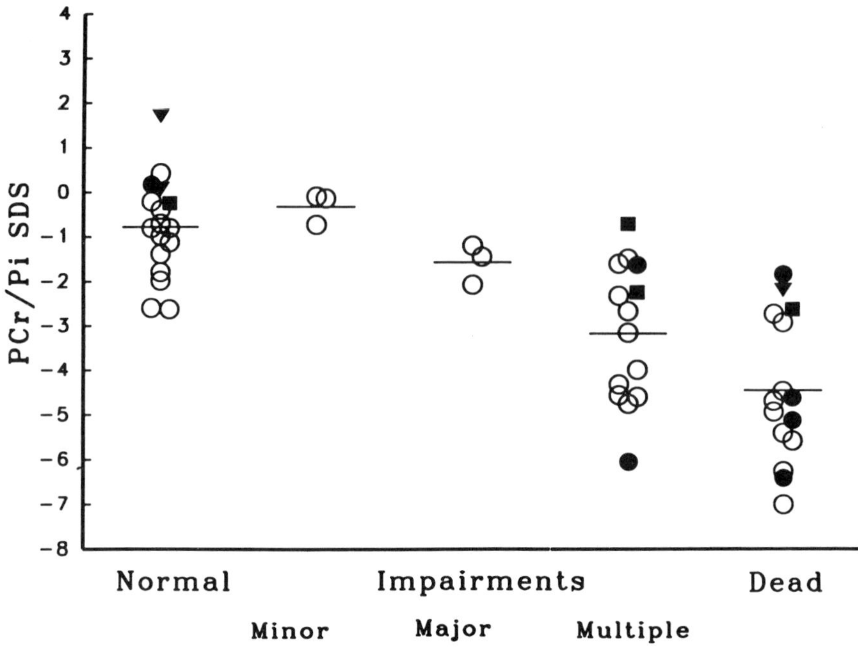

Fig 7-2.—The values for PCr-Pi standard deviation scores, according to the neurodevelopmental outcome group. *Open circles*, term appropriate-for-gestational-age (AGA) infants; *filled circles*, term small-for-gestational-age (SGA) infants; *triangles*, preterm AGA infants; *squares*, preterm SGA infants. (Courtesy of Roth SC, Azzopardi D, Edwards AD, et al: *Dev Med Child Neurol* 34:285-295, 1992.)

ports this method of predicting outcome. Although a 1-year follow-up will never satisfy the developmental purists, the extent of the neurologic abnormalities should salve their psyches.

The reasonable man adapts himself to the world; the unreasonable one persists in trying to adapt the world to himself. Therefore all progress depends on the unreasonable man.—George Bernard Shaw

A.A. Fanaroff, M.B.B.Ch.

References

1. 1987 Year Book of Neonatal and Perinatal Medicine, p 138.
2. 1990 Year Book of Neonatal and Perinatal Medicine, p 147.

Using Gross Motor Milestones to Identify Very Preterm Infants at Risk for Cerebral Palsy

Allen MC, Alexander GR (Johns Hopkins Hosp, Baltimore, Md; Univ of Minne-

sota, Minneapolis)
Dev Med Child Neurol 34:226–232, 1992 7–4

Background.—States have funding to provide coordinated family-oriented early intervention services to developmentally delayed infants and toddlers up to 2 years of age. Because of limited resources, many states have chosen to follow only at-risk infants. Motor milestones have been proposed as a simple, inexpensive way to monitor a child's motor development and to identify children with cerebral palsy. Ten gross motor milestones were evaluated to determine their efficacy in predicting cerebral palsy. Two research questions were considered: (1) whether to correct the age of milestone attainment for degree of preterm birth; and (2) whether race-specific development norms should be used to ascertain delay.

Method.—The milestones were analyzed in 173 high-risk preterm infants and included rollover from prone to supine; rollover from supine to prone; sit with arm-support in the middle of the floor; sit without arm-support; creep; crawl; come to a sitting position from prone or supine independently; pull to stand from crawl or sit; cruise; and walk independently. A standard 25% delay in motor milestone attainment was used to define risk. Calculations were made using total population and race-specific norms for white and nonwhite infants and chronological and term-age equivalent.

Findings.—Sensitivity was lower when correction was made for preterm birth, but there was dramatic improvement in both specificity and positive predictive value for every milestone. There was little difference in sensitivity, specificity, and positive predictive values when using population- vs. race-specific standards for white infants. For nonwhite infants, there was a slight disadvantage in specificity and positive predictive value using population-based standards, and increased sensitivity using race-specific standards. Delayed creep was associated with the highest prevalence of cerebral palsy.

Conclusion.—Gross motor milestone attainment is a simple, cost-effective way to identify high-risk infants. Screening on a sequential basis assists health-care providers in monitoring the development of high-risk infants.

► My knee jerk response to this manuscript was positive, but I was far from overwhelmed by the overall findings. The search for reliable neurologic indicators to identify which children are at greatest risk for cerebral palsy and other developmental disabilities is noble but far from complete. The statisticians may be satisfied with the findings, but the clinicians are not. "Delayed creep" emerged as the milestone associated with the highest prevalence of cerebral palsy, but this milestone frequently was not remembered by the family. The confounding issues of correcting for preterm birth and race cloud the picture, but they should not unequivocally mandate correction for preterm birth. How long to correct is disputed. We tend to do this for at least 2 years.

Following motor milestones should be a routine component of well-child care, not confined to infants at risk. Those with delayed milestones at any age require early referral for more comprehensive evaluation. Delayed milestones cause the infants to be at risk for a spectrum of disorders, including motor, cognitive, hearing, and visual loss. Early recognition and intervention may improve the outlook for these infants. High-technology ultrasound, CT scans, MRI, and electroencephalography all give some indicators of brain anatomy and function. In the meantime, the quest for simple methods of evaluating cortical function to predict outcome needs to continue (1).—A.A. Fanaroff, M.B.B.Ch.

Reference

1. 1990 Year Book of Neonatal and Perinatal Medicine, pp 162–163.

Role of Renal Sympathetic Nerves in Lambs During the Transition From Fetal to Newborn Life

Smith FG, Smith BA, Guillery EN, Robillard JE, Flansberg S, McWeeny OJ (Univ of Iowa, Iowa City)

J Clin Invest 88:1988–1994, 1991 7–5

Introduction.—Recent studies in immature animals have suggested that renal sympathetic nerves may regulate renin release and influence renal hemodynamics and function. The role of renal sympathetic innervation in renal and endocrine function during the transition from fetal to newborn life was studied in conscious, chronically instrumented fetal sheep.

Methods.—Studies were conducted at 3–6 days after bilateral renal denervation in 11 fetal sheep and after sham denervation in 12. Endocrine, renal, and cardiovascular parameters were measured before and after the delivery of lambs by cesarean section.

Results.—Blood pressure and heart rate were similar in intact and denervated fetuses, and they increased after delivery in both groups. In the immediate postnatal period, denervated lambs exhibited greater diuresis and natriuresis than intact lambs, despite a transient decrease in renal blood flow velocity in denervated lambs by 24 hours after birth. Fluid and electrolyte excretions were similar in both groups. The greater natriuresis in denervated lambs could not be explained by plasma levels of aldosterone, because these levels were similar in both groups—nor could they be explained by the plasma levels of natriuretic hormone, which, in fact, were much lower in denervated lambs (Fig 7–3). However, the normal increase in plasma renin activity at birth was attenuated in denervated lambs.

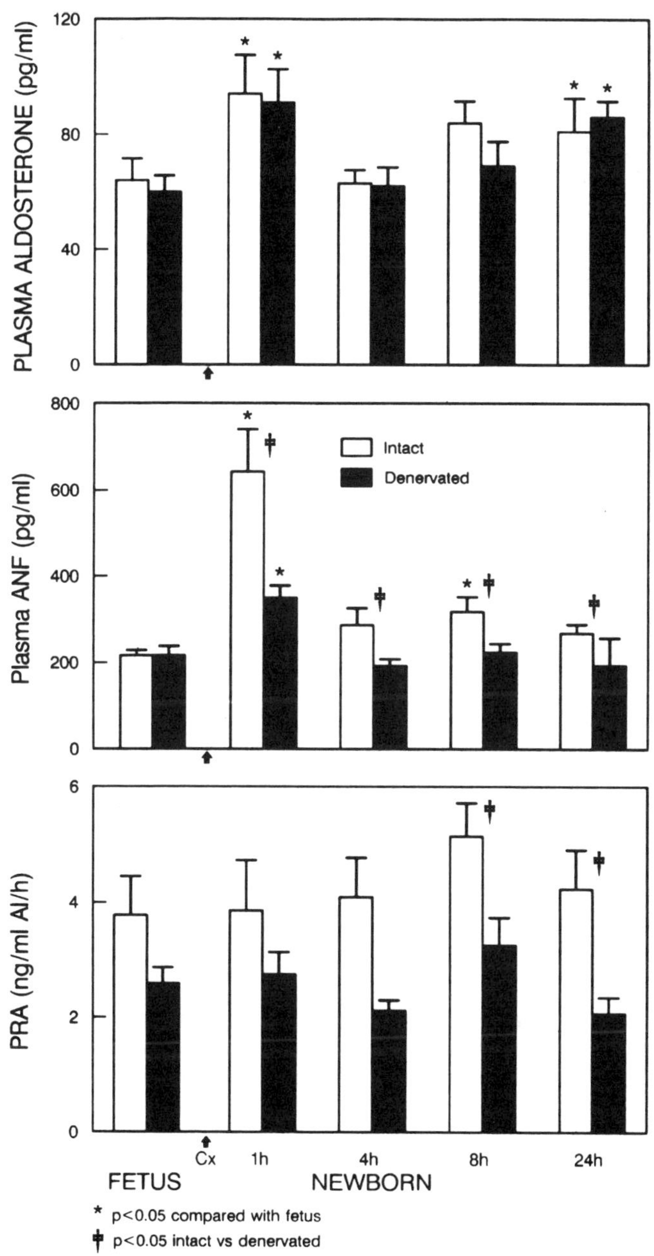

Fig 7–3.—The effects of cesarean delivery on endocrine function. Plasma aldosterone levels, plasma renin activity (PRA), and plasma atrial natriuretic factor (ANF) measured before (fetus) and 1, 4, 8, and 24 hours after cesarean delivery (newborn). (Courtesy of Smith FG, Smith BA, Guillery EN, et al: *J Clin Invest* 88:1988–1994, 1991.)

Conclusion.—These findings suggest that the renal sympathetic nerves play an important physiologic role during the transition from fetal to newborn life. This study provides the first evidence that birth is associated with stimulation of the renal sympathetic system. The renal sympathetic nerves regulate the fluid and electrolyte homeostasis during the adaptation of the kidney to postnatal demand.

▶ As in other organs of the neonate, the sympathetic nervous system of the kidney is implicated in the transition from fetal to newborn life. Perhaps in part because kidney function is not vital to the immediate survival of the neonate, our understanding of the mechanisms that alter renin and angiotensin at birth have lagged. The increase in renin and angiotensin II is important in influencing some of the circulatory adaptations that begin immediately after birth, including the rapid decrease in pulmonary vascular resistance. Further studies by this group have also demonstrated that the renal nerves play an important role in regulating renin gene expression during the transition from fetal to newborn life (1).—M.H. Klaus, M.D.

Reference

1. Page WV, et al: *Am J Physiol* 31:R459, 1992.

The Central New Jersey Neonatal Brain Haemorrhage Study: Design of the Study and Reliability of Ultrasound Diagnosis

Pinto-Martin J, Paneth N, Witomski T, Stein I, Schonfeld S, Rosenfeld D, Rose W, Kazam E, Kairam R, Katsikiotis V, Susser M (Univ of Pennsylvania, Philadelphia; Michigan State Univ, East Lansing; Jersey Shore Med Ctr, Neptune, NJ; et al)

Pediatr Perinat Epidemiol 6:273–284, 1992 7–6

Background.—Premature infants with a birth weight less than 1,500 g have a high incidence of germinal matrix/intraventricular hemorrhage (GM/IVH). The window of the anterior fontanelle makes it possible to examine the brains of these infants with ultrasonographic scanning. In this study of 1,105 premature infants, ultrasonographic screening was used to examine the etiology and consequences of neonatal brain hemorrhage.

Methods.—Infants eligible for the study weighed between 501 and 2,000 g and were born or transferred into 3 hospitals in central New Jersey between August 1984 and June 1987. For the 1,105 enrolled infants, the mean birth weight was 1,393 g and the mean gestational age was 30.9 weeks. Cranial ultrasonographic imaging was done at a mean age of 4.9 hours, 25.5 hours, and 7.2 days. The scans were read by 2 independent expert readers who were blind to all clinical information except the infant's birth weight.

Results.—When both readers made the initial diagnosis of either probable or definite GMH or IVH on the same ultrasonographic scan, concordance for the presence of GM/IVH was accepted; concordance for the absence was made if neither reader made a diagnosis on any scan. A third reader was called upon when readers disagreed. Concordance as to the presence or absence of GM/IVH was achieved at second readings in 82.4% of the infants. The first reading achieved a concordance of 76.3%. Reliability was affected by the perceived quality of the scan and the total number of scans available for review.

Conclusion.—The Kappa values obtained with ultrasound are comparable to those found in other diagnostic and imaging techniques, representing fair-to-good agreement.

▶ The advent of ultrasound has permitted a greater degree of precision with regard to the diagnosis of neonatal brain hemorrhage. Nonetheless, there is considerable room for variation when interpreting a specific study. This epidemiologic multicenter study, completed in the presurfactant era, documents the intercenter and inter-reader variability. From a practical standpoint, there is disagreement amongst the readers with 25% of the initial readings and 18% of the second readings. The Kappa value of .56 indicates that the readers are reliable, as values between .4 and .76 indicate fair-to-good agreement, according to Fleiss (1). Similar results were noted by Shankaran and collaborators (2, 3) during the intracranial observational study of the National Institute of Child Health and Development, in which a central reader was most likely to disagree with the local readers when making the diagnosis of periventricular leukomalacia.

The study was well-designed and had excellent compliance. It is not clear why a birth weight of up to 2,000 g was included, when the greatest risks are for those infants with a birth weight less than 1,500 g. The protocol required extensive chart reviews, questionnaires, and integration of a number of disciplines. The logistical side of the experiment was carried out flawlessly. However, there is a long gestation from the initiation of enrollment until manuscript acceptance and publication. The widespread introduction of surfactant has changed the population morbidity. Nonetheless, the authors can draw comfort by defining the optimal timing of the ultrasounds and establishing the ground rules for the diagnosis of intracranial bleeding.

I was impressed with the magnitude and efficiency of the task. The importance of the quality, timing and number of films, and standardization of technique were also driven home. The cost-effectiveness of studies such as this one are being closely observed by cost-conscious providers at all levels.—A.A. Fanaroff, M.B.B.Ch.

References

1. Fleiss JL: *Statistical Methods for Rates and Proportions.* New York, J Wiley, 1981, p 218.
2. Shankaran S, et al: *Pediatr Res* 29:266, 1990.
3. Shankaran S, et al: *Pediatr Res* 31:223, 1992.

Low Dose Intraventricular Fibrinolytic Treatment to Prevent Posthaemorrhagic Hydrocephalus

Whitelaw A, Rivers RPA, Creighton L, Gaffney P (Aker Univ Hosp, Oslo, Norway; Hammersmith Hosp, London; St Mary's Hosp Med School, London; et al)

Arch Dis Child 67:12–14, 1992 7–7

Background.—Post-hemorrhagic ventricular dilatation (PHVD) is secondary to intraventricular clot obstructing the CSF pathways responsible for fluid reabsorption. More than 60% of infants with progressive PHVD have required surgical placement of a shunt. All past treatment approaches have had major problems.

Study Plan.—In a pilot study, it was determined whether fibrinolysis could restore CSF pathways and thereby avoid the need for shunt surgery. Nine preterm infants with progressive PHVD received streptokinase intraventricularly for 12–72 hours. The infants received 20,000 to 25,000 units of streptokinase per 24 hours via a 20-gauge catheter in the temporal horn of the larger lateral ventricle.

Results.—All infants survived, and only 1 had progressive hydrocephalus develop, necessitating surgical shunt placement. Early catheter removal was required for technical reasons in 3 cases. In 1 infant, the infusion was stopped because of fresh intraventricular bleeding, but the infant stabilized after aspiration of blood from the ventricle. No infant had evidence of an effect of streptokinase in the circulating blood.

Conclusion.—Intraventricular fibrinolysis using streptokinase is the first direct therapeutic approach to PHVD, and it has been effective in preterm infants.

► Although fibrinolytic treatment was tried 25 years ago to prevent hydrocephalus in infants after meningitis, it was never used routinely. A small pilot study now suggests that further randomized controlled trials are the next step. The objective of the treatment is to destroy the multiple clots in the subarachnoid space that are blocking the reabsorption of CSF. We await further studies to determine whether this invasive treatment can prevent this devastating complication.—M.H. Klaus, M.D.

Postnatal Encephaloclastic Porencephaly: A New Lesion?

Cross JH, Harrison CJ, Preston PR, Rushton DI, Newell SJ, Morgan MEI, Durbin GM (Birmingham Maternity Hosp, England)

Arch Dis Child 67:307–311, 1992 7–8

Introduction.—It is well known that the brain in sick premature infants is susceptible to insult that can cause important morbidity and mortality. A new pattern of brain injury was recently discovered on the cerebral ultrasound scans of 15 preterm neonates treated at this institution.

The findings were confirmed at postmortem examination in 11 of the 14 infants who died. Such ultrasound patterns had not previously been reported in live-born infants.

Patients.—During a 20-month period, 15 preterm neonates in the intensive neonatal care unit showed a different pattern of severe brain injury compared with that previously described. The infants had a mean gestation of 27 weeks and a mean birth weight of 940 g. Fourteen infants required ventilation from birth for a mean of 15 days. Seven infants received colloid as treatment for a mean blood pressure of below 30 mm Hg in the first 24 hours of life; however, none had required inotropic agents. All infants underwent arterial cannulation. The 14 infants that died were profoundly abnormal neurologically, and 8 had required treatment for frank convulsions. At 12-month follow-up, the only surviving infant had a severe neurologic deficit.

Findings.—Cerebral ultrasound scans showed extensive, bilateral echodense and cystic lesions involving the periphery of the cerebrum. Postmortem examination showed full-thickness necrosis of the cerebral cortex and white matter, confirming the appearance on ultrasound scans. The presence of extensive necrosis strongly suggested ischemic injury, although no insult to the brain could be identified. It is suggested that these abnormalities represent the effects of an as yet unidentified postnatal event.

Conclusion.—A new, distinctive pattern of preterm brain injury that can be recognized on cerebral ultrasound scans is reported.

▶ Postnatal encephaloclastic porencephaly represents a new and devastating pathoneurologic disaster in the preterm infant. It is vital to quickly ascertain whether this is a local phenomenon in Birmingham, England, or (unlikely) a widespread phenomenon not previously recognized. In this instance, new is not better. At this point, postnatal encephaloclastic porencephaly is merely a descriptive title. It conjures up a "Pac-Man" type of image, with the cerebral cortex being consumed for unknown reasons. The shape of the lesion points to a vascular etiology, and MR angiography may cast some further light on these lesions.

The authors were unable to identify a specific etiology, and the hypotensive episodes were documented in only half the infants, occurring long before the lesions were detected ultrasonographically. The report lacks specific data concerning intrauterine events, including exposure to cocaine. Fetal blood-flow patterns may have been revealing (1), but they evidently were not documented. If further cases should be identified, they should be subjected to comprehensive neuroimaging studies to try to pinpoint the etiology of this mysterious lesion. Is it secondary to an insult initiated in utero, or is it a postnatal phenomenon?

Experience is a hard teacher. She gives the test first, the lesson afterward.—Anonymous

A.A. Fanaroff, M.B.B.Ch.

Reference

1. 1992 Year Book of Neonatal and Perinatal Medicine, pp 65–66.

Chiari III Malformation: Imaging Features

Castillo M, Quencer RM, Dominguez R (Univ of Texas, Houston; Univ of Miami, Fla)

Am J Neuroradiol 13:107–113, 1992 7–9

Background.—The finding of cervical spina bifida with multiple cerebellar and brain stem anomalies has traditionally been classified as a Chi-

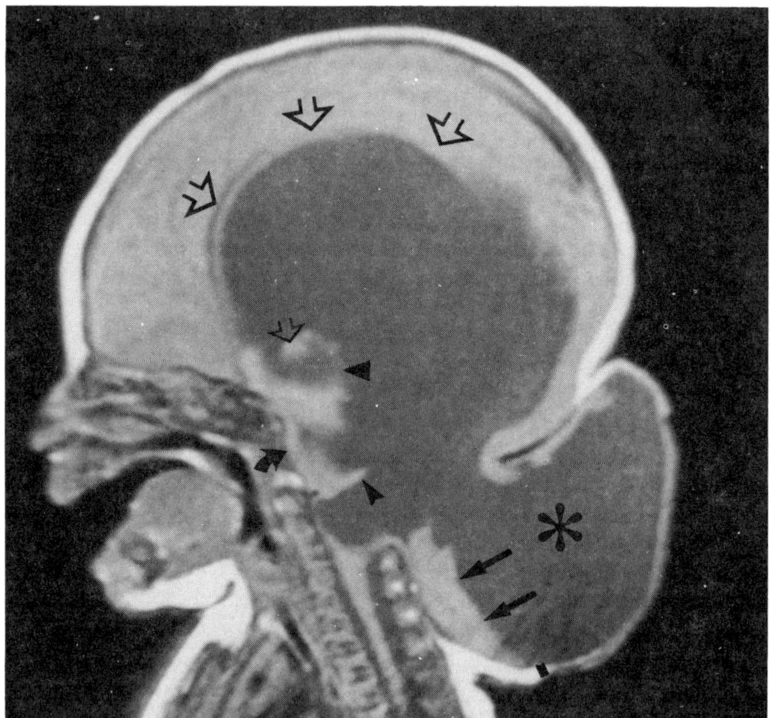

Fig 7–4.—Sagittal spin echo 750/20 slightly off-center image shows a large low occipital/high cervical encephalocele. The CSF density (*) inside the cephalocele is believed to be a markedly dilated fourth ventricle, with the roof of the fourth ventricle displaced superiorly (*small arrowhead*). The third ventricle (*large arrowhead*) and massa intermedia (*small open arrow*) are mildly prominent. The corpus callosum (*large open arrows*) is thin and the splenium is absent. Residual cerebellar tissue (*small arrows*) is present inside the encephalocele; posterior elements of C1, C2, and C3 are absent. Scalloping (*curved arrow*) of the clivus is present. There is marked dilatation of the lateral ventricles. (Courtesy of Castillo M, Quencer RM, Dominguez R: *Am J Neuroradiol* 13:107–113, 1992.)

ari III malformation. This definition has now been expanded to include herniation of the hindbrain into a low occipital and/or high cervical encephalocele, along with features of the Chiari II malformation. Magnetic resonance imaging (MRI) and CT were performed in 9 infants with Chiari III malformations.

Patients and Findings.—The patients were 6 girls and 3 boys, all of whom were born at term. Sonography showed encephalocele before birth in 5 cases. All had plain skull radiographs, 7 had MRI, and 2 had CT. All had high cervical to low occipital encephaloceles (Fig 7–4), and 4 had low and middle hypoplasia of the parietal bones. Varying amounts of brain tissue were found in the encephaloceles; 6 contained cerebellum and occipital lobes, and 3 contained cerebellum only. The fourth ventricle was included in 6 cases and the lateral in 3. Other findings included the cisterns, medulla, and pons.

There were 5 cases of petrous and clivus scalloping, 2 of overgrown cerebellar hemisphere, and 3 of cerebellar tonsillar herniation. All patients had deformation of the midbrain. Two patients had hydrocephalus, 6 had corpus callosum dysgenesis, 3 had agenesis of the posterior cervical vertebra, and 2 had spinal cord syrinxes. Aberrant deep draining veins and ectopic venous sinuses were found within the encephaloceles in 4 patients who underwent resection and closure. On pathologic examination of 4 encephaloceles, numerous abnormalities were found that could not be seen on imaging studies. These included necrosis, gliosis, heterotopias, and meningeal fibrosis.

Conclusion.—In newborns with Chiari III malformation, MRI can be used to determine the position of the medulla and pons before surgery. The surgeon must remember that venous anomalies are common. Magnetic resonance imaging cannot detect many possible abnormalities within the cephalocele, perhaps because of the marked disorganization of these tissues.

▶ Chiari III malformation, which has distinct clinical and imaging features that distinguish it from the more common Chiari I and II malformations, is, mercifully, a rare disorder. (Encephaloceles occur in 1 of every 4,000–5,000 deliveries.) The prognosis is poor, and maximum information concerning the contents of the cephalocele can be obtained by MRI. (Cephalocele is a skull defect associated with herniation of intracranial contents; if membranes are included, it is a meningoencephalocele; and if it includes brain only, it is an encephalocele.) Nonetheless, the gross anatomical distortion of the brain is also accompanied by multiple pathologic findings (e.g., necrosis, heterotopias, gliosis, fibrosis, and meningeal inflammation) that cannot be ascertained by MRI. This is inconsequential, as the treatment calls for surgical extirpation of the mass and its contents. It is key for the surgeon to know the location of the midbrain and medulla, as well as the site of aberrant venous channels. These data are readily supplied by MRI.

This otherwise-depressing manuscript (because of the nature of the subject) served to jog my memory regarding the terminology and classification of neural tube disorders. Furthermore, the accompanying illustrations bear testimony to how much detail can be obtained with the current imaging technology. Can we but hope that the antenatal administration of folic acid will sweep away these devastating neural tube disorders? See also Abstract 2–16.—A.A. Fanaroff, M.B.B.Ch.

Cerebral Venous Thrombosis in Neonates and Children

Barron TF, Gusnard DA, Zimmerman RA, Clancy RR (Children's Hosp of Philadelphia; Univ of Pennsylvania, Pa)

Pediatr Neurol 8:112–116, 1992 7–10

Purpose.—The clinical presentation, cause, treatment, and outcome of cerebral venous thromboses in 25 patients were reviewed retrospectively.

Findings.—There were 10 neonates (aged 2–30 days) and 15 children (aged 7 months–17 years). Seizures were the most common presenting sign in neonates, whereas headache or changes in mental status were more frequent in older children. In the neonatal group, cerebral venous thrombosis was commonly associated with an acute systemic illness, such

Results of MRI and CT Compared With Clinical Examination and Outcome

	Thrombosis		Thrombosis and Infarction	
	Neonates	**Children**	**Neonates**	**Children**
Clinical Examination				
Normal or signs of increased intracranial pressure	2*	9	2	0
Focal abnormality	0	1	3	6
Nonlateralizing abnormality	0	0	3	0
Outcome †				
Normal	2	10	3	4
Mild disability	0	0	2	1
Moderate disability	0	0	0	0
Severe disability	0	0	2	0

* None of the neonates showed signs of increased intracranial pressure.
† Excludes a patient who died secondary to congenital heart disease.
(Courtesy of Barron TF, Gusnard DA, Zimmerman RA, et al: *Pediatr Neurol* 8:112–116, 1992.)

as sepsis, shock, or dehydration. Thrombosis in the older group was most commonly associated with a hypercoagulable state (antithrombin III or protein C deficiency) or infection. Global or focal neurologic findings on initial examination that were unrelated to increased intracranial pressure correlated with the presence of an infarction on CT or MRI. Treatment consisted of conservative supportive measures; none of the patients was given anticoagulants specifically for the thrombosis. Outcome varied with age and location of the thrombus. Sequelae were relatively common in the neonatal group, but outcome was more favorable in the older children. Infants and children with thrombosis only had generally good outcome (table). Likewise, children and neonates in whom infarction was associated with a superficial venous thrombosis had uniformly good outcome. In contrast, patients with infarction associated with deep venous thrombosis had persistent neurologic disability.

Summary.—These findings suggest that acute anticoagulation may not be indicated as a specific treatment for cerebral venous thrombosis.

▶ It would be pushing my luck to call the 3 publications before this abstracted paper a flurry of activity related to neonatal cerebral venous thrombosis (1–3). Nonetheless, it is fair to state that there is renewed interest in this entity, which, with the improved imaging techniques, can be confirmed radiologically. Neonatal cerebral venous thrombosis should be added to the differential diagnosis of the critically ill, potentially septic neonate seen with seizures. Other entities to consider would include metabolic acidosis, congenital heart disease and hypercoagulable states such as protein C deficiency and polycythemia. Additionally, it is not uncommon to see evidence of venous thrombosis after ligation of the neck vessels for extracorporeal membrane oxygenation. The diagnosis can be made with enhanced CT; however, MRI is probably the imaging mode of choice. Cerebral venous thrombosis in neonates should not be regarded lightly, because sequelae are common. Expectant management with correction of dehydration and metabolic acidosis or polycythemia is recommended. Anticoagulation is not indicated and may lead to hemorrhage.

Behold the turtle. He makes progress only when he sticks his neck out.—James B. Conont

A.A. Fanaroff, M.B.B.Ch.

References

1. Wong VK, et al: *Pediatr Neurol* 3:235, 1987.
2. Hanigan WC, et al: *Pediatr Neurosci* 14:177, 1988.
3. Shevell MI, et al: *Pediatr Neurol* 5:161, 1989.

Intrauterine Growth and Spastic Cerebral Palsy II: The Association With Morphology at Birth

Blair E, Stanley F (Princess Margaret's Hosp, Subiaco, Western Australia)

Early Hum Dev 28:91–103, 1992 7–11

Introduction.—The association described between spastic cerebral palsy and a weight deficit may reflect a common cause—the factors impairing fetal growth also interfere with neuronal migration. Alternately, fetuses with a damaged or defective motor area may grow poorly in utero because of a paucity of fetal motion. A further possibility is that the cerebral motor centers in poorly growing fetuses may be vulnerable to further insult.

Objective.—An attempt was made to learn whether children with spastic cerebral palsy have growth characteristics at birth that differ from those of normal live-born infants. A total of 104 cases of spastic cerebral palsy were included in the study, which defined abnormality as beyond the 10th–90th percentile ranges of birth weight, length, head circumfer-

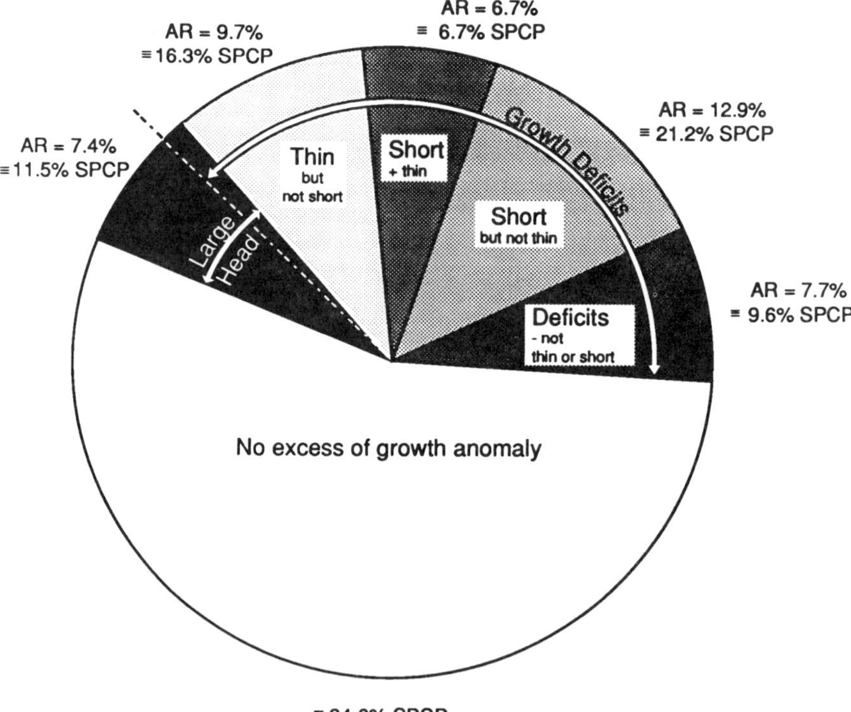

Fig 7–5.—Size anomaly and spastic cerebral palsy in infants born at ≥ 34 weeks of gestation: Attributable risks. *Abbreviations: AR,* attributable risk/excess proportion, *SPCP,* spastic cerebral palsied population (simple proportion of 104 cases, sum of attributable risks (= Σ AR = 7.4 + 9.7 + 19.6 + 7.7) = 44.4%. (Courtesy of Blair E, Stanley F: *Early Hum Dev* 28:91-103, 1992.)

ence, ponderal index, and length-to-head circumference ratio for control infants. Infants born before 34 weeks' gestation were excluded.

Results.—A 44% excess of "abnormal" measurements associated with increased risk was found in the study population (Fig 7–5). More than half of those excess cases were short for gestational age, and they tended to have more severe forms of cerebral palsy. Another 7% of infants had a head circumference above the 90th percentile; they generally had mild cerebral palsy.

Conclusion.—A strong association exists between spastic cerebral palsy in infants born after 33 weeks' gestation and the presence of morphologic abnormalities at birth. Further work should focus on the causative role of antenatal—especially early antenatal—events.

▶ The authors continue their expert detective work, and this report adds additional evidence that in infants with a gestational age greater than 34 weeks, cerebral palsy is (in most cases) not the result of birth asphyxia. This study is in agreement with the authors' previous work, which demonstrates an association between spastic cerebral palsy and low birth weight for gestational age. The next step is to uncover the insulting agent that is altering both physical growth and brain development. This is not a simple task considering the incidence of cerebral palsy is 2 in 1,000.—M.H. Klaus, M.D.

Special Senses

Effect of Prenatal Betamethasone/Thyrotropin Releasing Hormone Treatment on Somatosensory Evoked Potentials in Preterm Neonates

de Zegher F, de Vries L, Pierrat V, Daniels H, Spitz B, Casaer P, Devlieger H, Eggermont E (Univ Hosp Gasthuisberg, Leuven, Belgium)

Pediatr Res 32:212–214, 1992 7–12

Introduction.—The maternal administration of betamethasone and thyrotropin-releasing hormone (TRH) to accelerate fetal maturation is increasingly being used to prevent neonatal morbidity in preterm infants. The effect of prenatal treatment with betamethasone-TRH on the neural maturation of preterm infants was evaluated in a prospective, controlled, longitudinal study.

Methods.—Somatosensory evoked potentials (SEP) were measured in 26 preterm infants on the first postnatal day, at age 1 week, and before discharge. Gestational ages ranged from 29 to 36 weeks. The N1 latency values of the SEP were compared in 14 infants who were prenatally exposed to betamethasone-TRH and 12 who were not.

Findings.—On the first postnatal day, the control newborns had the previously reported longitudinal N1 latency pattern of "normal" low-risk preterm infants, with values that were strikingly elevated in 8 of 12 infants. In contrast, the N1 latencies in newborns exposed prenatally to betamethasone-TRH were strikingly shorter and were localized within the reference range in all 14 infants. Both groups had similar N1 latency values at age 1 week and at discharge.

Conclusion.—There is solid evidence that prenatal exposure to betamethasone-TRH accelerates the SEP-assessed neural maturation of the human fetus, followed by a compensatory relative deceleration during the early neonatal period. The subsequent SEP-assessed neural maturation then proceeds at a normal velocity.

▶ Not only is the lung altered by maternal hormone administration, but the fetal brain and gastrointestinal tract mature more rapidly. This paper supports the original clinical observation made several years ago by Claudine Amiel Tison and Louis Gluck, who presented evidence of more rapid neurologic maturation in infants of mothers who were given betamethasone. From the animal studies, it would appear that betamethasone alone would probably have this effect. Again we observe how sensitive the fetus is during some periods of its life.—M.H. Klaus, M.D.

Changes in the Sensory Processing of Olfactory Signals Induced by Birth in Sheep

Kendrick KM, Lévy F, Keverne ED (Inst of Animal Physiology and Genetics Research, Cambridge, England; Institut National de la Recherche Agronomique, Nouzilly, France; Univ of Cambridge, England)

Science 256:833–836, 1992 7–13

Background.—In ewes, interest in their lambs and the ability to recognize their own offspring rely on some effect of parturition to stimulate the lambs' sensory cues, which are mainly olfactory. With parturition, or with artificial stimulation of the vagina and cervix, the ewe's olfactory bulb undergoes profound neurochemical changes. The electrophysiologic and neurochemical changes in the organization of olfactory processing in the brain that allow ewes to recognize their own lambs were studied.

Methods.—Electrophysiologic recordings were made from olfactory bulb neurons in 4 conscious ewes before and after the animals gave birth. Glass-coated tungsten microelectrodes introduced into the olfactory bulbs were used to record single-cell activity. Various chemical and biological odors were presented before and after birth, and the responses were recorded. In another experiment, in vivo microdialysis was used in 9 ewes to measure the effect of mitral cells, the principal cells of the olfactory bulb, on the release of acetycholine, amino acid, and monoamine transmitters in the olfactory bulbs before and after birth.

Results.—Of the 188 cells responding differently to various odors, most were located in the mitral cell layer. None of those cells responded preferentially to lamb or amniotic fluid odors in the last 2 months of pregnancy. Three days to 4 weeks after birth, however, the proportion of cells responding preferentially to lamb odors increased significantly, to 60%. Thirty percent of those cells responded preferentially to the odor of the ewe's own lamb, with the smell of the lamb's wool being nearly as effective a stimulus as that of the whole lamb. Eleven percent of cells responded preferentially to amniotic fluid odors. In the second experiment, response to lamb odors was accompanied by increased cholinergic and noradrenergic neurotransmitter release. With selective recognition of the ewes' own lambs came increased activity of a subset of mitral cells and release of glutamate and gamma-aminobutyric acid (GABA) from the dendrodritic synapses between the mitral and granule cells.

Conclusion.—Ewes show a change in the olfactory bulb processing of biologically important odors after giving birth. More mitral cells respond to lamb odors after birth than before birth, some of which respond preferentially to the ewes' own offspring. These changes are associated with increased release of neurotransmitters, which suggests an increased efficacy of glutamate-evoked GABA release.

▶ There is suggestive evidence that portions of this response demonstrate, in part, how a human mother identifies her own infant. Kaitz et al. (1) recently reported that at 12 hours of life, mothers were more accurate when identifying their infants using the sense of smell and touch than when judging by the sound of the infant's cry or looking at a photograph of the infant. As noted by the authors, in the goat, this adaptive specialization was shaped by natural selection to solve specific problems posed by the environment. Why do we still observe remnants of this fascinating learning response in humans? How important is it in humans?—M.H. Klaus, M.D.

Reference

1. Kaitz M, et al: *Dev Psychobiol* 20:587, 1987.

Screening of Hearing Impairment in the Newborn Using the Auditory Response Cradle

Tucker SM, Bhattacharya J (Hillingdon Hosp, Uxbridge, Middlesex, England; Charing Cross Hosp, London)

Arch Dis Child 67:911–919, 1992 7–14

Introduction.—There is considerable belief—but limited scientific evidence—that early detection of hearing impairment and provision of hearing aids can aid a child's cognitive development and acquisition of language skills. Universal screening would be desirable, for many infants with hearing loss have none of the known risk factors. An experience with a new screening device, the Auditory Response Cradle (ARC), was reported.

Methods.—The ARC is a fully automatic microprocessor-controlled machine consisting of a trolley-mounted unit with a pressure-sensitive

Results of Auditory Response Cradle Trials

No of neonates tested	6000
Failed first ARC test	489 (8·1%)
Passed on retest	367
Could not be retested on the ARC:	20
1 severe bilateral S/N loss (a)	
1 severe bilateral high frequency S/N loss (b)	
15 cleared	
3 lost to follow up (1 died)	
Failed first and second ARC tests:	102 (1·7%)
7 severe bilateral S/N losses	
1 severe unilateral S/N loss	
1 severe bilateral S/N loss with conductive overlay	
2 moderate unilateral S/N losses (c, d)	
1 mild/moderate bilateral S/N loss	
5 middle ear pathologies (SOM) (moderate bilateral conductive losses)	
2 ABR abnormalities (mild/mioderate bilateral S/N losses)	
1 microcephalic	
1 spastic quadriplegic (severe bilateral S/N loss)	
2 lost to follow up (1 died)	
79 cleared (false positive rate =79/6000 = 1·3%)	

S/N represents sensorineural; SOM, serous otitis media.
(Courtesy of Tucker SM, Bhattacharya J: *Arch Dis Child* 67:911-919, 1992.)

mattress and headrest. Head turn, head startle, and body activity are monitored via the mattress and headrest, and respiratory activity is monitored by means of a transducer in a polyethylene band around the infant's abdomen. A high pass noise is presented to the infants through close-coupled ear phones. To evaluate the ARC, 6,000 infants were screened and followed up for 3 years.

Results.—The ARC screening was failed by 102 infants (1.7%). Twenty of these were found to have some hearing impairment—mild to moderate in 3 infants, moderate in 7, and severe in 10. Additional testing cleared 79 infants who failed the screening, giving the ARC a false positive rate of 1.3% (table). During the 3-year follow-up, 7 children who passed the screen were found to have a hearing loss. In 5 of these children, the loss was caused by postnatal factors or a hereditary progressive loss and was thus impossible to detect in the neonatal period.

Conclusion.—The ARC, which had a high rate of detection for hearing impairment in newborns, may be useful in universal screening programs. These findings also emphasize the need for follow-up screenings, because not all hearing loss is apparent at birth.

▶ This large, well-designed trial with a long follow-up suggests that routine testing of every newborn is possible with this device. The false positive rate is quite low (1.3%), and almost all severely and moderately impaired neonates were detected. It has the advantages of being noninvasive and having a short rating time (2–10 minutes). It also is easy to use and is acceptable to parents. With severe congenital hearing losses varying at 1 to 5 per 1,000 and a 50% pickup rate testing only high-risk infants, it is time the Committee of the Newborn of the American Academy of Pediatrics studies this interesting approach.—M.H. Klaus, M.D.

Prognostic Validity of Brainstem Electric Response Audiometry in Infants of a Neonatal Intensive Care Unit

Durieux-Smith A, Picton TW, Bernard P, MacMurray B, Goodman JT (Children's Hosp of Eastern Ontario, Ottawa, Canada)

Audiology 30:249–265, 1991 7–15

Background.—Brain stem electric response audiometry (BERA) using broad-band clicks is now an important tool in assessing hearing impairment in at-risk infants. There is little information on the validity of BERA. The ability of BERA to help identify children who are in need of audiologic management needs to be established.

Methods.—The results of BERA in infants in a neonatal intensive care unit were compared with those obtained in the same children with pure-tone audiometry 3 years later. Of the 600 infants tested initially, complete follow-up data were obtained for 333.

Findings.—The results of BERA accurately predicted hearing status at 3 years of age in 89% of the children followed up. Nine percent of the discrepancies were associated with conductive hearing losses. Seventeen children with a conductive hearing loss in the first few months of life had normal hearing at 3 years of age, and 12 with normal hearing in infancy had a conductive loss at 3 years of age. In 2 patients, BERA indicated a sensorineural hearing loss when hearing was normal. This may have been because of a conductive loss. Six children who were classified as normal by BERA had significant hearing losses at 3 years of age, and 5 of them had normal hearing at 1 frequency between 1,000 and 4,000 Hz. In the sixth child, a sensorineural hearing loss may have developed after birth. The sensitivities and specificities of BERA are shown in the table.

Conclusion.—Brain stem electric response audiometry is a powerful tool for assessing auditory function in high-risk infants. Normal BERA results in infancy predict normal hearing in the 2,000-Hz to 4,000-Hz frequency range.

▶ We are on the threshold of having universal hearing screening thrust upon us. After a March 1993 NIH consensus conference, the pressure to identify

Sensitivity and Specificity (%) of BERA for 3 Different Target Hearing Losses

	Condition 1 (all hearing losses including conductive)	Condition 2 (all sensorineural and mixed hearing losses)	Condition 3 (bilateral sensorineural and mixed hearing losses requiring amplification)
Sensitivity	43.3	61.5	86.0
Specificity	93.6	99.3	100.0
False-negative	56.7	38.5	14.0
False-positive	5.4	0.7	0.0

Sensitivity = $\frac{a}{a+c}$; specificity = $\frac{d}{b+d}$; false-negative = $\frac{c}{a+c}$; false-positive = $\frac{b}{b+d}$; a = disease present, test positive; b = disease absent, test positive; c = disease present, test negative; d = disease absent, test negative.

Neurologically abnormal results with BERA were excluded from analyses.

(Courtesy of Durieux-Smith A, Picton TW, Bernard P, et al: *Audiology* 30:249–265, 1991.)

everyone who is at risk for hearing problems began to be exerted, because the current screen is only capturing about 50% of those with hearing impairment. The ability to hear is critical for the acquisition of the spoken language, but the current average delay between birth and the detection of sensorineural hearing loss is 2.5 years. Because there are newer techniques of assisting the deaf, including cochlear implants, it is necessary to detect the infants after minimal auditory deprivation to obtain the maximal benefit from the device. Thus, the rationale of screening everyone may, at first glance, appear sound; however, implementation in the neonatal period, when there presumably is a captive audience, is flawed. With the current technology, too many neonates will fail the initial screen, placing an unnecessary burden on many families until it has been established that the child *does* hear normally.

Furthermore, even using the most sophisticated technology, some of the infants will be incorrectly classified, as noted in this report. For example, otoacoustic emission testing, which is high on the list for universal screening, is ineffectual when vernix remains in the auditory canal. Because many newborns are now discharged on the first day of life, the false positive rate, i.e., failed screening, will be unacceptably high with this otherwise promising innovative technique. Additionally, a number of hearing losses are secondary to conductive problems acquired during infancy. As I look at the road map for the implementation of universal screening, I detect a number of major potholes. There is still much gathering of data and cost accounting to be done before embarking on such an ambitious undertaking. For more on this topic, see Reference 1.—A.A. Fanaroff, M.B.B.Ch.

Reference

1. Mauk GW: *Ear Hear* 12:312, 1991.

Visual Recognition Memory in Drug-Exposed Infants
Struthers JM, Hansen RL (Univ of California, Sacramento)
J Dev Behav Pediatr 13:108–111, 1992 7–16

Background.—In high-risk infants, visual recognition memory testing has been shown to have significant predictive ability for later cognitive deficits. Cognition in infants who are prenatally exposed to illicit stimulant drugs was compared with that of nonexposed controls using a standardized test of visual recognition.

Methods.—The drug-exposed group included 36 healthy, full-term infants with prenatal exposure to cocaine and/or amphetamines. Those infants were matched by race and socioeconomic status to 26 infants who had not been exposed to drugs prenatally. The Fagan Test of Infant Intelligence (FTII) was used to test the 2 groups.

Findings.—The mean FTII scores were significantly lower in the drug-exposed group. In addition, the percentage testing at risk was significantly higher in the exposed group compared with the control group. Also differing between groups were the behaviors related to attention, distractibility, and activity level.

Conclusion.—These findings support recent longitudinal research results showing that infants who are prenatally exposed to drugs may be at risk for later subtle neurologic abnormalities. Such problems may be detected long before the children reach school age.

▶ We included this report not only to describe follow-up studies of infants exposed to cocaine, but also to demonstrate the potential of visual recognition memory testing (VRM) in infancy. Testing has shown more significant correlations between performance on infant VRM testing and IQ tests between 2 and 7 years of age (range, .33–.66; mean, .42) in 15 separate studies (1) compared with sensorimotor tests (mainly the Bailey tests), which have correlations of only .14 in the normal population and .21 in the abnormal population (2). In the test, the infant is given a specific time to become familiar with the picture of a face. The familiar and novel face are then placed on the screen. Looking through a peephole, the observer records how long the infant looks at each face by observing the infant's cornea. Normal infants prefer the novel face. A novelty preference scoring is obtained by dividing the time the infant looked at the new picture by the total time. Infants exposed to cocaine were noted by testers (who were blinded to infant status) to exhibit extreme activity, high distractibility, and exaggerated responses to stimuli, as well as staring spells. The authors suggest that VRM testing assesses processing skills, such as discrimination, categorization, retention, and retrieval. These observations do not bode well for their future development. In a follow-up report to appear shortly, the authors note that the visual-evoked responses were normal in these infants.—M.H. Klaus, M.D.

References

1. Fagan JF, Singer LT: Infant recognition memory as a measure of intelligence, in Lipsett LP(ed): *Advances in Infancy Research, vol 2.* Norwood, NJ, Ablex, 1983, pp 31-78.
2. Fagan JF, Montie JE: Behavioral assessment of cognitive well-being in the infant, in Kavanagh J(ed): *Understanding Mental Retardation: Research Accomplishments and New Frontiers.* Baltimore, Md, Paul H. Brookes, 1988, pp 207-221.

Severe Retinopathy of Prematurity and Steroid Exposure

Batton DG, Roberts C, Trese M, Maisels MJ (William Beaumont Hosp, Royal Oak, Mich)

Pediatrics 90:534–536, 1992 7–17

Introduction.—Severe retinopathy of prematurity (ROP) has become more common in recent years. At the study institution, the increase in this condition was not found to be related to improved survival of low-birth-weight infants. An attempt was made to determine what other factors might explain the significant increase in the number of infants requiring cryotherapy.

Methods.—Ninety-eight inborn infants with a gestational age of 23–26 weeks were admitted to the neonatal intensive care unit from 1988 through 1990. Forty-two of these infants died, and 4 had multiple anomalies. Of the remaining 52 infants, 9 required cryotherapy. The 43 infants who did not require cryotherapy served as controls.

Results.—The need for cryotherapy for severe ROP increased during the 3-year study: 0 of 20 surviving infants in 1988, 3 of 14 in 1989, and 6 of 18 in 1990. The control and study infants did not differ significantly in birth weight or gestational age. Those requiring cryotherapy were more likely to have had patent ductus arteriosus, mechanical ventilation for more than 21 days, and steroid treatment for lung disease. Multivariant logistic regression analysis confirmed exposure to steroids to be the single factor significantly related to cryotherapy. Steroids were started at a mean of 44 days after delivery and were continued for a mean of 38 days.

Conclusion.—In this neonatal intensive care unit, steroids are administered according to the attending neonatologist's preference. Animal studies have reported retinopathy after administration of steroids, but there has been no proof of steroid-induced retinopathy in human infants. The findings of this study, however, call into question the use of steroids for lung disease in infants of 23–26 weeks' gestation.

▶ Commenting on this article is David Durand, M.D., Neonatologist, Children's Hospital, Oakland, California:

▶ Some funny things are happening with the use of dexamethasone for infants with bronchopulmonary dysplasia. Although some groups are using it like water in their intensive care units, others are rarely using it at all. Both approaches can be justified; there is good evidence that dexamethasone improves pulmonary function, and there is good evidence that it is not without some risks. All of us are aware of the impact of chronic or semichronic administration of steroids on growth, glucose tolerance, and blood pressure. There is also some recent data suggesting that a hypertrophic cardiomyopathy occurs in some (most?) with bronchopulmonary dysplasia who are patients treated with dexamethasone (1). Now we have these data about the association between dexamethasone and severe ROP. Even granting all of the problems with uncontrolled or case-controlled studies such as this one, there may be some reason to worry about the impact of dexamethasone on severe ROP. Unfortunately, the picture is clouded by the fact that there are 2 other recent reports of the relationship between steroids and ROP. One suggests that dexamethasone is a significant risk factor for ROP ≥ 2 (2), whereas the other suggests that dexamethasone decreases the need for cryotherapy for severe ROP (3). Dr. Batton et al. should be congratulated for their cautious discussion section of this paper, which puts all of the data about dexamethasone and ROP into perspective. The bottom line: Be careful until we have better data.—D. Durand, M.D.

References

1. Werner JC, et al: *J Pediatr* 120:186, 1992.
2. Asztalos EV, et al: *Pediatr Res* 29:201, 1991.
3. Sobel DB, et al: *Pediatr Res* 209:235, 1991.

Retinal and Vitreal Neovascularization in Retinopathy of Prematurity: A Scanning Electron Microscopic Study in the Kitten

Yoneya S, Tso MOM (Univ of Illinois, Chicago)

Arch Ophthalmol 109:1744–1751, 1991 7–18

Introduction.—The retinopathy of prematurity (ROP) in the kitten is an established model of vitreal and retinal neovascularization. With the use of scanning electron microscopy the angioarchitecture of vitreal and retinal neovascularizations in the ROP induced in kittens was examined

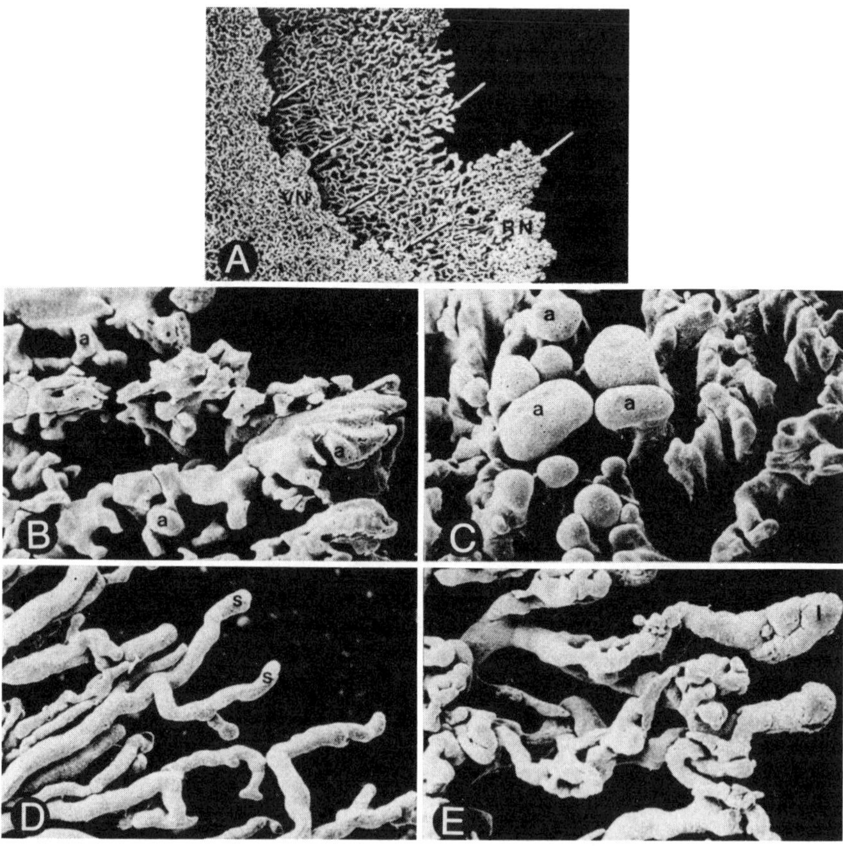

Fig 7–6.—Peripheral intraretinal neovascularization (RN) showing 3 morphologic forms. **A,** retinal vessels growing toward the vascular zone and forming a capillary frond (*white arrows*). Posterior to this frond, a second capillary frond (*black and white arrows*) is forming vitreous neovascular tuft (VN). Original magnification; ×50. **B** and **C,** neovascularization consisting of aneurysmal outgrowths (*a*) forms mushroom configuration. Original magnification; ×1,000. **D,** neovascularization consisting of bifurcating short vascular buds (*s*). Original magnification; ×3,000. **E,** neovascularization consisting of vascular loops (*l*). Original magnification; ×500. (Courtesy of Yoneya S, Tso MOM: *Arch Ophthalmol* 109:1744–1751, 1991.)

at different ages (2–9 weeks), at different stages of maturation, and in various topographic locations.

Findings.—The various forms of neovascularizations were noted, depending on the topographic locations. Intraretinal vessels advanced toward the avascular periphery in 3 morphologic forms: aneurysmal outgrowths, short vascular buds, and neovascular loops (Fig 7–6). Telangiectatic retinal vessels were observed posterior to this peripheral neovascularization frond. At the posterior pole, capillaries with microaneurysms extended toward the deeper layers of the retina from the vascular trunks at the nerve fiber layer. Vitreal neovascularization arose from aneurysmal dilatations of the branches of the main retinal vascular trunks to grow toward the internal limiting membrane. These vessels exhibited aneurysmal outgrowths, clusters of glomerular swellings, and sinusoidal vascular channels. At the optic disk, neovascularization consisted of aneurysmal outgrowths and long vascular buds.

Implications.—Vitreal neovascularization differs from intrarenal neovascularization in retinopathy of prematurity in the kitten. The topographic variation of the angioarchitecture of retinal and vitreal neovascularization depends on the maturity of the vessels and may be related to the hemodynamics at each site.

▶ The incorporation of gold into the vascular casts of the eye denotes this is a glittering study, by definition. The exquisite photographs from the scanning microscope clarify what could be a rather complex and confusing terminology. The differences between retinal and vitreal neurovascularization are striking. We must assume that the observations from a few subjects can be extrapolated to many. Because there have been no parallel studies on the circulation in the eye, the authors have free rein to speculate as to the underlying causes of the various findings. Their hypotheses are supported by fluorecein studies of the retina, which were reported by Flynn (1), and they are, empirically, all plausible. Thus, the sinusoidal vascular channels speak to slow flow with multiple connections, whereas the aneurysmal dilatations create the vivid image of "the blood current moving against a growing tip of a vascular cord, developing a whirlpool effect."

Ultimately, neovascularization will reflect the combined influences of angiogenic factors, tissue ischemia, the structure of surrounding tissues, and the maturation of the vasculature, as well as intravascular dynamics. Cryotherapy heads the arsenal to prevent visual loss in this common disorder. See also Abstract 7–19 and Reference 2.

A genius is one who shoots at something no one else can see and hits it.—Anonymous

A.A. Fanaroff, M.B.B.Ch.

References

1. Flynn JT, et al: *Arch Ophthalmol* 95:217, 1977.
2. 1992 Year Book of Neonatal and Perinatal Medicine, pp 302–303.

A Cohort Study of Transcutaneous Oxygen Tension and the Incidence and Severity of Retinopathy of Prematurity

Flynn JT, Bancalari E, Sim Snyder E, Goldberg RN, Feuer W, Cassady J, Schiffman J, Feldman HI, Bachynski B, Buckley E, Roberts J, Gillings D (Univ of Miami, Fla; Univ of Pennsylvania, Philadelphia; Univ of North Carolina, Chapel Hill)

N Engl J Med 326:1050–1054, 1992 7–19

Introduction.—Retinopathy of prematurity is a cause of visual impairment and blindness. An association between retinopathy of prematurity and the duration of exposure to supplemental oxygen in premature infants has been suggested, but a specific threshold level of arterial oxygen tension has not been identified. The incidence and severity of retinopathy of prematurity in preterm infants requiring supplemental oxygen was correlated with the duration of exposure to arterial oxygen levels of 80 mm Hg or higher, as measured transcutaneously ($tcPO_2$).

Methods.—The cohort included 101 premature infants (birth weights ranging from 500 to 1,300 g) who required supplemental oxygen administration. The number of hours during which the $tcPO_2$ was 80 mm Hg or higher during the first 4 weeks of life was tabulated for each infant.

Unadjusted and Adjusted Odds Ratios and 95% Confidence Intervals in the Ordinal Logistic-Regression Model for the 101 Infants Studied

Variable	Unadjusted	Adjusted
	odds ratio (95% CI)	
$tcPO_2$ ≥80 mm Hg (per 12-hr period)	3.0 (2.0–4.5)	1.9 (1.2–3.0)
Birth weight (per 100-g decrement)	2.4 (1.8–3.2)	2.3 (1.6–3.4)
5-Minute Apgar score (≤7 vs. >7)	5.3 (2.3–12.2)	7.2 (2.5–21)
Supplemental oxygen (FiO_2 ≥0.4) during entire hospitalization (per 72-hr period)	1.4 (1.1–1.8)	1.0 (0.97–1.05)

Note: The adjusted odds ratios were adjusted for the other variables shown.
Abbreviations: *CI,* confidence interval; Fio_2, fraction of inspired oxygen.
(Courtesy of Flynn JT, Bancalari E, Snyder ES, et al: *N Engl J Med* 326:1050–1054, 1992.)

Indirect ophthalmoscopy was performed as soon as the infant reached the postconceptional age of 32 weeks and was in stable clinical condition, and it was repeated every 2–4 weeks until discharge.

Results.—Retinopathy of prematurity developed in 52 of the 101 premature infants. The disease was present in 19 (86%) of 22 infants weighing less than 900 g. For weeks 1 through 4 of the study, retinopathy was moderate or severe in 15 infants and mild in 37 infants (of the 101 studied). Prolonged exposure to $tcPO_2$ of 80 mm Hg or higher during the first 4 weeks after birth was associated with an increase in both the incidence and the severity of retinopathy of prematurity. The odds ratio for each 12-hour period in which the $tcPO_2$ was 80 mm Hg or higher was 1.9. After adjusting the data for the confounding influence of low birth weight, low Apgar score, and exposure to inspired oxygen at a fractional concentration, the association remained significant (table). A precise threshold level of $tcPO_2$ that is toxic to the retina could not be identified and may not exist.

Conclusion.—The incidence and severity of retinopathy of prematurity in premature infants requiring supplemental oxygen are associated with the duration of exposure to arterial oxygen levels of 80 mm Hg or higher, as measured by continuous transcutaneous monitoring during the first 4 weeks of life.

▶ Although the past 10–12 years have focused on causes other than oxygen for retinopathy of prematurity, we are back to trying to fathom what levels of PaO_2 are safe. Although young prematures who had longer periods of PaO_2 greater than 80mm had more severe retinopathy. This trial demonstrated that continuous transcutaneous monitoring to prevent the occurrence of oxygen tensions greater than 80 mm Hg mercury was not effective in reducing the incidence of severe retinopathy in infants at higher risk. Back to the drawing boards!—M.H. Klaus, M.D.

8 Behavior and Pain Management

Novel Primitive Swallowing Reflex: Facial Receptor Distribution and Stimulus Characteristics

Orenstein SR, Bergman I, Proujansky R, Kocoshis SA, Giarrusso VS (Univ of Pittsburgh, Pa; Children's Hosp of Pittsburgh, Pa)

Dysphagia 7:150–154, 1992 8–1

Background.—A primitive swallowing reflex recently was described in young infants, as well as in neurologically compromised older individuals, in response to a puff of air to the face. A manometrically complete peristaltic sequence begins with a normal swallow within a few seconds of stimulus application.

Study Plan.—Twelve infants who had exhibited the reflex were studied at ages 1–9 months. A puff of 100–300 cc of air was administered to the face from about 30 cm, using a self-filling ventilating bag. An infant (age, 22 months) with carnitine deficiency also was studied. Four of the infants, including the neurologically abnormal one, were studied in conjunction with esophageal motility testing.

Findings.—The infants had consistently positive responses to stimulation of the maxillary-ophthalmic and maxillary-mandibular regions (Fig 8–1). Responses to stimulation of the ophthalmic branch alone were most often negative. Similarly, stimuli that excluded any of the perioral area usually did not elicit a swallow. The reflex was elicited with the mouth open or closed, and without blinking. It was not elicited during deep sleep, and was elicited only with difficulty during vigorous crying.

Discussion.—This swallow reflex probably requires stimulation of the perioral region via the maxillary and/or mandibular branches of the trigeminal nerve. The reflex has proved useful for passing tubes past the upper esophageal sphincter, and also for inducing swallowing of medication or food.

Primitive may be defined as the ". . . first point in time; existing in simple or early form; showing little evolution. Reflex indicates a reflected action or movement; the sum total of any particular involuntary activity."—Dorland's Medical Dictionary

▶ At first glance, the reader may decide that this whole concept belongs in a journal of irrelevant but novel facts. However, after closer inspection, I am

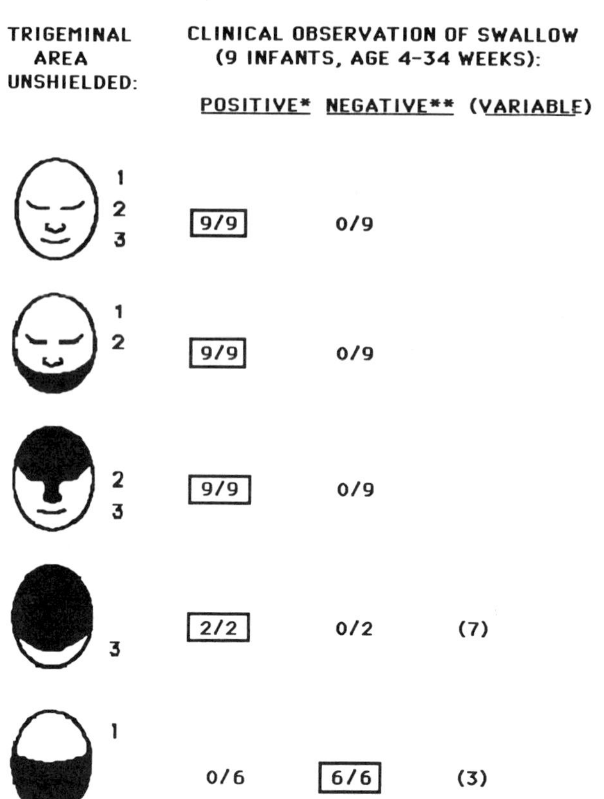

Fig 8–1.—The results of segmental trigeminal stimulation in 9 infants scored by clinical observation of swallowing. The *shaded areas* were shielded from stimulation. * Positive signifies the number of subjects with consistently positive responses, divided by the number of subjects with consistent responses (either positive or negative). **Negative indicates the number of subjects with consistently negative responses, divided by the number of subjects with consistent responses (either positive or negative). As shown, stimulation of the perioral area was needed for consistent positive responses; stimulation that did not involve this area was consistently negative in all subjects demonstrating a consistent response. (Courtesy of Orenstein SR, Bergman I, Proujansky R, et al: *Dysphagia* 7:150–154, 1992.)

confident that you will conclude that it may have some application in the care of the newborns requiring prolonged hospitalization.

The authors report the discovery of a new primitive reflex. The primitive component infers that it exists in simple or early form, showing little evolution, and that the sum total of involuntary activity defines the reflex. Whereas the precise pathways of the reflex are still being investigated, that it is triggered by thermal, rather than tactile, stimuli applied to the lower branches of the trigeminal nerve provides some clues as to the likely pathway. The reflex comprises relaxation of the upper esophagus and initiation of swallowing, which is best triggered by blowing air onto the lower face or lips. The reflex is attenuated by sleep and is difficult to elicit or is ablated by crying. Care givers can use this reflex to administer medications or pass nasogastric tubes in uncooperative patients. I wondered whether there was any relationship to the rooting reflex in the newborn in which stimulation of the side of the cheek or the upper or lower lip causes the infant to turn his mouth and face to the stimulus?

The truly civilized man is always skeptical and tolerant. . . His culture is based on "I am not too sure."—H.L. Mencken

A.A. Fanaroff, M.B.B.Ch.

The Development of Ultradian and Circadian Rhythms in Premature Babies Maintained in Constant Conditions

Tenreiro S, Dowse HB, D'Souza S, Minors D, Chiswick M, Simms D, Waterhouse J (St Mary's Hosp, Manchester, England; Univ of Manchester, England; Univ of Maine, Orono)

Early Hum Dev 27:33–52, 1991 8–2

Introduction.—During the last trimester of pregnancy, the fetus demonstrates some circadian rhythms that are believed to be imposed by the maternal environment. After birth, circadian rhythms develop slowly. To determine whether circadian rhythmicity arises from the neonates' own body clock or is imposed by environmental factors, the development of circadian rhythm was examined in very early premature infants who were kept in an unchanging intensive care environment.

Methods.—Within 24 hours of birth, 20 infants born at 24–29 weeks of gestation and maintained in an unchanging intensive care environment were monitored. Insulated skin temperature and heart rate were measured hourly for 6–17 weeks. The development of rhythms was assessed using maximum entropy spectral analysis and autocorrelation.

Results.—Circadian and ultradian rhythms could be detected, but they came and went erratically over time and did not increase with age. When some infants were placed in a ward where lighting was dimmed at night and regular feeding by mouth was instituted, there was some evidence for increases in rhythmicity.

Conclusion.—Rhythms were poorly developed in these preterm infants. Therefore, the rhythms detected during the last term of pregnancy are probably imposed by the maternal environment. As there is some evidence of rhythm in these neonates, although it is not maintained, it is possible that their immature suprachiasmatic nuclei produce a range of erratic and uncoordinated rhythms that eventually become coupled into a dominant frequency. It is not known whether external environmental cues are important to this process. If external cues play a role, then the maternal rhythms imposed in utero might play an important part. It has also been suggested that neonates benefit from a rhythmic environment.

The benefits to infants who require intensive care of a rhythmic environment should be investigated.

▶ A circadian rhythm pertains to the rhythmic repetition of certain phenomena in living organisms at about the same time each day, (i.e., in a 24-hour cycle), whereas an ultradian rhythm pertains to rhythmic repetition in a period of less than 24 hours. The circadian rhythm originates from the suprachiasmic nuclei, which are underdeveloped at term in the human.

There has been general acceptance of the concept that a circadian rhythm is present in the mother and fetus (driven from the maternal side) but not in the newborn (1). Evidence of elements of an active biological clock (notably body temperature) but none of the other physiologic variables were reported by Kok (2). This abstract represents a fine collaborative effort between biologists and clinical scientists. The data are stylishly presented, and the conclusions are essentially similar to those of Kok. It is nonetheless intriguing to speculate how the environment may influence the physiologic variables. The nursery at times represents a chaotic environment. It has been suggested that providing a rhythmic lighting environment, feeding schedule, and regular interaction with mother and nurse is beneficial for the neonate (3). Als has taken this a step further in proposing that an individualized care plan, cognizant of the infants' signals and rhythms, can reduce morbidity (4). Plans are already under way to review the optimal environment for the infant in the intensive care unit. The report of these task forces will need to be carefully scrutinized to determine which and how many circadian cues are essential for the optimal care of our tiny charges.—A.A. Fanaroff, M.B.B.Ch.

References

1. 1991 Year Book of Neonatal and Perinatal Medicine, pp 93–94.
2. 1991 Year Book of Neonatal and Perinatal Medicine, pp 169–170.
3. Mann NP, et al: *BMJ* 293:1265, 1986.
4. Als H: *Pediatrics* 78:1123, 1986.

Parturient Women Can Recognize Their Infants by Touch

Kaitz M, Lapidot P, Bronner R, Eidelman AI, (Hebrew Univ, Jerusalem; Shaare Zedek Med Ctr, Jerusalem)

Dev Psychol 28:35–39, 1992 8–3

Introduction.—Recognition of one's newborn infant is considered a very important part of maternal attachment, possibly a prerequisite. In addition to viewing and smelling their infants, mothers touch them frequently and, like nonhuman mothers, groom and clean their infants using their fingers.

Methods.—To establish the sensory basis of mother-infant bonding, mothers were tested for the ability to recognize their infants by touch early in the postpartum period. The mothers were instructed to stroke the dorsal surface of the hand of 3 infants, one of whom was her own. They then guessed which of the 3 was their own. The women were unaware that they would be asked to do this. The 46 women were tested 5–79 hours after giving birth vaginally. Most of the women were multiparous; the mean patient age was 28 years.

Results.—Most mothers were successful if they had been with their infant for at least 1 hour since childbirth. Control studies suggested that this ability was not based on olfactory or other nontactile cues. The findings were replicated in a further study of 36 parturient women.

Conclusion.—Mothers are able to learn the unique tactile features of their infants' skin in a short time, and to use these features to recognize their infants.

▶ This report continues the careful and well-designed studies of this group in exploring when the various sense organs of the mother permit her to recognize her own infant. Using several testing schemes and a proper design, they report that shortly after 1–2 hours of physical contact, the mother is able to recognize her own infant without prior intention. The women did not know before the testing that their ability with touch recognition would be studied. From their earlier work, it appears that human mothers are more quickly able to recognize their infants by the odor of the infants and the texture of their skin than by the auditory characteristics of the cry or their photograph. A mother's "more primitive senses" appear to quickly identify her own infant. Would a mother also quickly recognize her own infant if she first visited the infant at 3 or 4 days of age?—M.H. Klaus, M.D.

Parents' Knowledge of Neonatal Screening and Response to False-Positive Cystic Fibrosis Testing

Tluczek A, Mischler EH, Farrell PM, Fost N, Peterson NM, Carey P, Bruns WT, McCarthy C (Univ of Wisconsin, Madison; Med College of Wisconsin, Milwaukee)

J Dev Behav Pediatr 13:181–186, 1992 8–4

Introduction.—The immunoreactive trypsinogen assay now makes it possible to identify cystic fibrosis (CF) at an early stage, but false positive results are inevitable. Experience with screening for phenylketonuria showed that many parents become acutely or chronically anxious because of doubts about the test results and concern over their child's health. Conceivably, stress resulting from falsely positive tests could adversely influence the parent-child relationship.

Methods.—The parental responses to false positive CF screening results were examined in the Wisconsin neonatal screening program using a specially designed psychosocial assessment measure. The parents of 104 infants with false positive test results were assessed.

Response of Parents to Positive IRT and Negative Sweat Test Results

Question	Responses %			
	Agree	Disagree	Uncertain	No Response
Parental response to positive IRT test				
Thankful problem was found early	86	5	7	2
Concern	98	0	1	1
Shock	76	6	17	1
Disbelief	52	14	33	1
Depression	77	15	7	1
Anger	48	37	14	1
Confusion	61	21	16	2
No reaction	4	88	2	6
Parental response to negative sweat test				
Relief to know baby is "okay"	92	1	1	7

Abbreviation: IRT, immuoreactive trypsinogen.
(Courtesy of Tluczek A, Mischler EH, Farrell PM, et al: *J Dev Behav Pediatr* 13:181–186, 1992.)

Results.—Most understood that a positive test result meant that their child might have CF. Most parents had experienced strong emotional responses when learning of the positive result (table). Those parents who felt differently about their infants also expressed feelings of confusion, shock, and depression. At the same time, they were relieved that the sweat test result was negative. Slightly less than 10% of families definitely changed their minds about having more children, but another 20% were uncertain.

Conclusion.—A face-to-face encounter will be more informative about screening measures than a phone conversation. The potential psychological effects of misunderstanding test results can have significant consequences.

▶ Although severe adverse parental reactions were observed 25 years ago, just 1½ years after neonatal testing first began, the care takers of young infants generally are not aware of the significant number of parents with false positive results who continue to misunderstand the meaning of the normal test results long after a discussion. It should be emphasized that, in this study, as much as an hour's worth of time was used to explain the final result, a much longer time than is often now given for these discussions. Parents who hadn't finished high school whose infant had a low Apgar score, and who were informed by telephone rather than in person were most likely to misunderstand the problem. To reduce possible significant after-effects, including the vulnerable child syndrome, greater public education concerning neonatal screening is required both in the media and in school.—M.H. Klaus, M.D.

Psychological and Social Consequences of Community Carrier Screening Programme for Cystic Fibrosis

Watson EK, Mayall ES, Lamb J, Chapple J, Williamson R (St Mary's Hosp, London)

Lancet 340:217–220, 1992 8–5

Background.—With the identification and characterization of the cystic fibrosis (CF) gene, it is now possible to determine carriers in the general population. Testing for the most common mutation and 3 additional mutations would identify 72% of carrier couples in Britain. The results of a pilot study to assess the effects of screening for CF carrier status were evaluated.

Methods.—Volunteers for the screening were recruited through primary health-care services and family-planning clinics. A mouthwash sample was collected for DNA analysis and screened for 4 CF mutations. Those volunteers testing negative were told that the possibility of being a carrier was not completely ruled out. Carriers were given more detailed information and offered a counseling appointment. A questionnaire was designed to assess the impact of screening on carriers and on a sample of those testing negative.

Results.—Of 3,176 individuals screened, 100 carriers with no known family history of CF were identified. Most (81%) of the carriers said they were glad they had been tested, even though positive results had been a shock. More than half (64%) of those who attended counseling said the session had eased their concerns. When carriers suggested testing to their partners, 87% of those partners were tested. Individuals who tested positive indicated that knowledge of carrier status would influence their future reproductive decisions. Follow-up questionnaires at 6 months showed that most participants retained an understanding of CF and its inheritance.

Conclusion.—The mouthwash sample test for CF carrier status is reliable and would identify more than 70% of reproductive age carriers with the most common mutation in north European countries and the United States. It is not certain, however, whether benefits of screening outweigh its financial and social costs. These results suggest that screening will not stigmatize or cause lasting psychological damage to those testing positive.

The Psychological Consequences of Predictive Testing for Huntington's Disease

Hayden MR, for the Canadian Collaborative Study of Predictive Testing (Univ of British Columbia, Vancouver, Canada)

N Engl J Med 327:1401–1405, 1992 8–6

Introduction.—It is possible through DNA analysis to predict a person's risk of inheriting the gene for a number of usually adult-onset diseases, including Huntington's disease; however, the impact of such tests on the subjects and their families is not known. The results of the Canadian Collaborative Study of Predictive Testing, established in 1988 to determine the psychological effects of testing for the gene for Huntington's disease, were reviewed.

Methods.—The study cohort included 208 participants (from 14 genetic centers) who had a positive family history of Huntington's disease and requested predictive testing. Fifty-five did not complete the baseline assessment, and 18 were excluded when they were found to have clinical symptoms of Huntington's disease. Thirty-seven of the remaining 135 individuals found their risk for the disease to be 75% or more (an increase in risk), 58 had a risk of 25% or less (a decrease in risk), and 40 had no change in risk (the test was inconclusive or they declined to take the test). The participants were evaluated by standard measures of psychological distress before genetic testing and at post-test intervals of 7 to 10 days, 6 months, and 12 months.

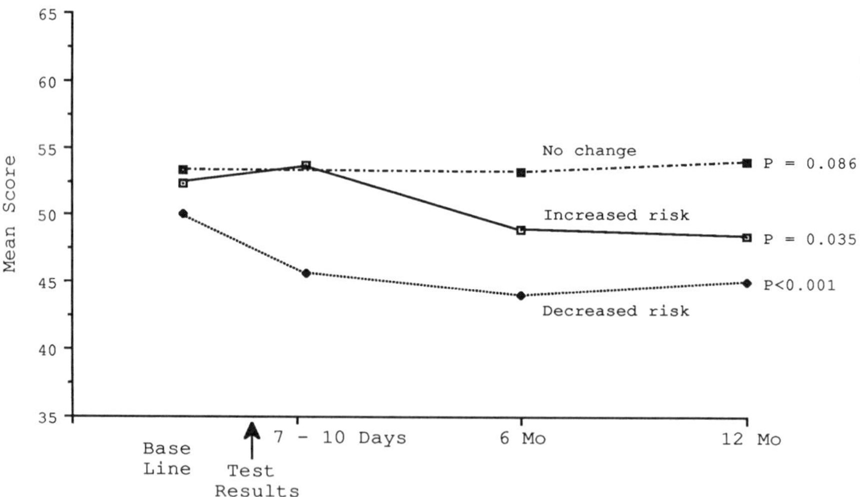

Fig 8–2.—The mean scores on the General Severity Index for the 3 study groups at each assessment. Lower scores indicate less psychological distress. The overall difference in scores during 1-year follow-up was detected for increased-risk group and for the decreased-risk group, but not for the no-change group. (Courtesy of Hayden MR, for the Canadian Collaborative Study of Predictive Testing: *N Engl J Med* 327:1401–1405, 1992.)

Results.—The mean age of the 90 women and 45 men was 37.5 years. More than two thirds were married. At 7- to 10-day assessment, the decreased-risk group showed an increase in general well-being and reductions in distress and depression. Those who found their risk to be increased had decreased scores in general well-being but little change on the other measures. During the study year, the increased-risk group showed small linear declines for distress and depression. Both groups whose risk changed after testing had lower scores for depression and higher scores for well-being at 12 months compared with the no-change group (Fig 8–2).

Conclusion.—There is some concern that knowledge of increased risk for a serious disease such as Huntington's may precipitate emotional breakdown or suicide. These results, however, suggest that such information may actually improve the psychological well-being of many people at risk. When provided as part of an intensive protocol with counseling and psychological support, predictive testing can prove beneficial.

▶ Commenting on Abstracts 8–5 and 8–6 is Laurie Zoloth-Dorfman, Ph.D., Bioethics Consultation Group, Berkeley, California:

▶ In the paradigm of mythic literature, winning the treasure invariably results in the most complex sort of challenges. Abstracts 8–5 and 8–6 record the complicated reaction to the glittering prize of medical science, genetic literacy. They may well serve as a cautionary moral tale for our age, for in the leap from research to clinical application, a difficult route must be traversed, and the way is fraught with dilemmas raised by the needs of therapy, the demands of the marketplace, and the basic morality of the quest itself.

Soon after the identification of the genes associated with Huntington's disease (HD) and cystic fibrosis (CF), what had been an interesting research achievement became a compelling therapeutic technique. Families with histories of these devastating diseases wanted to know whether the clinical applications of such information could lead to cures, or at least to screening and detection. The implication of many such requests was that such information, if available to couples at risk, would influence reproductive decisions. In individuals with HD, the implications were more complex, centering around the resolution of the uncertainty that presumptive family history brought.

Linked to the interest in the general population was a marketplace interest: soon after the gene mutation sequences were published, several biotechnology companies enthusiastically offered screening testing services to physicians (1). Such analysis can provide information about the likelihood that the manifestations of the disease will appear at some time in the future, but they do not provide information about the age of symptom onset or the severity of the illness (Abstract 8–6).

Calls for screening have aroused similar concerns for these 2 very different diseases (HD and CF). The concerns have been centered around the possible psychological effects on individuals who screen positive (HD) or who screen as having carrier status (CF). In both cases, pilot studies with careful controls have been recommended in advance of screening programs that are aimed at a wider public. The American Society of Human Genetics (2) and the National Institutes of Health (3) have both called for a moratorium on population screening for the CF gene.

The 2 articles (Abstracts 8–5 and 8–6) published in 1992 and selected for inclusion in this YEAR BOOK are reports of the first of such pilot studies. They can be critically reflected on, and the problems that they raise can be seen as anticipatory deliberations on the virtual flood of such DNA sequencing screening tests that will become available in the future, including familial Alzheimer's disease and some types of familiar cancer (Abstract 8–6).

The Wiggins study (Abstract 8–6) details a testing program that was undertaken in Canada to follow 135 participants at high familial risk for HD. The aim was to determine whether predictive testing for this adult-onset neurologic disease would be beneficial or would result in harmful, even fatal, psychological consequences for the participants. It is reported in the article—and in the first-person narrative that accompanies it (4)—that predictive testing for HD has potential *benefits* for the psychological health of individuals who receive results indicating either an increased *or* decreased risk of inheriting the gene for the disease.

The use of the HD screening test is markedly different from the use of other genetic screening tests. In the initial use of genetic tests, prenatal genetic screening was available to assist couples (often couples who already had an affected child) in making their decision as to whether to continue a pregnancy that would result in a child born with severe and unrelenting handicaps. The prototypical example was the trisomic child. Later, increasingly sensitive tests led to the identification of a wider range of genetic abnormalities, which ranged from severe and fatal (Lesch-Nyhan syndrome) to ones that resulted in more mild handicaps (Turners' Syndrome).

In screening for HD, the emphasis has been to identify adults who are at risk for the disease. In some cases, these adults have not yet made their reproductive decisions; however, in many cases, the test is administered to give warning of the disease before onset of symptoms. The rationale for the test is based on the notion that it is better to know one's health status than not to know, an assumption that seems to be borne out in practice.

It is important to reflect on some aspects of this study. First, were the participants better able to adjust to the devastating nature of their impending illness because they lived in Canada, a country with fully funded long-term health-care provisions? What would be the effect of such disclosure in an American context, where, in many states, not only is coverage for long-term care unobtainable, but a predictive diagnosis calls into question the very presumption of private health insurance, that health risk is mutually unknowable?

It is important to reflect on the reaction of those who were identified as being at risk. Once designated as "ill," there "was a new focus on physical symptoms, with frequent requests for physical examination and a need for continued support and reassurance." The individuals had been named as patients, and they began to act in their new "sick role." Once the intervention has been made in the lives of tested individuals, it seems imperative that the

Moving?

I'd like to receive my ***Year Book of Neonatal and Perinatal Medicine*** without interruption. Please not the following change of address, effective:

Name: ______________________________

New Address: ______________________________

____

City: ____________________ State: ________ Zip: ________

Old Address: ______________________________

____

City: ____________________ State: ________ Zip: ________

Reservation Card

Yes, I would like my own copy of ***Year Book of Neonatal and Perinatal Medicine***. Please begin my subscription with the current edition according to the terms described below.* I understand that I will have 30 days to examine each annual edition. If satisfied, I will pay just $64.95 plus sales tax, postage and handling (price subject to change without notice).

Name: ______________________________

Address: ______________________________

City: ____________________ State: ________ Zip: ________

Method of Payment

❍ Visa ❍ Mastercard ❍ AmEx ❍ Bill me ❍ Check (in US dollars, payable to Mosby, Inc.)

Card number: ____________________ Exp date: ____________

Signature: ______________________________

LS-0908

*Your *Year Book* Service Guarantee:

When you subscribe to the *Year Book*, we'll send you an advance notice of future volumes about two months before they publish. This automatic notice system is designed to take up as little of your time as possible. If you do not want the *Year Book*, the advance notice makes it quick and easy for you to let us know your decision, and you will always have at least 20 days to decide. If we don't hear from you, we'll send you the new volume as soon as it's available. And, of course, the *Year Book* is yours to examine free of charge for 30 days (postage, handling and applicable sales tax are added to each shipment.).

NO POSTAGE
NECESSARY
IF MAILED
IN THE
UNITED STATES

BUSINESS REPLY MAIL

FIRST CLASS MAIL PERMIT No. 762 CHICAGO, IL

POSTAGE WILL BE PAID BY ADDRESSEE

Chris Hughes
Mosby-Year Book, Inc.
200 N. LaSalle Street
Suite 2600
Chicago, IL 60601-9981

NO POSTAGE
NECESSARY
IF MAILED
IN THE
UNITED STATES

BUSINESS REPLY MAIL

FIRST CLASS MAIL PERMIT No. 762 CHICAGO, IL

POSTAGE WILL BE PAID BY ADDRESSEE

Chris Hughes
Mosby-Year Book, Inc.
200 N. LaSalle Street
Suite 2600
Chicago, IL 60601-9981

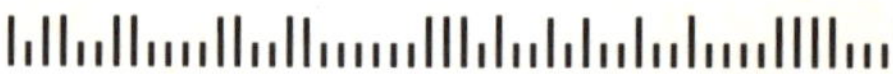

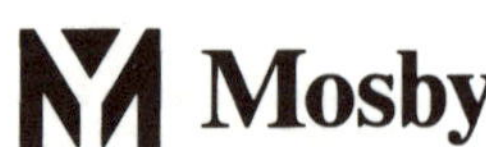

Dedicated to publishing excellence

medical profession not abandon them. Where there is no cure for the disease, there must be provision for support. To simply name and define one as being ill and then to neglect to take responsibility for what follows may be the only response that is currently offered, especially in the experimental context. We ought to acknowledge that this is an ethically unacceptable response. Although there is as yet no genetic intervention—no cure for HD, there *is* care. Such expensive care calls on the community for vast amounts of social support and demands that we give attention to the problem of funding for long-term and dignified care.

What of those individuals who do not carry the HD gene in the study population? Once renamed as having a diminished risk, one might assume that there would be a universal cheerfullness. It is interesting to note that this is not the case. The researchers correctly note that "the major hurdle for them appears to be the realization that they are facing an unplanned future." Like most of us, individuals who are newly considered not at risk do not now know what it is that they will die of, and the defining construct of their lives is now altered.

The researchers do not mention another issue that may lead to this ambivalent reaction, one that is eloquently noted by the first-person account of such testing. Huntington's disease is a familial disease. There is no "freedom," no guiltless, autonomous escape from this. The newly not-at-risk individual is, in all likelihood, surrounded by a family and has obligations to that family in which the cruel lottery of genetics is still being played out.

The study by Watson et al. on the effects of testing and screening for the CF gene (Abstract 8–5), was also carried out in England, and it similarly raises the issue of the impact of negative outcomes in an American society in which there is no guaranteed health care for the afflicted. The anxiety raised by this problem does not seem inconsiderable; however, the results are still informative. If "the central ethical dilemma is how to balance the benefit to persons who may wish to avoid the birth of a child with CF against the potential harm that would result from the confusion, stigmatization, and discrimination associated with testing" (1), then this study addresses the issue of potential harm directly. Watson (Abstract 8–5) finds no adverse psychological consequences, at least in British society among the population so examined.

To some extent, this seems to be based on the rather remarkable ability of the individuals in the study to deny the implication of the findings: "One in five believed that there was no risk they could be a carrier despite being told to the contrary both verbally and by letter."

Carriers and noncarriers in this large (3,000-person) study appear both to approve of screening and to be glad to have been tested. Thus, the major concerns raised in previous speculative academic articles may be "ill founded" in the clinical world so examined.

The changes in the perception and reality of the commonly occurring disease CF have themselves been dramatic, which may ultimately affect our understanding of such screening programs. Cystic fibrosis has been understood as a fatal disease of early childhood, associated with an agonizing death and costly and exhausting treatment regimens. Changes in treatment have meant that some affected children can live into their fourth decade. Testing larger numbers of the population has revealed CF in less affected individuals, and in individuals that manifest no symptoms until adolescence or early adulthood (1). Finally, new therapies and experimental lung transplants offer the first possibilities for therapeutic cures. The issues of cost remain. If widespread screening and supportive counseling is called for, this represents the appearance of an enormous new market in health care at just the moment where health-care costs are being scrutinized.

The ethical implications are equally haunting. What benefit are we looking for as a society? What would constitute a successful medical outcome? For what should a physician wish? We are at an odd stage in genetic research. We can see the future, or at least some outlines of it, but we cannot change it (some wishes can be granted, but not all). This may well change in the next generation of genetic science. In the case of CF, trials have already been approved for treatment (not just testing) using gene transfer vector therapy. In the meantime, is the goal eradication of diseases such as CF and HD by an enthusiastic testing and reproductive counseling program (i.e., urging carriers to either not reproduce or to abort affected fetuses)? For families whose lives have been defined by their love for and the love of individuals with such chronic diseases, the answer is not so simple. Hayes, in her first person account, states: "We are accustomed to the changes that the disease brings about, and although we may be fearful, we live and value our affected relatives. For many of us, abortion might be the best option when there is a risk of some *other* medical condition, but not *our own* " (emphasis added). If some families choose to continue pregnancies to term, will their reproductive decision be supported by public policy and public funds? Will insurance companies support this decision? There have already been disturbing reports of denial of coverage based on predictive testing (1), and many ethicists (5) have raised questions regarding the meaning of care for the handicapped if this is perceived as a willful choice rather than an act of God. The assumption of many theoretical studies is that couples would be less likely to consider having children at risk for CF, but the Watson article reminds us that, according to the research data, this has not been proven to be the case.

Deep cultural differences are at the heart of all reproductive decision-making. What is "normal," what is "acceptable risk," and who can be loved are all relative to the chance, abundance, and social solidarity expressive of life in different cultures. Many such constructions of "normal" and "healthy" will have to be critically examined in light of this. Furthermore, the inherent bias of physicians and researchers will have to be similarly examined (6). The central ethical question at the centerpiece of all genetic therapy ought not to be "Can we afford it?" but, rather, "Are there any limits on our moral ability to know, to name, and to reconstruct human persons?"

Finally, the social context for reflecting on cost-benefit analysis, which is so mesmerizing in the research on CF population screening, must be examined. At stake here are 3 classic ethical principles. First, is it a reflection of the autonomous rights of any individual to know as much as possible about his or her own gene structure? Can the medical profession decide what risk is considered "low" and, hence, acceptable or what information might be too worrisome to provide? Also, can consideration of justice overrule the demands of any one individual? This last problem is linked to the cost of the testing and counseling itself. These studies show that, in the pilot studies that were called for by geneticists and ethicists, the subjects, despite dire predictions, were not adversely affected by such testing; in most cases, they seemed to benefit from it. This was true despite outcome, and it was generally true for both HD and CF. Does this now make it epidemiologically acceptable to offer the testing and attendant counseling? An intervention such as this, which makes widespread counseling available to prospective parents, offers a curious "side effect" with fascinating possibilities. It could well offer the only time that parents reflect on the meaning of parenting itself, a task that is both so basic and complex, this bringing of a new person and his or her own constellation of grief and triumph into the social world. If parents' real fears and real hopes could be heard, it would change not only the incidence of genetically transmitted diseases, but what we make of parenting itself—not just for the most vulnerable, but for all our children. As dramatic as the genetic screening is, an intervention such as this would have an even more dramatic effect on the lives of the handicapped. The prize reached for, genetic certainty, may be far diminished by the one that is finally grasped.—L. Zoloth-Dorfman, Ph.D.

References

1. Wilfond B, Fost N: *Milbank Q* 70:629, 1992.
2. Caskey CT, et al: *Am J Hum Genet* 46:393, 1990.
3. National Institutes of Health Workshop: N *Engl J Med* 323:70, 1990.
4. Hayes CV: N *Engl J Med* 327:1449, 1992.
5. Hauerwas S: *Suffering Presence.* Notre Dame, Ind, Univ of Notre Dame Press, 1986.
6. Bosk C: *All God's Mistakes: Genetic Counseling in a Pediatric Hospital.* Chicago, Univ of Chicago Press, 1992.

Communicating Medical Bad News: Parents' Experiences and Preferences

Sharp MC, Strauss RP, Lorch SC (Univ of North Carolina, Chapel Hill)
J Pediatr 121:539–546, 1992 8–7

Introduction.—Numerous studies have dealt with the ways physicians communicate medical bad news. It is clear that parents want to be given such information in a realistic, sympathetic, positive, and timely manner. Parents are dissatisfied when physicians control the interaction and offer an overly pessimistic view of a child's future. Parents' experiences and preferences and the ways in which social class influences communication were examined.

Methods.—A questionnaire sent to parents who had children in developmental day care centers in North Carolina examined the experience of being told bad news and elicited preferences for physician behavior in a hypothetical situation. The survey was completed by 189 parents, the majority (64.9%) of whom were white; nearly all (93%) respondents were women.

Results.—Most (79%) of the informing professionals were male. Fewer than half of the parents believed that the physician allowed them to show their feelings (47%) or made an effort to make them feel better (41%). Parents also complained about the lack of information offered at the time of diagnosis. About one third of the physicians showed little of their own feelings when telling the bad news. Parents with less than a college education were generally better satisfied with the amount of information given and the manner the news was communicated. Although most parents (87%) wanted to be referred to parents of children with similar problems, few such referrals (19%) were given.

Conclusion.—Most physicians learn to tell bad news by observation or by trial and error. At this critical time, physicians must inspire trust and communicate effectively. This survey confirms that parents want a physician to have a caring and confident attitude, to share information, and to allow the parents to talk and show their own feelings.

► This sensitive and perceptive report of a survey of parental experiences and preferences can help all care givers meet the needs of their patients at this difficult time. Sadly, in a large proportion of instances, the behaviors of the physician did not match the parents' desires. Focused training of personnel using videotaped role-playing techniques can markedly improve our effectiveness in this area.—M.H. Klaus, M.D.

Avoidance of Emergency Surgery in Newborn Infants With Trisomy 18

Bos AP, Broers CJM, Hazebroek FWJ, van Hemel JO, Tibboel D, Wesby-van Swaay E, Molenaar JC (Sophia Children's Hosp, Rotterdam, The Netherlands)
Lancet 339:913–917, 1992 8–8

Introduction.—Trisomy 18, or Edwards' syndrome, shows both external signs and life-threatening abnormalities that can require immediate surgical care in the newborn. A quick identification method for trisomy 18 is needed because the surgery may then be withheld in the neonate with a short life-expectancy. Karyotyping in lymphocytes, a 3-day method, was evaluated in 7 patients with this genetic condition.

Methods.—Chromosomal analysis of peripheral blood lymphocytes identified 7 of 84 patients with structural congenital anomalies as having the karyotype 47, XX/XY, +18. All 7 had at least 1 life-threatening malformation.

Case Report.—Girl, born at 42 weeks' gestation and weighing 2,010 g, had Edwards' syndrome that included micrognathia, low-set ears, short palpebral fissures, hypoplastic nails, and clenched fists. In addition, she had esophageal atresia and respiratory distress. She underwent a gastrostomy before the failure of the lymphocyte culture. She continued receiving life support until a second successful karyotyping cell culture confirmed the clinical diagnosis on day 8, after which support measures were slowly discontinued. She died at 11 days of age.

Results.—The treatment policy for the 7 patients with clinical Edwards' syndrome showed that karyotyping of a bone-marrow aspirate shortened the diagnosis period for 3 patients. Four other patients underwent surgery before the diagnosis of trisomy 18 could be confirmed by routine karyotyping.

Conclusion.—The most conservative treatment should be used in neonates with a clinical suspicion of Edwards' syndrome while awaiting the results of karyotyping in the peripheral lymphocytes. Because of the limited life expectancy and profound mental retardation for infants with trisomy 18, these patients should be transferred to an intensive care unit and allowed to die rather than undergo attempts at surgery and life-saving medical support. Active euthanasia is not recommended but, rather, comforting care for the terminal state of these newborns.

▶ As some areas of perinatal care become more intensive, it is necessary that we do not lose sight of the overall goal of medicine. With new techniques of cytogenetics, there does not appear to be any justification for extensive surgery. Our major task regarding infants with trisomy 18 is to help the parents understand physical abnormalities, to listen to the parents as they begin to integrate the disaster into their family, and to work with them on a reasonable plan for the baby. This sometimes is difficult, because many parents have an unrealistic view of what physicians can correct.—M.H. Klaus, M.D.

9 Gastroenterology and Nutrition

Randomised Trial of Continuous Nasogastric, Bolus Nasogastric, and Transpyloric Feeding in Infants of Birth Weight Under 1400 g

Macdonald PD, Skeoch CH, Carse H, Dryburgh F, Alroomi LG, Galea P, Gettinby G (Glasgow Royal Maternity Hosp, Scotland; Univ of Strathclyde, Scotland)

Arch Dis Child 67:429–431, 1992 9–1

Introduction.—Feeding tiny preterm infants is most important but may be very difficult. Growth was compared in 43 infants (birth weight, less than 1,400 g) who were randomly assigned to hourly bolus nasogastric (NG) feeding, continuous NG feeding, or continuous transpyloric (TP) feeding.

Methods.—The infants initially received total parenteral nutrition and were randomized on day 2. Milk feeds were begun at 1 mL/hr and were increased incrementally as tolerated. After reaching a weight of 1,600 g, the infants all received bolus NG feeding.

Results.—More complications occurred with TP feeding than when the NG route was used, without apparent benefits in growth rate or oral energy input. The time to full enteral feeding did not differ significantly between the various groups. Growth patterns also did not differ significantly. Four of 10 infants in the TP group required treatment for gastric bleeding.

Conclusion.—Nasogastric feeding of small preterm infants, using either a continuous or a bolus approach, can be as effective as TP and is safer. Transpyloric feeding may be used in infants who persistently fail to tolerate NG feeding.

▶ The timing and technique of feeding sick low-birth-weight infants continues to be a fruitful area for research. I thought that the issue of TP feeding had been put to rest. It is partially resurrected in this report, although the authors' recommendation that TP feedings be "reserved for those infants who persistently fail to tolerate nasogastric feeding" requires a major leap of faith, as it cannot be justified from the data generated.

The above trial, which was carried out in Glasgow over the period of a year, is limited in size, and the power analysis to justify the group sizes is not presented. There is major attrition from the TP group, with 33% of subjects not completing the study. Three died before milk feeding was established, one was transferred out, and the pylorus was not successfully negotiated with a tube in one infant, despite 5 attempts. The high rate of complications without documented clinical or biochemical benefit renders TP feeding too risky. Furthermore, the need for radiologic confirmation of TP tube placement unnecessarily exposes the infants to irradiation. The investigators had methodologic problems with prealbumin determinations and concluded that skinfold measurements were not helpful in these subjects because of interobserver variability. The trial did not distinguish between continuous and intermittent NG feeding, but both were considered superior to TP feeds. As has become customary with studies of nutrition in low-birth-weight infants, the conclusions are unsatisfactory, and more questions have been raised than answered.—A.A. Fanaroff, M.B.B.Ch.

Role of Delayed Feeding and of Feeding Increments in Necrotizing Enterocolitis

McKeown RE, Marsh TD, Amarnath U, Garrison CZ, Addy CL, Thompson SJ, Austin TL (Univ of South Carolina, Columbia)

J Pediatr 121:764–770, 1992 9–2

Objective.—The cause of necrotizing enterocolitis remains unclear, and there is still controversy about the prevention regimens for this condition, particularly with regard to enteral alimentation. In a matched-case control study, the relationship of necrotizing enterocolitis with timing of first feeding, size of feeding volumes and increments, and a risk factor index based on the system of Ostertag et al. was evaluated.

Patients.—Fifty-nine case patients with stage 2 or higher necrotizing enterocolitis using Bell's staging and 59 matched controls were studied.

Findings.—The case patients were fed earlier, received full-strength formula sooner, and received larger feeding volumes and increments than did controls. Infants with higher risk scores were more vulnerable to larger feeding increments than were infants with a low score. In case patients, age at first feeding correlated significantly with age at diagnosis, even after adjustment for the effects of birth weight and risk index, indicating that delayed feeding was related to delayed onset of disease.

Conclusion.—Both timing of initial feeding and size of feeding increments may be important in the pathogenesis of necrotizing enterocolitis. Earlier, more rapid feeding places stress on infants at greater risk for the development of this condition, and more severely ill infants are more vulnerable to aggressive feeding practices.

▶ If attitude were a felony, a number of my colleagues in neonatal medicine would be serving prolonged sentences because of their attitude toward this concept of delayed feeding and necrotizing enterocolitis (NEC). The etiology of NEC, the major gastrointestinal disorder in the neonatal period, remains elusive. Teams of investigators have been titillated by the copious epidemiologic database but have yet to emerge with a substantial breakthrough. (1, 2) How many times is it necessary to document that NEC is more prevalent in low-birth-weight infants? Lucas and Cole (3) reported that breast milk protected infants against NEC, and Carrion and Egan (4) suggested that lowering the gastric pH would have a similar effect.

It has become fashionable to provide even the most immature infant with small volumes of milk soon after birth. The purpose is to prime the gut, and these "hypocaloric feeds" or "gut stimulation" protocols appear to enhance enteral feeds. The role of early feeding in NEC is unclear, as the controlled trials have only randomized a total of approximately 150 patients. There is no "apparent" increase in NEC; however, McKeown's findings that infants become vulnerable to NEC when their feeds are advanced too rapidly is in accord with the data of Anderson (5) and the larger case-matched study of the National Institute of Child Health and Development (6), which involved almost 250 patients with NEC.

A moments' insight is sometimes worth a life's experience.—Oliver Wendell Holmes

A.A. Fanaroff, M.B.B.Ch.

References

1. McClead RE Jr: *J Pediatr* 117:S1, 1990.
2. Uauy RD, et al: *J Pediatr* 119:630, 1991.
3. 1992 Year Book of Neonatal and Perinatal Medicine, pp 170–172.
4. 1992 Year Book of Neonatal and Perinatal Medicine, pp 172–173.
5. Anderson DM, Kliegman RM: *Am J Perinatol* 8:62, 1991.
6. Wright L: *Pediatr Res* 33:313A, 1993.

Maturation of Antroduodenal Motor Activity in Preterm and Term Infants

Ittmann PI, Amarnath R, Berseth CL (Mayo Clinic and Found, Rochester, Minn)

Dig Dis Sci 37:14–19, 1992 9–3

Introduction.—Low-compliance, continuous-perfusion manometric techniques that permit prolonged studies of antral and duodenal motor activity in preterm and term infants were used to compare antral and duodenal activity and the coordination of these activities in 19 preterm and 9 term infants.

Results.—In both term and preterm infants, antral activity consisted of isolated single contractions and clustered phasic contractions (Fig 9–1). There were no significant differences between the groups with regard to antral activity. Intestinal motor contractions varied significantly between the groups. Clustered phasic contractions occurred more frequently and

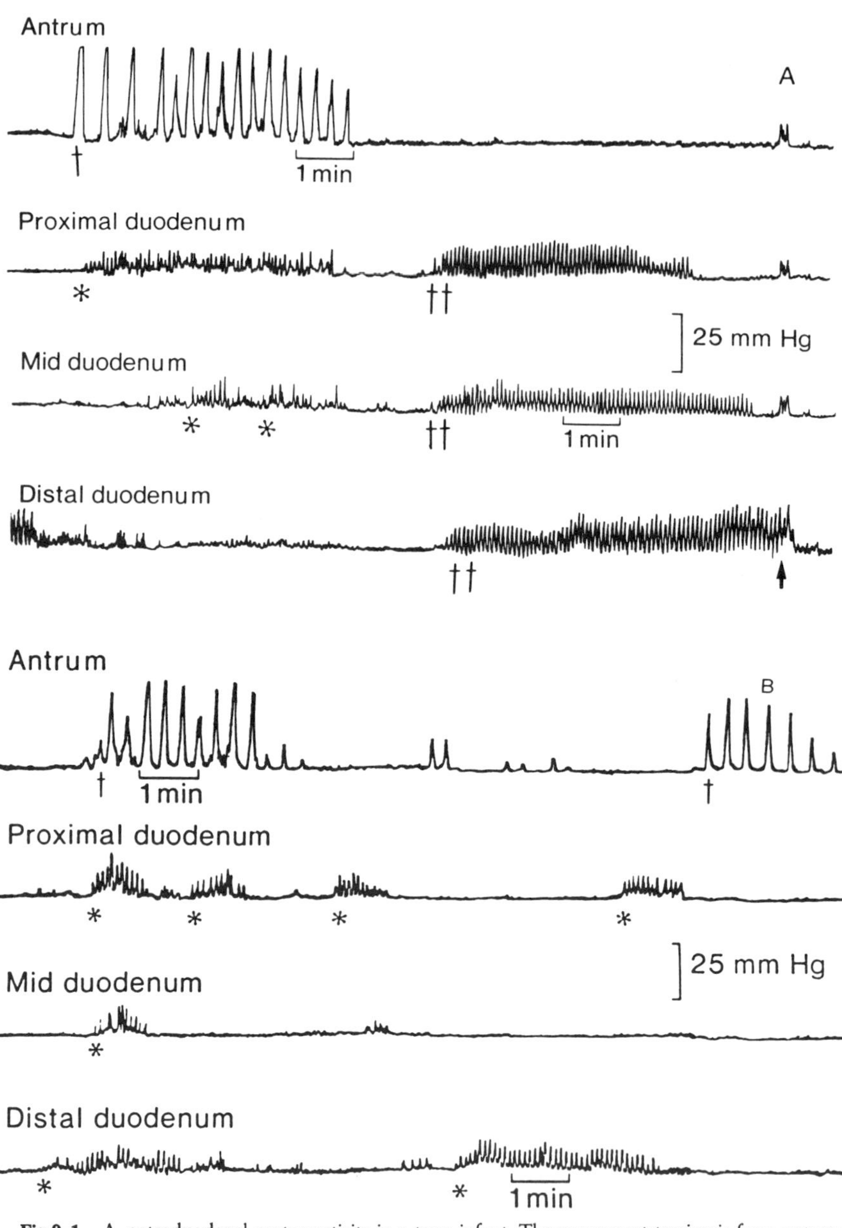

Fig 9–1.—A, antroduodenal motor activity in a term infant. The uppermost tracing is from antrum and the lower 3 are from duodenum. Phasic activity is present in the antrum (*dagger*) and it is temporally coordinated with migratory phasic activity in all 3 duodenal sites (2 *daggers*); 3 other duodenal clusters (*asterisk*) fail to migrate. *Arrow* indicates the presence of movement artifact. B, antroduodenal motor activity in a preterm infant. Two antral clusters (*dagger*) are present: phasic activity occurs only in the first and third middle duodenal sites (*asterisk*), whereas the second duodenal site contains little activity. None of the duodenal phasic clustered activity migrates and occurs asynchronously with respect to the 2 antral clusters. (Courtesy of Ittmann PI, Amarnath R, Berseth CL: *Dig Dis Sci* 37:14–19, 1992.)

were of shorter duration and lower amplitude in preterm infants. Duodenal clusters were significantly less frequent and had increased amplitude with increasing age. The coordination of antral and duodenal activity increased with increasing age.

Conclusion.—Although antral activity is similar in the preterm and term infant, duodenal activity is significantly different. When manometrics are used to determine the readiness of a preterm infant for feeding, attention should be focused on the maturity of intestinal motor activity.

▶ These investigators have provided us with a steady stream of publications on gastrointestinal motility and function. They've compared term and preterm infants under conditions of health, disease, fasting, and feeding. This report amplifies previous findings of diminished duodenal activity in the preterm infant by simultaneously measuring antral and duodenal activity in the fasting period. These studies were all done in the fasting state at the time feedings were to be initiated.

Antral activity is equivalent in preterm and term infants. However, coordinated/duodenal activity is infrequent in preterm infants. Also, duodenal motor activity is quantitatively reduced and lacks propulsion in the preterm infants.

The clinical implications of these findings remain the subject of conjecture and speculation that regrettably lack supportive data. In adults, coordinated antraduodenal activity is associated with gastric emptying, as evidenced by duodenal acidification. Gastric emptying of liquids, the exclusive diet in term and preterm neonates, is initiated by gastric fundal motor activity. Berseth reported that gastrointestinal peptides (GIP) enhance gastrointestinal motility (1). Enteroglucogen, gastrin, motilin, and neurotensin, are additional factors that may enhance motility. Gastrointestinal motility follows an orderly maturational process. When the neurologic and humoral factors dictating this maturation are better understood, the tools will be available to hasten this process. In the meantime, challenging the gut with very small feeds (minimal enteral nutrition) or "hypocaloric feeds" may accelerate maturation (2, 3). Any practical nurse with experience feeding premature infants would have concluded that preterm infants have problems with motility. They would not have quantitated the antroduodenal activity so elegantly.—A.A. Fanaroff, M.B.B.Ch.

References

1. Berseth CL: *Pediatr Res* 31:587, 1992.
2. Berseth CL: *Pediatr Res* 29:291, 1991.
3. Dunn L, et al: *J Pediatr* 112:622, 1988.

Plasma Gastrin-34 Increases During and Immediately After Breast-Feeding in 3-Day-Old Infants

Marchini G, Redham I, Uvnäs-Moberg K (Karolinska Hosp, Stockholm; Karolinska Inst, Stockholm)

J Pediatr Gastroenterol Nutr 14:140–145, 1992 9–4

Introduction.—The ability of newborn infants to secrete gastrin has not been documented. However, it is possible that previous studies have failed to detect transient increases that occur during feeding.

Methods.—The plasma concentration of gastrin was monitored by radioimmunoassay before, during, and after breast-feeding in 72 healthy infants 3 days after birth. Concentration of somatostatin also was estimated, and both peptides were further characterized by high-performance liquid chromatography.

Findings.—The mean level of gastrin increased significantly 5 and 10 minutes after the start of sucking and just after breast-feeding. The level of somatostatin did not change. The level of gastrin did not relate either to the amount of milk taken or to the duration of feeding in infants, fed to satiety. A single peak of gastrin activity coeluted with nonsulfated gastrin-34. Most somatostatin activity coeluted with somatostatin-14.

Conclusion.—Plasma gastrin activity increases during and immediately after breast-feeding in neonates.

▶ This report continues a long-term investigation by this Swedish team. They note a marked increase in a specific form of gastrin in the neonate during breast-feeding. It is of special interest that this group reported similar changes in maternal gastrointestinal hormones shortly after initiation of suckling, also without any change in somatostatin (1). They postulated that breast-feeding induces a reflex activation of the release of maternal gastrointestinal hormones that is analogous to the reflex-induced output of pituitary hormones (oxytocin and prolactin). Because gastrin stimulates gastric acid secretion and the growth of the intestinal tract, this would fit the need of a breast-feeding mother to take in more food to produce adequate milk. Thus, both the mother's and the infant's gastrointestinal hormones are responding to breast-feeding in a similar fashion. This is a most reasonable design.—M.H. Klaus, M.D.

Reference

1. Widström AM, et al: *Early Hum Dev* 16:293, 1988.

Intestinal Development and Fatty Acid Binding Protein Activity of Newborn Pigs Fed Colostrum or Milk

Reinhart GA, Simmen FA, Mahan DC, White ME, Roehrig KL (Ohio State

Univ, Columbus)
Biol Neonate 62:155–163, 1992 9–5

Background.—Increased intestinal weight in the nursing pig has been associated with mucosal incorporation of milk proteins. Fatty acid-binding proteins (FABPs) are abundant low-molecular-weight proteins pres-

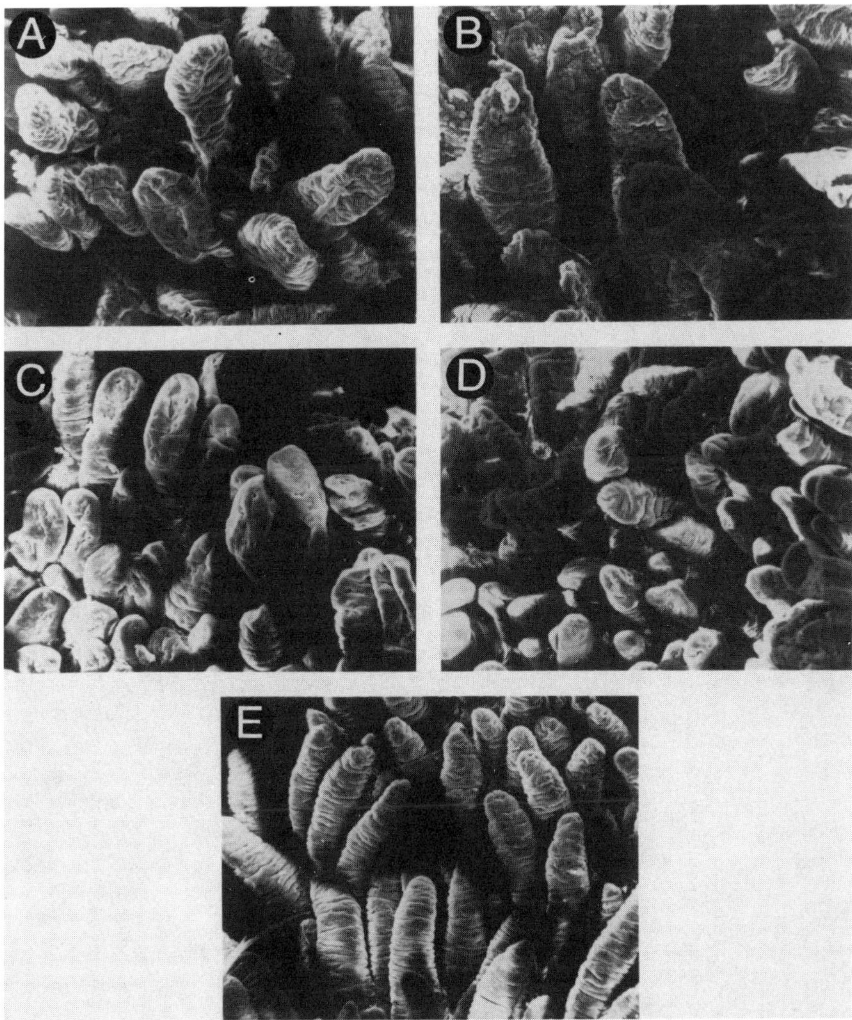

Fig 9–2.—The effect of feeding colostrum or mature milk on morphologic characteristics of small intestinal villi. Scanning electron microscopy at 25% of small intestinal length in neonatal pigs after feeding of 1 of the following diets for a 24-hour period: whole colostrum (**A**), defatted colostrum (**B**), whole day 21 milk (**C**), defatted day 21 milk (**D**), 5% lactose/electrolyte solution (**E**). Three pigs per treatment were examined with representative views presented. Original magnification, ×150. (Courtesy of Reinhart GA, Simmen FA, Mahan DC, et al: *Biol Neonate* 62:155–163, 1992.)

ent in the soluble fraction of enterocytes, and they are known to bind long-chain fatty acids and their coenzyme A derivatives.

Objective and Methods.—Colostrum-deprived newborn pigs were gavage-fed with sow's colostrum, defatted colostrum, whole milk, defatted milk, or 5% lactose solution over 24 hours, after which they were killed and the small intestine was removed. High-molecular-weight proteins were removed from the cytosol fraction of intestinal mucosa before quantifying FABP activity.

Findings.—Those animals fed colostrum had a greater mucosal mass in the proximal small bowel than did those fed milk or lactose. Total FABP activity and activity per milligram of DNA in the proximal bowel also were higher in colostrum-fed pigs than in those given lactose solution. Feeding defatted material lowered the consequent FABP activity in small bowel samples. The intestinal villi from colostrum-fed pigs were tongue-shaped and plicated, whereas those from milk-fed animals were shorter and broadly ridged (Fig 9–2).

Conclusion.—Colostrum stimulates differentiation of the proximal small bowel in newborn pigs. Analyzing FABPs may prove helpful in understanding the relationship between maternal mammary gland secretions and perinatal development of the gut.

▶ Cross-species studies help us gain insight into many areas of development that cannot easily be studied in the human. The pig has proved to be a hardy model, and it is rapidly becoming the favorite neonatal animal model. This study will provide food for thought for the many investigators who desire rapid gratification. A 24-hour period suffices to determine the intestinal development and FABP of pigs fed pure or modified colostrum, or milk or lactose solution only. Much useful information is garnered from a well-designed experiment. The electron microscope pictures are beautiful, even if the findings cannot all be easily explained. The DNA measurements permit differentiation between increases in cell size and cell number. The investigators ultimately conclude that the changes in the mucosal mass induced by colostrum and, to a lesser extent, the milk, are the result of an uptake of protein and water by preexisting cells. This reaffirms the findings of that remarkable nutritional expert Dame Elsie Widdowson (1). Was she ever wrong?

The benefits of colostrum feeding continue to emerge. It remains for clinicians to ensure that all newborns become recipients of this multifunctional fluid.

No other solution will provide the premature infant with nutrients, micronutrients, growth factors, hormones, and immunologic protection, all in the correct doses.—A.A. Fanaroff, M.B.B.Ch.

Reference

1. Widdowson EM, et al: *Biol Neonate* 28:272, 1976.

Tumor Necrosis Factor-α in Human Milk

Rudloff HE, Schmalstieg FC Jr, Mushtaha AA, Palkowetz KH, Liu SK, Goldman AS (Univ of Texas, Galveston)

Pediatr Res 31:29–33, 1992 9–6

Background.—Much of the protective effect of human milk is ascribed to an antimicrobial system comprising both humoral and cellular components. Leukocytes are of particular relevance. Previous work suggests that some biological activities of human milk are partly blocked by antibodies against human tumor necrosis factor-α (TNF-α).

Objective.—Immunochemical methods were used to confirm the presence of TNF-α in human milk taken early in the course of lactation. Specimens were taken from healthy women aged 18–35 years.

Findings.—Gel filtration studies demonstrated the presence of TNF-α in molecular-weight fractions of 80–195 kD. The factor was detected by

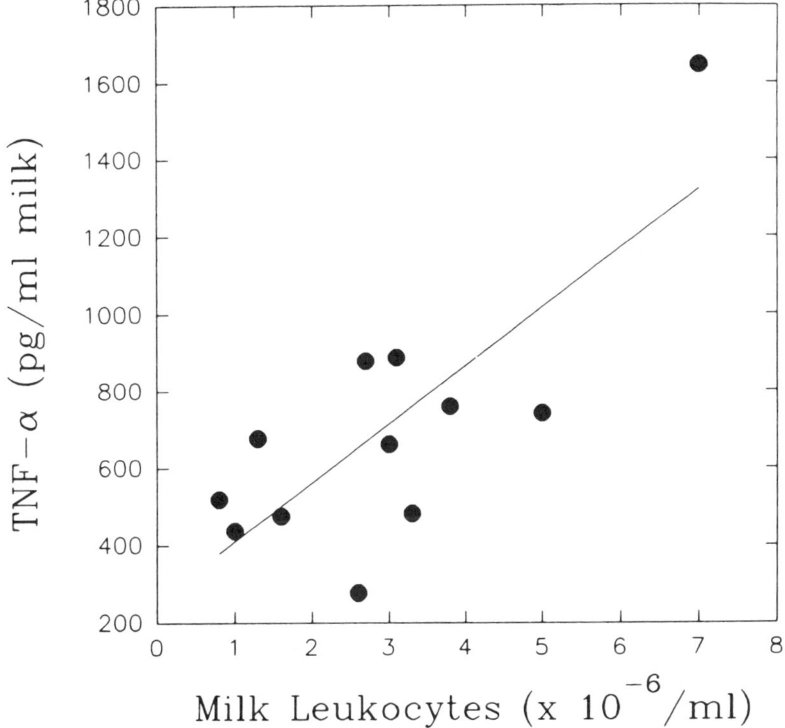

Fig 9–3.—Correlation between the concentrations of TNF-α and the numbers of leukocytes in human milk. Tumor necrosis factor-α and the total number of leukocytes were quantified in the same specimens. The correlation between the concentrations of TNF-α and total leukocytes in human milk was significant ($r^2 = .59$; $P < .01$). (Courtesy of Rudloff HE, Schmalstieg FC Jr, Mushtaha AA, et al: *Pediatr Res* 31:29–33, 1992.)

a competitive radioimmunoassay, but not consistently by Western blotting or cytotoxic assays. The mean concentration of TNF-α by radioimmunoassay was 25 pg per mg of total protein, or 620 pg per mL of milk. The level of TNF-α in the fluid phase of milk correlated with total cells (Fig 9–3), but not with the number of macrophages.

Implication.—Tumor necrosis factor-α is present in human milk early in the course of lactation, in concentrations high enough to be physiologically active.

▶ This is the fifth year that the YEAR BOOK OF NEONATAL AND PERINATAL MEDICINE has described the discovery of a new component of breast milk. The authors note that the cytokine activity previously observed in breast milk could be the result of tumor necrosis factor-α. Their evidence suggests that the necrosis factor is produced in the breast by macrophages and is present in sufficient amounts to have a significant biological effect. With the multiple actions that this factor has on various immunologic components, it may be significant in the maturation of the defense systems of the infant. As part of a long-term investigation of breast milk, this unit has attempted to track which component of breast milk increases the mobility of macrophages. Several lines of evidence suggest that it may be tumor necrosis factor. Again, we observe why breast milk substitutes are no match for the real product.—M.H. Klaus, M.D.

Influence of Breast Versus Formula Milk on Physiological Gastroesophageal Reflux in Healthy, Newborn Infants

Heacock HJ, Jeffrey HE, Baker JL, Page M (King George V Hosp for Mothers and Infants, Camperdown, Australia)

J Pediatr Gastroenterol Nutr 14:41–46, 1992 9–7

Introduction.—There is great variability in physiologic gastroesophageal reflux (GER) in healthy newborn infants. One variable that might influence GER is the type of milk fed. The effects of breast-feeding compared with bottle feeding on GER has not been examined. The differences in the number and duration of physiologic GER episodes were monitored in 37 healthy breast-fed and 37 healthy formula-fed infants, aged 2–8 days.

Methods.—Neonates were randomly selected from a public maternity ward and were studied for 4 hours after their morning feed. A pH microelectrode was placed 6 cm above the gastroesophageal junction, and the GER was recorded during the third and fourth postprandial hours. Sleep state was defined by EEG, electrooculogram, electromyogram, and breathing and behavioral observations. Movement was recorded from a piezoelectric transducer.

Results.—During active sleep, breast-fed neonates had significantly shorter episodes of GER than formula-fed neonates (table). This differ-

Mean and 95% Confidence Intervals for All Reflux Parameters for All States and Feed Types

	AW	AS	IS	QS
State time (min/h)				
BF	7.3 (4.7,9.9)	30.4 (27.1,33.7)*	7.8 (6.2,9.4)	14.5 (10.0,19.0)*
AF	6.3 (4.2,8.4)	34.7 (32.5,36.9)	8.3 (6.8,9.8)	10.7 (9.0,12.4)
Episodes (per h)				
BF	1.8 (0.5,3.0)	1.5 (0.8,2.1)	0.7 (0.7,0.7)	0.1 (0.1,0.3)
AF	3.6 (1.8,5.3)	2.3 (1.8,2.8)	1.4 (0.2,2.5)	0.3 (0.1,0.8)
Duration (min/h)				
BF	1.4 (0.5,2.9)	3.0 (1.6,5.2) *	1.1 (0.3,2.4)	0.5 (0.0,1.2)
AF	3.1 (1.5,5.6)	8.3 (5.0,13.3)	1.8 (0.8,3.6)	1.2 (0.5,2.3)
Episodes (>5 min/h)				
BF	0.6 (0.0,1.3)	0.5 (0.3,0.8) *	0.4 (0.0,0.8)	0.2 (0.0,0.4)
AF	0.5 (0.1,0.9)	1.3 (0.8,1.7)	0.4 (0.0,0.7)	0.4 (0.0,0.8)

Abbreviations: AW, wakefulness; AS, active sleep; IS, indeterminate sleep; QS, quiet sleep; BR, breast fed; AF, artificial or formula fed.

* $P < .05$ (significant differences between breast-feeding and artificial feeding), using analysis of covariance with age as the covariant for each reflux parameter between BF vs. AF (in that sleep state only).

(Courtesy of Heacock HJ, Jeffrey HE, Baker JL, et al: *J Pediatr Gastroenterol Nutr* 14:41–46, 1992.)

ence could not be explained by differences in milk volume or movement between the groups. There was also a significantly lower median pH value for GER in breast-fed infants. This difference may reflect more rapid gastric emptying in breast-fed neonates.

Conclusion.—Feed type appears to be an important variable to consider in the evaluation of physiologic GER.

▶ Add diminished reflux to the already crammed scorecard documenting the advantages of breast-feeding. For good measure, also keep in mind that breast-fed infants spend more time in quiet sleep than do formula-fed infants. There were no differences in the volume of milk consumed. More reflux has been reported with increased fat content (1). The fat content of breast milk was not measured, but it usually is equal to or in excess of the 3.5 grams of fat present in the formula. Although the pH of breast milk was initially higher than that of formula, at the time of reflux, the pH of the gastric contents was lower in the breast-fed infants and the duration of reflux shorter. This is consistent with adult data, which show that a lower pH on reflux induces peristalsis and clears the esophagus more rapidly.

This was a well-organized and implemented protocol, and the results are logically presented. The next phase of the study will test the "container." Is it breast milk or is it the manner in which milk is presented?—A.A. Fanaroff, M.B.B.Ch.

Reference

1. Vandenplas Y, et al: *Eur J Pediatr* 148:152, 1988.

The Effect of Diet on Feces and Jaundice During the First 3 Weeks of Life

Gourley GR, Kreamer B, Arend R (Univ of Wisconsin, Madison; Waisman Ctr on Mental Retardation and Human Development, Madison, Wis)
Gastroenterology 103:660–667, 1992 9–8

Background.—Serum bilirubin levels are higher in breast-fed than in formula-fed infants. Because bilirubin and its conjugates are primarily excreted in the feces, the relationship between fecal output and neonatal jaundice was evaluated in infants fed only human milk or 1 of 3 commercial infant formulas.

Setting.—During the first 3 weeks of life, stool output was quantitated in full-term infants fed ad libitum with either human breast milk or 1 of 3 infant formulas—whey-predominant, Enfamil; casein hydrosylate, Nutramigen; or casein-predominant, 3305H. Neonatal jaundice was assessed by measuring serum bilirubin levels and the transcutaneous "jaundice index" on days 3 and 21.

Results.—After day 4, the individual wet and dry stools in breast-fed infants weighed less than those in formula-fed infants. Similarly, cumulative wet and dry stool output was also lowest in breast-fed infants. After the first week, breast-fed infants produced more stools per week than formula-fed infants. After day 3, the jaundice index, which correlated positively with serum bilirubin levels, was higher in breast-fed infants than in formula-fed infants. The jaundice index of infants fed casein hydrosylate was significantly lower than in other-formula-fed infants on days 10–18. In breast-fed infants, the change in serum bilirubin levels and jaundice index from day 3 to day 21 strongly correlated with both total wet and total dry cumulative stool weights on day 21. No similar correlation was observed in any of the formula-fed infants.

Conclusion.—In infants who are fed human milk, the quantity of stool excreted is related to decreases in serum bilirubin levels. These findings are consistent with previous reports that hyperbilirubinemia in infants fed human milk may be related in part to delayed bilirubin clearance, which results from low stool output.

▶ M. Jeffrey Maisels, M.D., Clinical Director of Pediatrics at William Beaumont Hospital, Royal Oak, Michigan, and Clinical Professor of Pediatrics at Wayne State University and University of Michigan Medical Center, who is always eager to express an opinion on anything related to bilirubin, says:

▶ Dr. Gourley and his colleagues continue to conduct meticulous clinical measurements that help us to understand the physiology of neonatal jaundice and its relationship to breast- and formula-feeding. They have confirmed and extended previous observations in humans and in animals, which show quite convincingly that the major factor accounting for both early and late hyperbilirubinemia in breast-fed newborns is an increase in the intestinal absorption of bilirubin. Why does this occur? When compared with formula-fed infants, breast-fed newborns have (1) a significant decrease in stool output throughout the first 3 weeks of life; (2) an increased activity of beta-glucuronidase, which hydrolyses bilirubin glucuronide (conjugated bilirubin) and converts it back to its unconjugated form, which can be easily absorbed by the intestine; and (3) a delayed excretion of urobilin in their stools (perhaps as a result of the effect of breast milk on intestinal flora, which delays the formation of urobilin), further enhancing the possibility of intestinal reabsorption of bilirubin. There also is some evidence that breast-fed infants may have a mild degree of cholestasis.

Gourley and colleagues speculate that one explanation for the greater stool weights and lower serum bilirubin levels in infants who are fed formula rather than breast milk is related to differences in fat absorption. Breast-fed infants absorb more fat than do formula-fed infants. Because bilirubin is lipophilic, any increase in fat absorption will increase bilirubin absorption (and decrease bilirubin clearance). The decline in serum bilirubin levels from day 3 to day 21 was strongly associated with the cumulative stool excretion in breast-fed, but not in formula-fed, infants. Fat and bile salt-stimulated lipase levels vary considerably in human milk, and the variable effect that this has on fat absorption (and, hence, bilirubin absorption) might explain the relationship found between stool output and the decline in bilirubin levels in breast-fed infants.—M.J. Maisels, M.D.

Breast Milk and Subsequent Intelligence Quotient in Children Born Preterm

Lucas A, Morley R, Cole TJ, Lister G, Leeson-Payne C (MRC Dunn Nutrition Unit, Cambridge; Norfolk and Norwich Hosp, Norwich; Jessop Hosp for Women, Sheffield, England)

Lancet 339:261–264, 1992 9–9

Introduction.—Research into the effect of nutrition on neurodevelopment in early life has been inconclusive. In a previous study, mothers' decisions to provide breast milk for their preterm infants were associated with higher developmental scores at 18 months. Intelligence quotients (IQs) were determined in the same group of children at age 7½–8 years.

Methods.—The follow-up study included 300 of 313 children from the original study. All weighed less than 1,850 g at birth. Whether to provide breast milk was decided by the mother within 72 hours of delivery; 210 infants received mother's milk and 90 did not. The IQs of the children were assessed by an abbreviated version of the Wechsler Intelligence Scale for Children, revised Anglicized version.

Findings.—The mean IQs at age 7½–8 years were 92.8 for children who received no mother's milk and 103.7 for those who did receive mother's milk. The advantage in overall IQ was 8.3 points, which represented more than half of a standard deviation. That advantage persisted

Intelligence Quotient at 7½–8 Years in the 2 Groups

	Mean (SEM) scores		Advantage for group II
	Group I	Group II	babies (95% CI)
Abbreviated WISC-R			
Verbal scale	92·0 (2·0)	102·1 (1·3)	10·1 (4·7, 15·5)*
Performance scale	93·2 (1·7)	103·3 (1·2)	10·1 (6·0, 14·2)*
Overall IQ	92·8 (1·6)	103·0 (1·2)	10·2 (6·3, 14·1)*

Abbreviation: CI, confidence interval.
* $P < .001$, group I vs. group II.
(Courtesy of Lucas A, Morley R, Cole TJ, et al: *Lancet* 339:261–264, 1992.)

after adjustment for differences in maternal education and social class and was the strongest of several factors (table). The association was with tube feeding of mother's milk rather than breast-feeding, and IQ was related in dose-dependent fashion to the proportion of mother's milk in the diet. Seventeen mothers elected to provide milk but could not do so; their children's IQs were the same as those whose mothers chose not to provide breast milk.

Conclusion.—Intelligence quotient is higher at age 7½–8 years in preterm children who received mother's milk than it is in those who did not. Furthermore, there appears to be a significant dose-response relationship between the proportion of mother's milk consumed and the child's subsequent IQ. Human milk apparently has a beneficial effect on neurodevelopment; however, the results could be explained by group differences in parenting skills or genetic potential.

▶ In a previous YEAR BOOK, we cautiously presented the striking results at 18 months which are now confirmed at 7½ years. In a most conservative discussion of the results, the authors aggressively attempt to find a flaw in their study, such as mothers who breast-feed coming from a different population, etc. Luckily, there were mothers who had wanted to breast-feed but couldn't, and the IQs of their infants were similar to those of infants who were fed formula. The higher IQ did not appear to be related to actual sucking of the breast milk, because infants who were fed breast milk by tube also had the IQ advantage. That the increased IQ was related to the dose and remained a strong correlation after adjusting for confounding variables also supports these striking findings. All care takers of neonates should read this report closely, because it forces a complete reevaluation of our present feeding practices.—M.H. Klaus, M.D.

Effect of Discharge Samples on Duration of Breast-Feeding

Dungy CI, Christensen-Szalanski J, Losch M, Russell D (Univ of Iowa, Iowa

City)
Pediatrics 90:233–237, 1992 9–10

Introduction.—Previous studies have suggested that both free distribution of infant formula samples to mothers of newborns at the time of discharge from the postpartum unit and maternal breast-feeding attitudes contribute to the declining rate of breast-feeding in the United States. The roles of hospital discharge samples and maternal attitudes were investigated as predictors of breast-feeding duration.

Setting.—A total of 146 women who initiated breast-feeding during their stay in a community hospital serving predominantly white, middle-class, well-educated, urban-rural population were evaluated. At discharge, the women received, at random, either a specially prepared pack containing a manual breast pump but no infant formula or a commercial discharge pack containing infant formula. The women were interviewed while in the hospital and at 2-week intervals until 8 weeks post discharge.

Findings.—At each time point, follow-up data were available for 85% of the eligible women. Overall, the rate of exclusive breast-feeding decreased from 68% at 2 weeks to 30% at 8 weeks post partum. Women who received the breast pump continued exclusive breast-feeding for a significantly longer period of time (mean, 4.18 weeks) than did women who received discharge packs containing infant formula (mean, 2.78 weeks) (Fig 9–4). Ease of feeding was the only significant predictor of

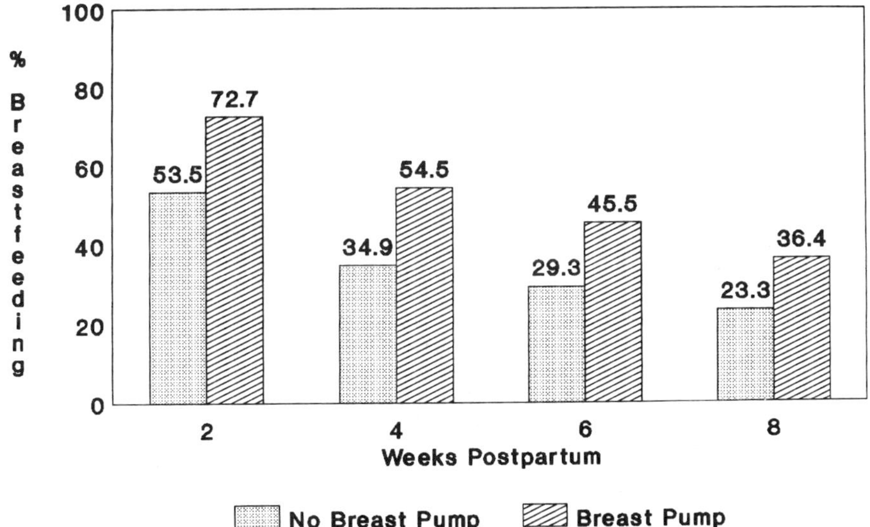

Fig 9–4.—Rates of exclusive breast-feeding among women receiving a breast pump (n = 43) and those not receiving a breast pump (n = 44). (Courtesy of Dungy CI, Christensen-Szalanski J, Losch M, et al: *Pediatrics* 90:233–237, 1992.)

whether a woman exclusively breast-fed her infant. In particular, women who indicated that ease of nighttime feeding was an important factor were significantly more likely to breast-feed their infant over the entire 8 weeks if they received the breast pump rather than the infant formula.

Implications.—The provision of a breast pump in the hospital discharge package is an easily implemented, low-cost intervention that may increase the duration of exclusive breast-feeding. Furthermore, maternal attitudes are important predictors of duration of breast-feeding, and ease of nighttime feeding may interact with the provision of manual breast pumps in predicting breast-feeding behavior.

▶ As researchers continue to record the powerful effects of breast-feeding in reducing the incidence of acute infections in infancy as well as possibly lessening the prevalence of chronic disease in adults, it is imperative that we explore procedures to increase the relatively low incidence of breast-feeding in the United States compared with other countries in the Western world. Sweden, with one of the highest rates of breast-feeding, has specific interventions that have been demonstrated to contribute to a much larger percentage of women who breast-feed for a longer time. These include discussing with both parents during pregnancy the importance to the infant of breast-feeding, routine suckling in the first hour of life, breast-feeding classes in the hospital, and strong lactation support after discharge. Of special interest in this report is that mothers who benefitted the most from receiving a breast pump were those who believed that bottle feeding made nighttime feeding easier. If these women received a breast pump, 33% breast-fed for the entire 8 weeks of the study, whereas if they were given infant formula, 8.3% exclusively breast-fed their infants for 8 weeks ($P < .05$). Each move, gesture, gift, and discussion carries a meta-message.—M.H. Klaus, M.D.

Early Infant Diet and Risk of IDDM in Blacks and Whites: A Matched Case-Control Study

Kostraba JN, Steenkiste AR, Dorman JS, Gloninger M, LaPorte RE, Drash AL, Scott FW (Univ of Pittsburgh, Pa; Health and Welfare Canada, Ottawa, Ont, Canada)

Diabetes Care 15:626–631, 1992 9–11

Introduction.—It has been suggested that breast-feeding offers a protective effect against the development of insulin-dependent diabetes mellitus (IDDM), but other reports are contradictory. Diabetic children and their nondiabetic siblings were studied to determine the relationship between early infant feeding and IDDM.

Methods.—The study included both black and white participants. Black Americans have a lower incidence of IDDM and markedly different infant nutrition practices compared with white Americans. Individuals recruited for the study had IDDM diagnosed between 1965 and 1989 and were younger than 17 years of age at the time of diagnosis. Infant

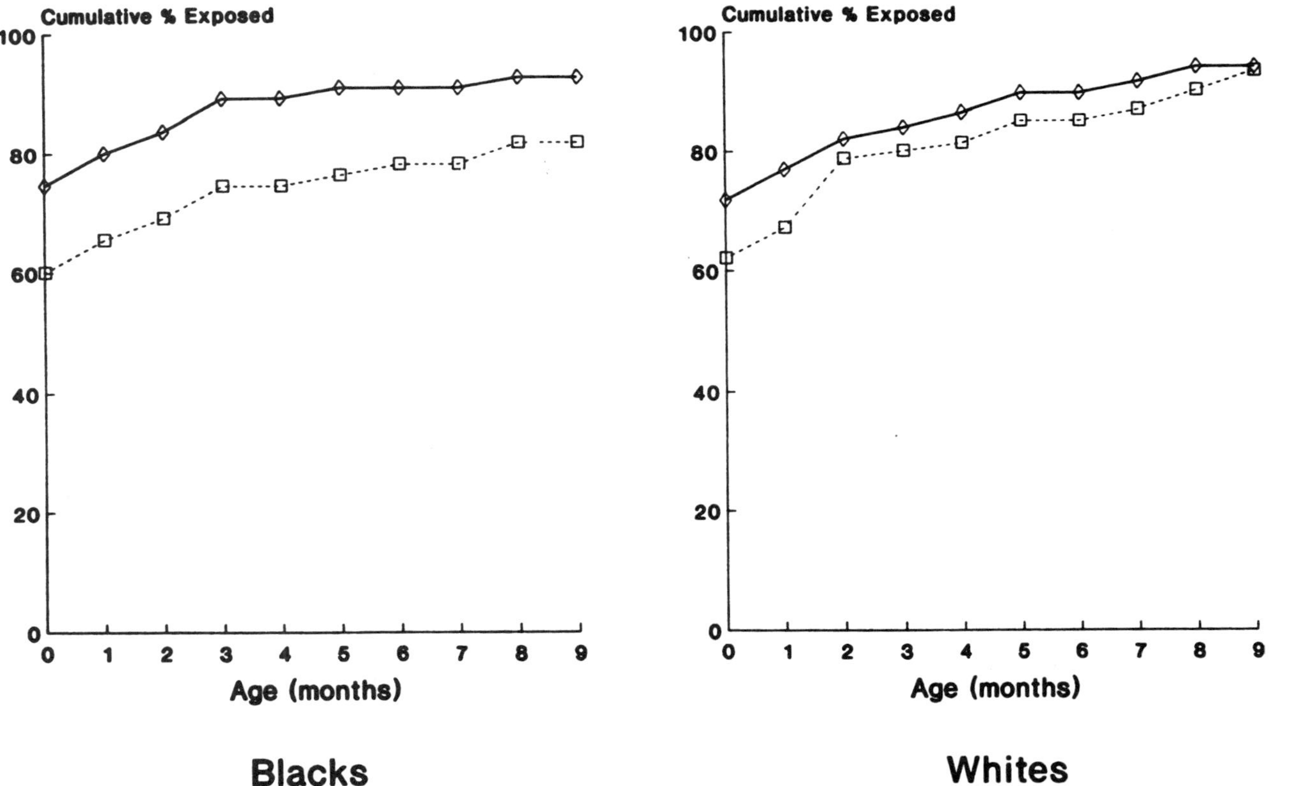

Fig 9–5.—Cumulative percentage of exposure to breast milk substitutes (*diamond*, diabetic; *square*, nondiabetic control) in blacks (54 diabetic and 54 control subjects) and whites (151 diabetic and 151 control subjects). The curves are significantly different by case-control status in blacks (P = .04, Wilcoxon's test) but not in whites (P = .33). (Courtesy of Kostraba JN, Steenkiste AR, Dorman JS, et al: *Diabetes Care* 15:626–631, 1992.)

nutrition data were collected by questionnaires mailed to the mothers. The medical records of the diabetic patients were also reviewed.

Results.—White diabetic subjects were less likely to have been breast-fed than control subjects. In blacks, breast-feeding status did not differ significantly between IDDM and control subjects. For both racial cohorts, duration of overall and exclusive breast-feeding did not differ between diabetics and controls. White diabetics and controls were exposed at a similar age to breast-milk substitutes and cow's milk-based substitutes. Black diabetics were exposed significantly earlier than black controls to breast milk substitutes (Fig 9–5).

Conclusion.—In this study cohort, the protective effect of breast-feeding on the risk of IDDM was related to the age at first exposure to breast milk substitutes in blacks, but not in whites. It is possible that low-risk populations, such as blacks, have a smaller genetic influence and may be more strongly affected by environmental factors. The growing trend in breast-feeding has not resulted in a decline in IDDM incidence, suggesting that breast milk alone is not protective.

▶ Although the editors of the YEAR BOOK OF NEONATAL AND PERINATAL MEDICINE are especially interested in the advantages of breast milk, we have stayed clear of an ongoing discussion as to whether complete and extended breast-feeding in infancy reduces the incidence of diabetes. This study was stimulated in part by animal studies noting that early exposure to cow's milk protein at weaning could trigger diabetes, as well as by a Finnish study that noted that diabetic children, as infants, had an earlier introduction of supplementary milk feeding. The inclusion of this inconclusive report begins a closer reporting of this interesting question. We await further evidence.—M.H. Klaus, M.D.

Infant Cerebral Cortex Phospholipid Fatty-Acid Composition and Diet

Farquharson J, Cockburn F, Patrick WA, Jamieson EC, Logan RW (Royal Hosp for Sick Children, Glasgow, Scotland)

Lancet 340:810–813, 1992 9–12

Background.—Growth of the brain is accompanied by an increase in incorporation of long-chain polyunsaturated fatty acids (PUFAs) into the phospholipid of the cerebral cortex, but it is not clear that nutrition in early infancy influences later neurologic development and function. If so, it is likely that essential fatty acids and their metabolites are most susceptible.

Objective and Methods.—Gas chromatographic methods were used to determine the phospholipid fatty acid composition of cortical gray matter in 20 term infants and 2 preterm infants who had died "cot deaths." The findings were related to the milk diet that had been given. All were

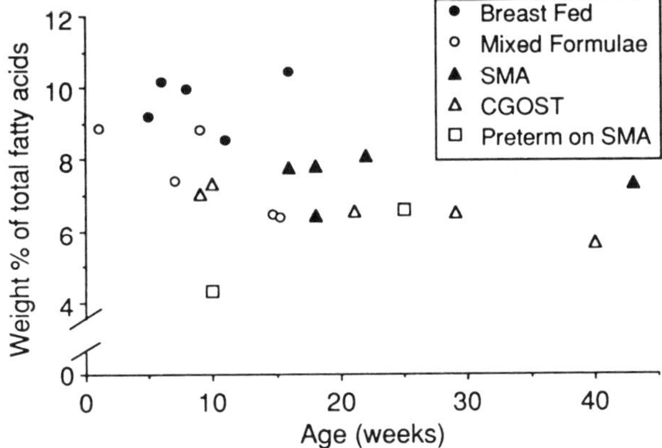

Fig 9–6.—Cerebral cortex phospholipid docosahexaenoic acid (C22L6n-3) in relation to infants' diet and age. (Courtesy of Farquharson J, Cockburn F, Patrick WA, et al: *Lancet* 340:810–813, 1992.)

previously healthy infants who had died suddenly at home, within 43 weeks of birth.

Findings.—The mean percent of docosahexaenoic acid was significantly greater in infants fed breast milk than in those of comparable age who received formula (Fig 9–6). In formula-fed infants, the percentage of long-chain PUFAs was maintained through increased incorporation of major n-6 series fatty acids.

Recommendations.—At least trace amounts of docosahexaenoic acid should be included in artificial formulas. Those formulas designed specifically for preterm infants should contain arachidonic acid as well.

▶ Commenting on this article is Art D'Harlingue, M.D., Neonatologist, Children's Hospital, Oakland, California:

▶ This article demonstrates that variations in dietary PUFAs alter the composition of PUFAs in infant cerebral cortex phospholipids. Previous articles have found comparable results with respect to other human tissues, including plasma and red blood cell membrane. Past studies of fatty acid composition primarily focused on linoleic and linoleic acids (the first fatty acids in the n-6 and n-3 series, respectively). Linoleic acid has clearly been shown to be an essential fatty acid. Whether linoleic acid is essential has remained unanswered. Linoleic and linoleic acids can be metabolized in vivo to longer chain (— 20 C) PUFA's. Two particular long-chain PUFAs, arachidonic acid and docosahexaenoic acid (DHA), are incorporated in large amounts into developing brain and retinal phospholipids. However, the human infant may be limited in its ability to synthesize longer chain PUFAs from linoleic and linoleic acid. For the rapidly growing newborn, dietary DHA may be conditionally essential for normal neural development. The premature infant may be especially at risk because of interruption in the normal transfer of long-chain

PUFAs across the placenta. Currently available infant formulas and techniques of total parenteral nutrition do not provide dietary DHA, arachidonic acid, or other long-chain PUFAs. This is particularly important in light of the observed negative effects of dietary deficiency of DHA on visual function in animals and humans. Further work is needed to define the function of DHA and other long-chain PUFAs in the brain and retina. The enteral and parenteral dietary requirements for DHA, arachidonic acid, and other long-chain PUFAs need to be defined for premature and term infants. New infant formulas and intravenous lipid emulsions containing DHA and other long-chain PUFAs will likely need to be developed.—A. D'Harlingue, M.D.

Changes in the Plasma Aminogram of Parenterally Fed Infants Treated With Dexamethasone for Bronchopulmonary Dysplasia

Ng PC, Brownlee KG, Kelly EJ, Henderson MJ, Smith M, Dear PRF (St James's Univ Hosp, Leeds, England)

Arch Dis Child 67:1193–1195, 1992 9–13

Background.—Some amino acids, such as phenylalanine, have a potentially toxic effect. The plasma aminogram in parenterally fed preterm infants was monitored before and during dexamethasone treatment for bronchopulmonary dysplasia (BPD).

Methods.—From 1987 to 1990, 59 parenterally fed preterm infants receiving dexamethasone for BPD were studied. Steroids were started at a mean of 20 days of age. All infants received a 3-week course of dexamethasone, beginning at .6 mg/kg/day, then dropping to .3 mg/kg/day in the second week and .15 mg/kg/day in the third week. As a matter of protocol, the infants were given parenteral nutrition on the second day of life. Plasma aminograms were checked weekly for as long as the infants were receiving parenteral nutrition.

Findings.—There was a marked increase in the plasma concentration of most amino acids in the infants shortly after dexamethasone treatment was begun. The size of the increase seemed to be related to dose. However, neither phenylalanine nor tyrosine concentrations were significantly elevated.

Conclusion.—In a group of infants with chronic lung disease, a substantial, apparently dose-related increase in plasma concentration of most amino acids occurred soon after dexamethasone treatment was begun. This phenomenon probably resulted from steroid-induced protein catabolism.

▶ Commenting on this article is Art D'Harlingue, M.D., Neonatologist, Children's Hospital, Oakland, California:

▶ Glucocorticoids have been shown to be beneficial in the treatment of bronchopulmonary dysplasia (BPD). Various studies have shown improved pulmonary compliance, shortened duration of mechanical ventilation, reduced oxygen requirements, and improved neurodevelopmental outcome in steroid-treated patients as compared with controls. Although one study showed a decrease in the number of days of supplemental oxygen administration, this effect was not found in other studies. The lengths of hospitalization and survival generally have not been affected by the use of steroids in BPD. With the wider use of steroids for BPD, a number of complications have been identified, including sepsis, hypertension, hyperglycemia, cardiomyopathy, gastrointestinal bleeding, suppressed adrenal function, and impaired growth. High-dose glucocorticoids also increase protein catabolism and urinary nitrogen excretion. Impairment of growth by high-dose steroids is especially worrisome for small premature infants, who should be growing postnatally at roughly the intrauterine third-trimester growth rate of 10–15 g/kg/day.

This study by Ng et al. provides further insight into the growth problems of infants with BPD who are treated with high-dose steroids. The generalized hyperaminoacidemia demonstrated in this study is probably secondary to an increase in protein catabolism. The combination of poor growth, hyperaminoacidemia, and presumed increased urinary nitrogen excretion during administration of high-dose steroids for BPD raises several issues in the nutritional management of these infants. Would an increase in caloric and protein intake, above the usual requirements calories alone, be demanded in light of a mostly generalized hyperaminoacidemia on steroids? Would the provision of an anabolic hormone such as exogenous insulin (concurrent with increased administration of glucose, as needed) or growth hormone maintain normal weight gain and improve nitrogen retention during administration of high-dose steroids? Perhaps some of the failure of steroid therapy for BPD in reducing the time of oxygen and supplementation length of hospitalization is a result of impaired lung growth, increased protein catabolism of respiratory muscle, and other effects on general growth.—A. D'Harlingue, M.D.

Low Bone Mineral Content in Summer-Born Compared With Winter-Born Infants

Namgung R, Mimouni F, Campaigne BN, Ho ML, Tsang RC (Univ of Cincinnati, Ohio; Children's Hosp Research Found, Cincinnati, Ohio; Yonsei Univ, Seoul, Korea; Magee-Women's Hosp, Pittsburgh, Pa)

J Pediatr Gastroenterol Nutr 15:285–288, 1992 9–14

Background.—Several studies of adults have shown a trend toward lower bone mineral content (BMC) during the winter months, perhaps the result of seasonal changes in vitamin D metabolism or seasonal variations in bone remodeling activity. With the assumption that variations in BMC are related to vitamin D status, the hypothesis that BMC in newborns would be lower in winter than in summer was examined.

Methods.—The study subjects were 55 healthy newborns enrolled for a longitudinal nutrition study during summer (July–September 1988) or

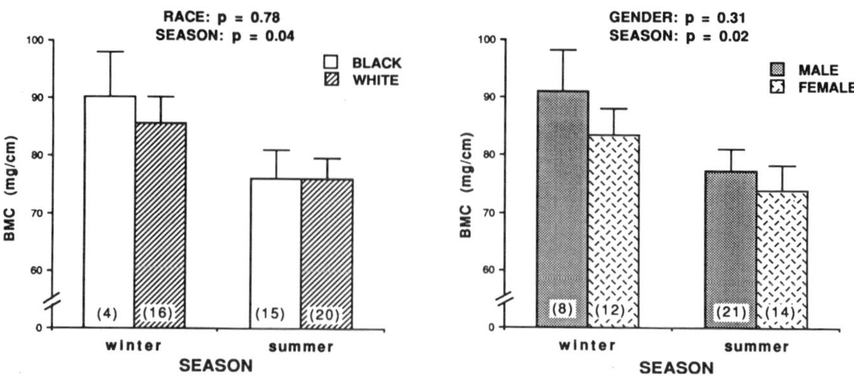

Fig 9–7.—Newborn BMC in winter and summer by race and gender. Values are mean ± standard deviation and are expressed as milligram per centimeter of bone. Number of newborns is shown in parentheses. Seasonal differences in BMC were statistically significant even when controlling for race and gender individually or together. (Courtesy of Namgung R, Mimouni F, Campaigne BN, et al: *J Pediatr Gastroenterol Nutr* 15:285–288, 1992.)

winter (January–March 1989). The group included 36 white infants and 19 black infants; 29 were boys and 26 were girls. A single-beam photon absorptiometer suitable for infant measurement was used to determine BMC. At least 3 scans of the distal radius were obtained, and the mean value was used for analysis.

Results.—The summer- and winter-born newborns did not differ in birth weight or gestational age. Summer-born newborns had a significantly lower mean BMC value than did infants born during winter months (75.94 mg/cm vs. 86.55 mg/cm). There were no significant race or gender differences in the mean values of BMC. Seasonal differences in BMC remained significant after controlling for race or gender, or both (Fig 9–7). Mean bone width also showed a significantly lower value in summer, compared with winter (.467 cm vs. .521 cm).

Conclusion.—In adult studies, BMC has usually been lower in winter than in summer. The opposite finding in newborns suggests that maternal sunshine deprivation in winter may operate especially in early pregnancy, resulting in lower BMC at birth approximately 6 months later.

▶ Bone mineral content (BMC), as assessed via photon absorptiometry, has become a widely used yardstick for assessing the adequacy of bone mineralization in neonates. Using this procedure, Dr. Namgung et al. measured a significantly ($P = .035$) lower BMC among infants born during summer months than among those delivered during winter months. Dr. Namgung speculates that maternal vitamin D status in early pregnancy (during the winter months for the summer-born infants in his study) may have been low secondary to reduced exposure to the sun, resulting in a lower BMC 6 months later for the summer-born infants. No maternal vitamin D data are presented to support or refute this proposed first-trimester effect on the fetus. Furthermore, much accretion data are published that indicate calcium is retained by the fetus (presumably for bone mineralization) primarily during the third trimester of pregnancy.

The dietary intake of calcium and phosphorus in neonates appears to dictate the skeletal accretion of minerals. To date, no significant correlation has been reported between neonatal BMC and either neonatal or maternal serum vitamin D or any other calcium homeostatic factor or marker. Nevertheless, because calcium homeostasis is clearly maintained by these hormonal regulators, bone mineralization must also be related to them. Similarly, although maternal calcium regulating hormones may, in part, control fetal bone mineralization, no report of this relationship has been published.

Dr. Namgung et al. have described a unique observation and speculated on its etiology. This report represents a piece in the puzzle that requires further study to determine how it fits into the picture entitled "fetal bone mineralization."—W.B. Pittard, III, M.D., Professor and Vice-Chairman, University of South Carolina Medical School, Charleston

---

Prevalence of Cystic Fibrosis in Fetuses With Dilated Bowel

Estroff JA, Parad RB, Benacerraf BR (Children's Hosp, Boston; Brigham and Women's Hosp, Boston)

Radiology 183:677–680, 1992 9–15

Introduction.—The finding of a dilated fetal bowel on sonography is usually a nonspecific result that can suggest a variety of intestinal abnormalities. Fetuses with cystic fibrosis have demonstrated dilated intestinal loops sonographically, but the incidence of this condition among these fetuses remains unknown. Findings were presented on the prevalence of cystic fibrosis in fetuses with bowel dilatation and any associated sonographic data in those who are so affected.

Methods.—A retrospective review of the medical records of all intra-abdominal dilated loops cases between February 1988 and October 1991 found 15 fetuses with these conditions. Cystic fibrosis was diagnosed using the quantitative pilocarpine iontophoresis sweat test.

Results.—Review of the 15 patients with fetal signs of intra-abdominal dilated loops showed that most had undergone initial scanning in the third trimester. Five of the 15 fetuses had cystic fibrosis, for a prevalence rate of 33%. Eleven of the neonates had bowel dilatation at birth based on abdominal radiographs, contrast material studies, or surgery; 4 of these infants had cystic fibrosis. Seven of the 11 had small bowel atresia or stenosis; 3 of these 7 had cystic fibrosis. In 6 of the 15 pregnancies, polyhydramnios developed, with 3 of the 6 occurring in cystic fibrosis fetuses. No overt sonographic characteristics for bowel dilatation differentiated the cystic fibrosis fetuses from those without this genetic disorder.

Conclusion.—Because cystic fibrosis has a high prevalence rate among infants with bowel obstruction, these results support the suggestion that the presence of dilated loops of bowel within the fetal abdomen should require prenatal parental testing for cystic fibrosis. The patient should then undergo ultrasound monitoring until delivery of the infant. This experience indicates that dilated loops persisting in the neonatal period always require surgery.

▶ These observations can now be added to the many other findings of fetal physiology derived from ultrasound. A dilated bowel in a fetus joins several other abdominal problems that require a sweat test at birth for ruling out cystic fibrosis, including meconium plug and meconium ileus. A total of 80% of infants with meconium ileus and 25% of those with meconium plug have cystic fibrosis.—M.H. Klaus, M.D.

Biliary Atresia: A 25-Year Survey

Engelskirchen R, Holschneider AM, Gharib M, Vente C (Kinderchirurgische Klinik, Köln, Germany)

Eur J Pediatr Surg 1:154–160, 1991 9–16

Objective.—The role of operative treatment of biliary atresia has been questioned in view of the improved recovery and survival with liver transplantation. A 25-year experience with biliary atresia, with emphasis on hepatoporto-jejunostomies was reviewed.

Patients.—From 1963 to 1988, a total of 90 children were treated for biliary atresia. Forty-seven had purely extrahepatic bile duct lesions, 21 had purely intrahepatic bile duct lesions, and 22 had both. Forty-five children had no surgery or simply had a diagnostic laparotomy. The other 45 underwent a drainage procedure, including implantation of artificial bile ducts in 12, cholecystoduodenostomy in 4, or hepatoportojejunostomy with or without an enterostomy in 29.

Outcome.—Twenty-seven patients (30%) survived, including 8 of 29 patients (27.5%) who underwent hepatoportojejunostomy. However, even after introduction of the hepatoportojejunostomy, hepatic failure accounted for 52% of deaths. Current data for 23 surviving patients were studied. Only 10 children had normal liver function. Only 5 of the 29 patients who underwent hepatoportojejunostomy achieved a lasting postoperative biliary flow, and only 1 was completely healthy with regard to his liver function.

Discussion.—Although a 5-year survival rate of 25% to 30% can be achieved with hepatoportojejunostomy, complete recovery from the underlying disease is rare. In view of the encouraging results of transplantation in children with extrahepatic biliary atresia, liver transplantation appears to be the best rationally substantiated causal therapy, even if a hepatoportojejunostomy has been performed. In patients who manifest cirrhosis of the liver, a liver transplantation should be the method of choice.

► This article should satisfy even the most ardent linguists, as the manuscript is abstracted in French, German, and English. The series of 90 patients collected over 25 years had a 70% mortality rate, which indicates the severity of the disorder. The reader also gets a bird's-eye view of the change in the approach to therapy. The era commences with therapeutic nihilism; therefore, before 1971, diagnostic laparotomy without an operative bile drainage was performed in many of the patients (34). Most (31) were deemed inoperative, contributing to the high mortality rate. Before 1966, surgery was essentially comprised of a hepatogenostomy with implantation of artificial bile ducts. The Kasai-Kimura procedure (hepatoportojejunostomy) held count until the 1980s, when, with the availability of cyclosporine, hepatic transplantation emerged as the treatment of choice.

Since the introduction of cyclosporine, the survival rates for liver transplantation have ranged from 57% to 80%. The goals are to establish cholestasis within the first 4 weeks of life. The Kasai operation may be used as a temporary procedure but, ultimately, liver transplantation becomes necessary. Advanced imaging techniques have demystified the diagnosis of biliary atresia, which represents the end stage of a hepatic inflammatory process. See also References 1–3.

The excellent is new forever.—Ralph Waldo Emerson

A.A. Fanaroff, M.B.B.Ch.

References

1. Otte JB, et al: Z *Kinderchir* 43:99, 1988.
2. Starzl TE, et al: *Transplant Proc* 19:3230, 1987.
3. Pett S, et al: *Transplant Proc* 19:3256, 1987.

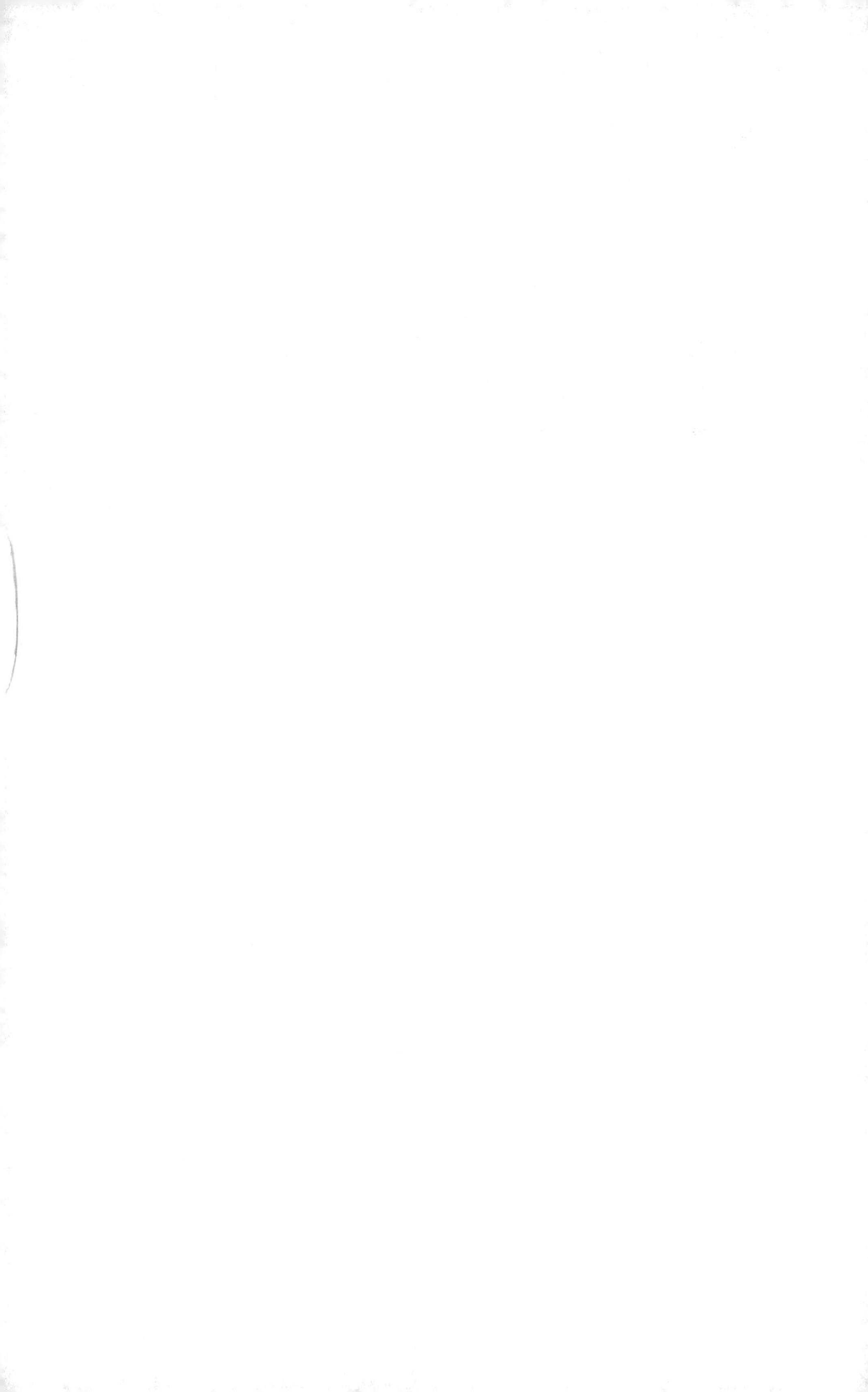

10 The Respiratory Tract

Respiratory Disease in Very-Low-Birthweight Infants After Prenatal Thyrotropin-Releasing Hormone and Glucocorticoid

Ballard RA, Ballard PL, Creasy RK, Padbury J, Polk DH, Bracken M, Moya FR, Gross I, and the TRH Study Group (Mount Zion Hosp and Med Ctr, San Francisco; Yale Univ, New Haven, Conn; Univ of Texas Health Science Ctr, Houston; et al)

Lancet 339:510–515, 1992 10–1

Background.—Despite prenatal glucocorticoid therapy, respiratory distress syndrome (RDS) and chronic lung disease (CLD) may develop in very-low-birth-weight (VLWB) infants. In a multicenter, blinded, randomized trial, researchers investigated the effect of additional prenatal treatment with thyrotropin-releasing hormone (TRH).

Methods.—Eligible participants were women with threatened preterm delivery at less than 32 weeks' gestation. Of the 404 women enrolled, 198 received betamethasone plus TRH (4 doses of 400 μg each given every 8 hours), and 206 were given betamethasone plus placebo. Complete data were available for 114 infants delivered to 99 women in the treatment group and for 117 infants of 105 women in the control group.

Results.—The 2 groups had no significant differences in birth weight, gestational age, mortality, gender, or racial distribution. In neonates with a birth weight less than 1,500 g, TRH treatment did not affect the total incidence of RDS (47% vs. 58% in control infants) or of severe RDS (13% vs. 25% in control infants). Chronic lung disease developed in significantly fewer TRH-treated infants (18%) than control infants (44%). The TRH group had significantly fewer adverse outcomes, defined as death or continuing oxygen requirement, than did the steroid-alone group both at 28 days and at 36 weeks after conception (Fig 10–1; table). Other complications of prematurity occurred at similar rates in the 2 groups. The women in the TRH group experienced more side effects (nausea, vomiting, and flushing) than did those in the steroid-alone group.

Conclusion.—Prenatal treatment with TRH plus glucocorticoid substantially reduced the occurrence of CLD in VLBW infants. There were no fetal deaths associated with TRH therapy and only minor maternal side effects.

▶ The obstetric team now has another weapon that significantly reduces infant morbidity. Again, this resulted from many years of laboratory studies,

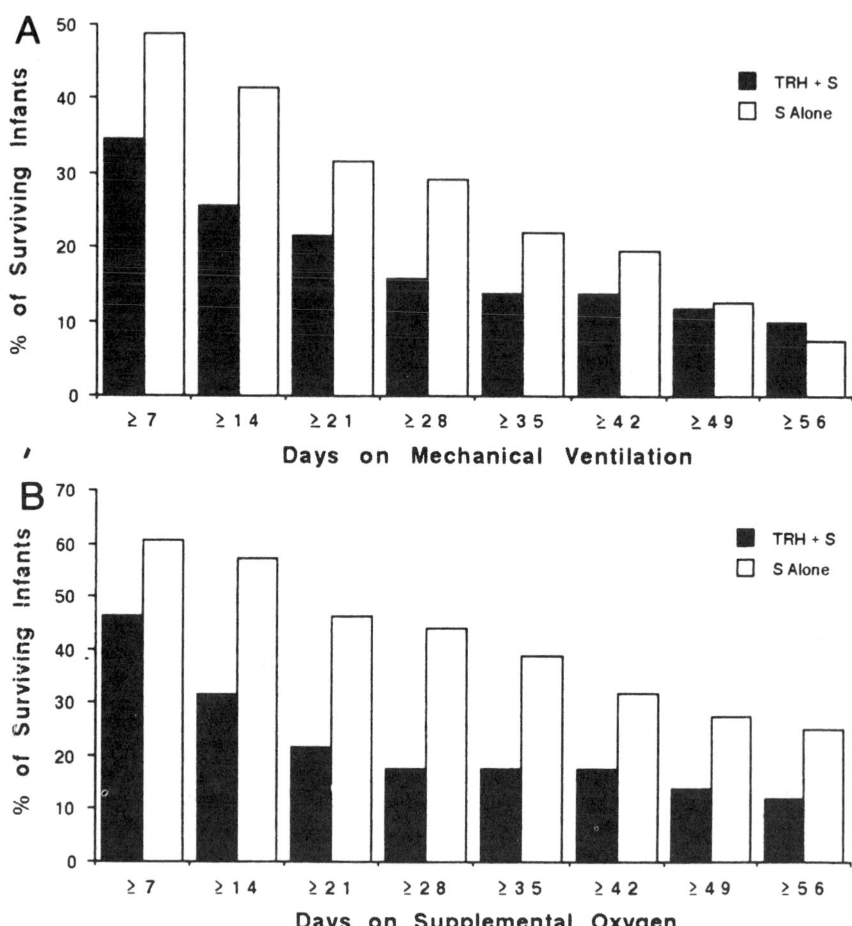

Fig 10–1.—Percentage of surviving, fully treated infants in each treatment group requiring assisted ventilation **(A)** and supplemental oxygen **(B)** during the first 8 weeks of life. (Courtesy of Ballard RA, Ballard PL, Creasy RK, et al: *Lancet* 339:510–515, 1992.)

and it emphasizes how important bench research is to clinical care. The real question is whether this approach will be applied? Sadly, there is evidence that a majority of mothers in premature labor will not receive antenatal prevention. It is well known that a course of maternal steroids started more than 24 hours before birth for infants less than 33 weeks' gestation significantly reduces the mortality from RDS and the incidence of chronic lung disease as well as necrotizing enterocolitis. Less than a quarter of the mothers in a recent large (6,744 infants) surfactant trial had been started on steroids. One measure of the quality of care on any obstetric floor should be whether every mother in premature labor is given both betamethasone and thyrotropin at an appropriate time.—M.H. Klaus, M.D.

Survival and Respiratory Status 28 Days After Birth and at 36 Weeks After Conception

Live-born infants	All treated infants* TRH+S (n=78)	All treated infants* S-alone (n=74)	Fully treated infants† TRH+S (n=55)	Fully treated infants† S-alone (n=48)
28 days				
Survivors *(%)*	72 *(92·3)*	66 *(89·2)*	51 *(92·7)*	41 *(85·4)*
O_2 requirement *(%)*	16/72 *(22·2)*	24/66 *(36·4)*	9/51 *(17·6)*	18/41 *(43·9)*‡
Adverse outcome *(%)*§	22/78 *(28·2)*	32/74 *(43·2)*	13/55 *(23·6)*	25/48 *(52·1)*‡
36 weeks' postconception				
Survivors *(%)*	72 *(92·3)*	65 *(87·8)*	51 *(92·7)*	40 *(83·3)*
O_2 requirement *(%)*	10/72 *(13·9)*	13/65 *(20·0)*	6/51 *(11·8)*	10/40 *(25·0)*¶
Adverse outcome *(%)*§	16/78 *(20·5)*	22/74 *(29·7)*	10/55 *(18·2)*	18/48 *(37·5)*‡

* Three or fewer doses of TRH or placebo.
† Four doses of TRH or placebo.
‡ $P < .01$.
§ Adverse outcome is defined as death or chronic lung disease (requirement for supplemental oxygen).
¶ $P = .1$.
(Courtesy of Ballard RA, Ballard PL Creasy RK, et al: *Lancet* 339:510–515, 1992.)

Inositol Supplementation in Premature Infants With Respiratory Distress Syndrome

Hallman M, Bry K, Hoppu K, Lappi M, Pohjavuori M (Children's Hosp, Helsinki, Finland; Univ of California, Irvine)
N Engl J Med 326:1233–1239, 1992 10–2

Background.—Serum concentrations of inositol increase in premature infants fed breast milk, but they tend to decrease in infants receiving parenteral nutrition. Studies have shown that inositol administered to immature animals increases levels of pulmonary surfactant. The results of a trial in which infants with respiratory distress syndrome who were receiving parenteral nutrition and were treated with inositol during the first 5 days of life were evaluated.

Methods.—The placebo-controlled, randomized, double-blind trial was carried out between 1985 and 1989. Two hundred twenty-one infants with a gestational age of 24–32 weeks and a birth weight of less than 2,000 g were included in the trial. All were treated with mechanical ventilation, and some were treated with human surfactant as well. The 114 infants randomized to inositol received 80 mg per kg of body weight per day. The infusions were first given from 4 to 12 hours after birth and subsequently at 12-hour intervals.

Primary Outcomes in the Study Groups at the Age of 28 Days

Outcome	Placebo (N = 107)	Inositol (N = 114)	P Value
	no. of infants (%)		
Death during first 28 days	26 (24)	13 (11)	0.012
Survival up to 28 days			
With bronchopulmonary dysplasia	26 (24)	20 (18)	0.22
Without bronchopulmonary dysplasia	55 (51)	81 (71)	0.005

* There was a significant difference in the distribution of the infants in the study groups in relation to the 3 outcomes ($P = .002$ by the Wilcoxon-Mann-Whitney test). Neonatal mortality was significantly lower in the inositol group, after adjustment for the infants' characteristics by logistic regression ($P = .015$).

(Courtesy of Hallman M, Bry K, Hoppu K, et al: *N Engl J Med* 326:1233–1239, 1992.)

Results.—The primary end point of the study was survival at 28 days without bronchopulmonary dysplasia. Significantly more infants given inosital achieved this outcome (table). Infants receiving inositol had lower mortality resulting from pulmonary causes (6%) than infants in the placebo group (16%). Compared with placebo, inositol resulted in significantly lower mean requirements for inspiratory oxygen and mean airway pressure from the 12th through the 144th hour of life. Retinopathy of prematurity occurred in 13% of the infants who were given inositol and 26% of those given placebo. Among the infants given placebo, there was an association between poor outcome and lower serum inositol concentrations during days 2 through 7.

Conclusion.—Inositol treatment increased serum inositol concentrations in premature infants with respiratory distress syndrome and decreased the likelihood of severe, chronic injury of the lung and the retina. Inositol supplementation is recommended for premature infants.

▶ There is a portion of the equation that must be missing. If the simple addition of inositol during the early days of life enhances endogenous surfactant production, reduces the incidence of chronic lung disease and, as an unanticipated bonus, also decreases the rate of retinopathy, why aren't more infants with respiratory problems receiving inositol supplementation? The answer did not jump out at me from this manuscript, although it did become apparent that the inositol supplementation was only worthwhile in the first week of life. Furthermore, inositol did not seem to potentiate the effect of exogenous surfactant, and the precise mechanism of action is unknown.

The small print sometimes makes for interesting reading. The laborious but necessary methodology concludes with the statistical analysis. The purpose of this study, to increase survival without bronchopulmonary dysplasia by

15% (above an anticipated rate of 50% in the placebo group) required 220 infants in each limb, for an alpha error of 2% and a power of 80%. Interim looks were scheduled after every 100 patients, and the monitoring committee recommended stopping the trial after the second look because of the increased survival, without BPD and no trend to serious morbidity. (The actual rate of death of BPD was 49%. Thus, we have a well-designed study.

The interrelationships between nutrition and pulmonary disorders is coming under closer scrutiny. Inositol is a component of membrane phospholipids, and it is abundantly present in colostrum. It is absent from currently used neonatal intravenous solutions and is present in small amounts in formula. Nutritional deprivation may impair surfactant synthesis, decrease respiratory center activity, and decrease respiratory muscle strength. Oxygen toxicity is enhanced by undernutrition and modified by lipid status; vitamins A, C, and E are an integral part of the antioxidant defense team (1). An integrated approach to nutrition and pulmonary management is needed to resolve these many complicated issues. Perhaps then the role of inositol will be clarified.—A.A. Fanaroff, M.B.B.Ch.

Reference

1. Frank L, Sosenko IR: *Am Rev Resp Dis* 138:725, 1988.

A Cohort Study of Transcutaneous Oxygen Tension and the Incidence and Severity of Retinopathy of Prematurity

Flynn JT, Bancalari E, Snyder ES, Goldberg RN, Feuer W, Cassady J, Schiffman J, Feldman HI, Bachynski B, Buckley E, Roberts J, Gillings D (Univ of Miami, Fla; Univ of Pennsylvania, Philadelphia; Univ of North Carolina, Chapel Hill)

N Engl J Med 326:1050-1054, 1992 10–3

Introduction.—Retinopathy of prematurity is a cause of visual impairment and blindness. An association between retinopathy of prematurity and the duration of exposure to supplemental oxygen in premature infants has been suggested, but a specific threshold level of arterial oxygen tension has not been identified. The incidence and severity of retinopathy of prematurity in preterm infants requiring supplemental oxygen were correlated with the duration of exposure to arterial oxygen levels of 80 mm Hg or higher measured transcutaneously ($tcPo_2$).

Methods.—The study cohort included 101 premature infants with birth weights ranging from 500 to 1,300 g who required supplemental oxygen administration. The number of hours during which the $tcPo_2$ was 80 mm Hg or higher during the first 4 weeks of life was tabulated for each infant. Indirect ophthalmoscopy was performed as soon as the infant reached the postconceptional age of 32 weeks and was in stable clinical condition, and it was repeated every 2–4 weeks until discharge.

Results.—Retinopathy of prematurity developed in 52 of the 101 premature infants. The disease occurred in 19 (86%) of 22 infants weighing less than 900 g. Retinopathy was moderate or severe in 15 infants and mild in the other 37 infants. Prolonged exposure to $tcPo_2$ of 80 mm Hg or higher during the first 4 weeks after birth was associated with an increase in both the incidence and the severity of retinopathy of prematurity. The odds ratio for each 12-hour period in which the $tcPo_2$ was 80 mm Hg or higher was 1.9 after adjusting the data for the confounding influence of low birth weight, low Apgar score, and exposure to inspired oxygen at a fractional concentration. The association remained significant. A precise threshold level of $tcPo_2$ that is toxic to the retina could not be identified and may not exist.

Conclusion.—The incidence and severity of retinopathy of prematurity in premature infants requiring supplemental oxygen are associated with the duration of exposure to arterial oxygen levels of 80 mm Hg or higher as measured by continuous transcutaneous monitoring during the first 4 weeks of life.

Early Versus Delayed Neonatal Administration of a Synthetic Surfactant: The Judgment of OSIRIS

The OSIRIS Collaborative Group (Radcliffe Infirmary, Oxford, England)

Lancet 340:1363–1369, 1992 10–4

Introduction.—The administration of exogenous surfactant can greatly reduce the morbidity and mortality of infants at risk for or with signs of respiratory distress syndrome (RDS). In the OSIRIS trial (Open Study of Infants at High Risk of or With Respiratory Insufficiency, The Role of

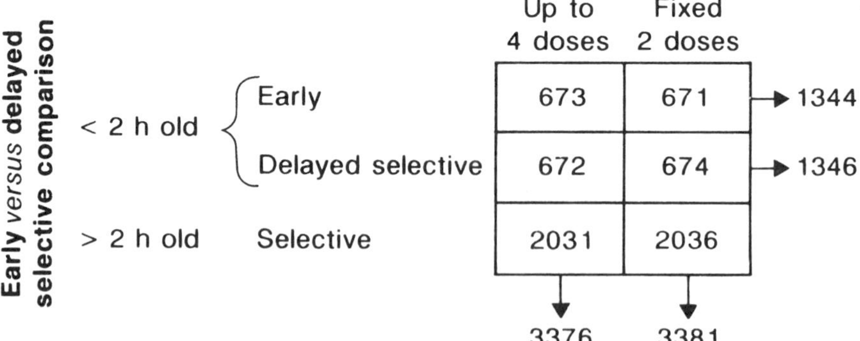

Fig 10–2.—Derivation of study groups. (Courtesy of the OSIRIS Collaborative Group: *Lancet* 340:1363–1369, 1992.)

Surfactant), attention was focused on when the surfactant should be started and how often it should be given.

Methods.—The trial began when surfactant was introduced into clinical practice. Data were gathered from 229 centers in 21 countries between April 1990 and December 1991 when 6,774 infants were recruited to the trial. Randomization was to early vs. delayed administration of Exosurf, a synthetic surfactant, and to 1 of 2 dosing protocols (Fig 10–2). Exosurf was given either in 2 doses 12 hours apart or with the option of third and fourth doses at 12- to 36-hour intervals if signs of RDS persisted or recurred.

Results.—Information on outcome was available for 6,757 infants (99.7%). Those allocated to early administration of surfactant had a better outcome than those allocated to delayed selective administration. Exosurf significantly reduced the risk of oxygen dependence or death when given to infants at high risk of RDS before age 2 hours. Early administration to an estimated 32 infants, when compared with treatment of established RDS, would prevent 1 infant's death and another infant from having long-term dependence on extra oxygen. The risk of pneumothorax was 32% lower with early administration. Similar outcomes were reported for the 2 dosing regimens in terms of death, long-term oxygen dependence, and other major morbidity.

Conclusion.—The early administration of exogenous surfactant to infants at high risk of RDS prevents both chronic lung disease and death. There is no evidence of benefit from continued administration of surfactant to infants who continue to show signs of RDS after the standard 2-dose regimen.

▶ This report is another example of how valuable and influential the Oxford Perinatal Group has been under the direction of Dr. Iain Chalmers in organizing large, well-assigned trials. Wide collaboration on an international scale has led to the recruitment of nearly 7,000 infants, making this the largest randomized control trial conducted in neontal medicine. Unfortunately, the results of the group's extensive evaluations of obstetric and neonatal care during the past 15 years have had less of an influence on perinatal care. As an example, less than 25% of the mothers in this large trial had been given antenatal corticosteroid to prevent the respiratory distress syndrome, a far less expensive and a most useful intervention. This report should be closely read by anyone working in the intensive care nursery.—M.H. Klaus, M.D.

Calf Lung Surfactant Extract Prophylaxis and Retinopathy of Prematurity

Repka MX, Hudak ML, Parsa CF, Tielsch JM (Johns Hopkins Univ, Baltimore)

Ophthalmology 99:531–536, 1992 10–5

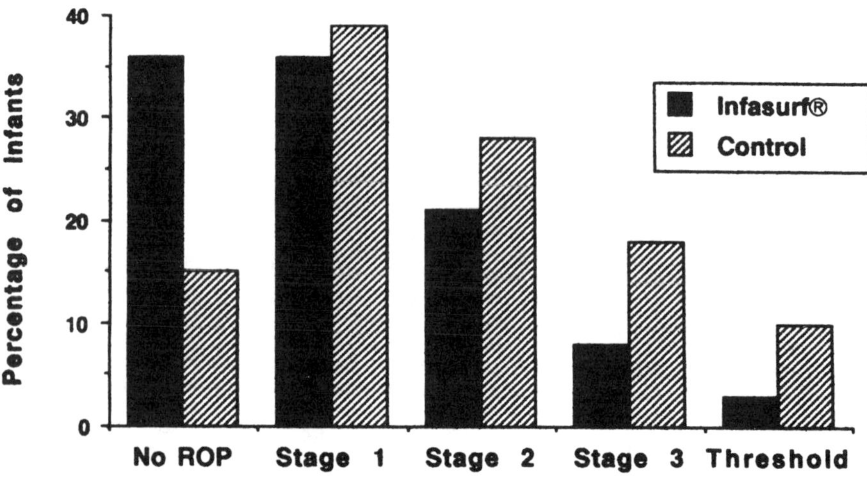

Fig 10–3.—Histogram of the percentages of the most advanced stage of active ROP achieved by control and Infasurf-treated infants. (Courtesy of Repka MX, Hudak ML, Parsa CF, et al: *Ophthalmology* 99:531–536, 1992.)

Background.—Despite advances in neonatal care and surgical interventions, retinopathy of prematurity (ROM) remains an important cause of blindness in extremely low-birth-weight (≤ 1,000 g) infants. Surfactant therapy, which reduces the severity of respiratory distress syndrome in these infants, may also lessen the incidence of ROP. The effect of prophylactic treatment with calf lung surfactant extract (Infasurf) on the ophthalmologic and pulmonary outcomes of extremely-low-birth-weight infants was examined retrospectively.

Methods.—A prophylactic surfactant protocol was introduced at Johns Hopkins Hospital in May 1988. The records of extremely-low-birth-weight infants born at the hospital during 1986 and 1987 and between May 1988 and May 1990, intervals before and immediately after initiation of the protocol, were reviewed.

Results.—There were 131 eligible infants in the 2-year presurfactant period and 112 in the surfactant period. The 2 groups did not differ with respect to birth weight, gestational age, race, or gender. The introduction of Infasurf was associated with reduced mortality (21% vs. 37%) and increased intact cardiopulmonary survival (39% vs. 18%). The incidence of total ROP was signficantly less in the infants treated with surfactant (64%) than in the control group (85%); threshold ROP was substantially reduced (3.4% vs. 10%) (Fig 10–3). Survival to discharge was 79% in the surfactant-treated group and 63% in controls.

Conclusion.—The prophylactic use of surfactant in extremely low-birth-weight infants has no significant side effects and reduces the extent of lung disease. The findings, although not significant, suggest that surfactant may reduce the incidence and severity of retinopathy of prematurity.

▶ As we observe the remarkable improvement with pulmonary surfactant, several other important outcome measures are of special interest in relation to the quality of survival. However, this small trial was not randomized. The report gives me the opportunity to introduce all readers to a new volume entitled *Effective Care of the Newborn Infant,* edited by John Sinclair and Michael Bracken (1), a book that should be in every hospital that cares for infants. The authors of this most important volume have collected all properly done randomized trials in the field of neonatal medicine and evaluated the results using a metanalysis. On the question at hand, they note that "prophylactics administered surfactant had no effect on the incidence of retinopathy in individual studies or assessed together." Much larger clinical trials and longer follow-up will be required to determine the effect of surfactant on the retinopathy of prematurity.—M.H. Klaus, M.D.

Reference

1. Sinclair JC, Bracken M: *Effective Care of the Newborn Infant.* Oxford Publishing, 1992.

Intratracheal Suctioning, Systemic Infection, and the Meconium Aspiration Syndrome

Wiswell TE, Henley MA (Walter Reed Army Med Ctr, Washington, DC)

Pediatrics 89:203–206, 1992 10–6

Introduction.—As many as 15% of all deliveries are complicated by the presence of meconium in the amniotic fluid, and approximately 5% of the infants will have meconium aspiration syndrome (MAS). The rate of death and infection from MAS has significantly decreased with the practice of immediate intratracheal suctioning of these neonates. Infants with MAS were retrospectively studied to determine the percentage that required resuscitation, the clinical outcomes of these newborns, and the types of cultured infections that occurred.

Methods.—After the medical records of all meconium-stained newborns seen from 1985 through 1989 were reviewed, infants requiring resuscitation were identified. Their data were assessed for meconium consistency, the need for intratracheal suctioning or intubation, hospital course, and outcome.

Results.—Seven hundred forty-one of the 5,697 liveborn infants (43%) had meconium staining, with 36 having MAS. Six hundred eight of the meconium-stained group, required intubation in the delivery room and underwent suctioning without complications. Five of the 46 culture-proved cases of bacteremia had been meconium-stained. Only 1 of the 36 newborns with MAS (2.8%) had bacteremia. Twenty of the 36 infants did not require positive-pressure ventilation during delivery. Those treated with positive-pressure ventilation immediately after birth had significantly lower 1- and 5-minute Apgar scores. Infants not suctioned had a significantly longer mean duration of oxygen treatment and experienced significantly more detrimental pulmonary sequelae than those who were suctioned promptly after birth.

Conclusion.—A substantial proportion of newborns with MAS have not depressed and do not require positive pressure ventilation immediately after birth. Neonates who have MAS after not being intubated may be at high risk for serious sequelae.

▶ Commenting on this article is David Durand, M.D., Neonatologist, Children's Hospital, Oakland, California:

▶ I like this paper; it confirms several things I have been saying to residents and general pediatricians for a number of years. Suctioning meconium is good. Not only does it build character for the suctioner, but it also is associated with a low incidence of complications and does not appear to be associated with a significantly increased risk of bacteremia. Furthermore, suctioned infants were at less risk for severe meconium aspiration syndrome, needing extracorporeal membrane oxygenation, or dying than were their nonsuctioned counterparts.

We all know that many meconium-stained infants do well without being suctioned. However, this is a dangerous thing to admit in public. There seems to be a natural tendency among pediatricians to avoid intubation and suctioning if at all possible. As this paper shows, this occasionally results in an infant who is not suctioned and in whom severe MAS develops. Be cautious—suction all of 'em!—D. Durand, M.D.

Lung Function and the Hering Breuer Reflex in the Neonatal Period
Chan V, Greenough A (King's College Hosp, London)
Early Hum Dev 28:111–118, 1992 10–7

Introduction.—The Hering Breuer reflex is readily elicited perinatally, even in premature infants. It has an important role in controlling lung volume, and it can influence both respiratory rate and tidal volume. Little is known of the process by which the reflex matures.

Methods.—The effects of intrauterine and extrauterine maturation on the Hering Breuer reflex were studied in premature infants weighing less than 2,000 g at birth. In addition, term infants with mild respiratory distress were studied in the first week of life. The 10 preterm infants had a median gestational age of 29.5 weeks; 8 were initially ventilator-dependent.

Results.—The Hering Breuer reflex was elicited in all infants throughout the neonatal period. The strength of the reflex did not correlate with postconceptional or postnatal age; it correlated inversely with static compliance and directly with tidal volume. The preterm infants had lung function similar to that of term infants when related to body weight.

Conclusion.—This study gave no evidence of intrauterine or extrauterine maturation of the Hering Breuer reflex in the neonatal period in infants with noncompliant lungs.

▶ The Hering Breuer reflex is mediated via stretch receptors in the lung. They are useful to study, because they, in part, control respiratory rate and tidal volume. Stimulation of these receptors decreases respiratory rate by lengthening the time of expiration. The reflex is especially responsive in the first hours of life, and it might be helpful in opening the alveoli of the neonate with their wide range of alveolar sizes. The reduced compliance or increased lung stiffness appears to be the most likely explanation for the similar responses over time.—M.H. Klaus, M.D.

Rate of Bronchopulmonary Dysplasia as a Function of Neonatal Intensive Care Practices

Van Marter LJ, Pagano M, Allred EN, Leviton A, Kuban KCK (Children's Hosp, Boston; Harvard School of Public Health, Boston)

J Pediatr 120:938–946, 1992 10–8

Introduction.—Neonates surviving the intensive care unit often have repeated bouts of bronchopulmonary dysplasia (BPD). The rates of occurrence of BPD differ among tertiary care centers. The BPD incidence results recorded as part of a prospective, randomized clinical trial on the effects of phenobarbital prophylaxis against intracranial hemorrhage in these infants were reported.

Methods.—A total of 280 infants were prospectively enrolled in the neonatal intensive care units of 3 Harvard-associated hospitals. The infants required intubation within the first 12 hours of birth, weighed less than 1,751 g, and had no intracranial hemorrhage. Seventy-six subjects had both clinical and radiographic evidence of BPD. Those with the highest inherent risk of BPD were assumed to be at the greatest risk for exposure to medical care practices influencing this BPD risk. The medical practices observed included oxygen toxicity, barotrauma, and fluid overload.

Results.—Using step-wise logic regression to follow prenatal and perinatal occurrences, the birth weight, gestational age, prebirth maternal glucocorticoid use, tracheal intubation, material toxemia, and neonatal intensive care unit admittance all significantly contributed to the model. The 3 neonatal intensive care units did not differ for birth weight, gestational age, or gender distribution, but they did differ significantly for toxemia during pregnancy, prenatal maternal glucocorticoid treatment, and delivery room intubation. Intensive care unit 1 used higher-than-expected colloidal volumes during the first 4 days whereas unit 3 used significantly lower amounts. Unit 1 had higher patent ductus arteriosus, but unit 2 had lower numbers than predicted. Maximum arterial oxygen tension was significantly less than expected at unit 3, which had the lowest bronchopulmonary dysplasia rate.

Conclusion.—These results did not support oxygen toxicity or the barotrauma hypothesis in the etiology of bronchopulmonary dysplasia in neonates in intensive care units. The data do show significant associations for 3 correlates of fluid therapy: birth-weight–adjusted intake of crystalloid and of colloidal fluids and signs of patent ductus arteriosus.

▶ Commenting on this article is David Durand, M.D., Neonatologist, Children's Hospital, Oakland, California:

▶ This is another study suggesting that we should not let our infants get too soggy. It agrees with the results of many other studies that tell us that high fluid loads are associated with an increased incidence of patent ductus arteriosus and BPD. The authors used some elegant statistics to tease out the impact of fluid intake from other confounding variables. However, it is important to realize that these are old, retrospective data. These patients were all treated from 1981 to 1984, and they were not enrolled in a study primarily looking at factors associated with BPD. How relevant these data are to the current era of surfactant treatment and conservative use of fluids is debatable.—D. Durand, M.D.

Spirometric and Endoscopic Evaluation of Airway Collapse in Infants With Bronchopulmonary Dysplasia

McCoy KS, Bagwell CE, Wagner M, Sallent J, O'Keefe M, Kosch PC (Univ of Florida, Gainesville)

Pediatr Pulmonol 14:23–27, 1992 10–9

Introduction.—Infants with bronchopulmonary dysplasia (BPD) sometimes have repetitive episodes of clinical deterioration with marked oxygen desaturation and cyanosis, termed "twit spells" or "pulmonary seizures." They have been ascribed to a wide range of possible causes, including airway hyperreactivity, gastroesophageal reflux, aspiration, seizures, laryngospasm, and tracheomalacia.

Objective and Methods.—Bedside spirometric monitoring was carried out in 8 infants with BPD and recurring episodes of agitation, cyanosis, and tachycardia or bradycardia not attributable to seizures, sepsis, or heart disease. Air flow was monitored using a pneumotachograph. Six infants were examined endoscopically during episodes that were elicited by toe pinching.

Findings.—Expirations were followed by the nearly complete cessation of air flow (Fig 10–4). Oxygen saturation declined rapidly, by as much as 20%. Electromyographic (EMG) activity, recorded from the abdomen and diaphragm, was very high. The episode ended with an inspiration. Exhaled volume during the episode appeared to be less than the

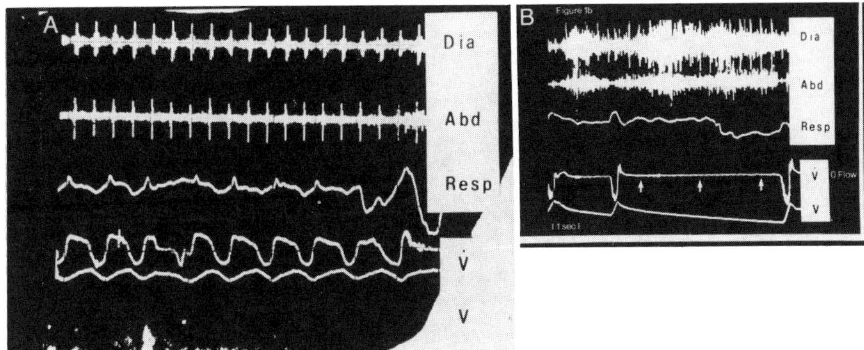

Fig 10–4.—**A,** a baseline tracing. The horizontal axis is time. *Abbreviations: Dia,* diaphragmatic EMG; *Abd,* abdominal EMG; *RESP,* Respitrace®; V̇, airflow; V, volume. Inspiration is an upward deflection for Resp and V and downward for V̇. The diaphragm EMG is contaminated with some expiratory abdominal signal. **B,** components are labeled as at baseline. This tracing demonstrates stimulation of the same infant, with recording made while the infant is agitated by toe pinch. Near complete, prolonged expiratory airflow cessation (marked by *arrows*) and extremely active expiratory EMG activity are evident. (Courtesy of McCoy KS, Bagwell CE, Wagner M, et al: *Pediatr Pulmonol* 14:23–27, 1992.)

inhaled tidal volume. The episodes resembled a prolonged Valsalva maneuver. Endoscopy revealed collapse of the tracheal walls during forced exhalation after elicitation of an episode. Both the anterior and posterior tracheal walls collapsed.

Interpretation.—Dynamic tracheal collapse during forced exhalation appears to underlie acute episodes of deterioration in infants with BPD. Acquired tracheomalacia probably is responsible.

Management.—Five of the more seriously affected infants underwent aortopexy. In all of them, extubation was possible shortly after surgery, although 4 infants had never been successfully extubated before. Four of the patients had no further BPD spells. There were no perioperative complications.

▶ Reading about infants with BPD who are still dependent on ventilators at 7 months or thereabouts brings to the surface a whole gamut of emotions: (1) the anger and frustration engendered by the inability to solve the seemingly daily setbacks of these complex chronically ventilator-dependent infants; (2) the empathy with and admiration for the courage and devotion shown by the families and nurses who are constantly trying to meet the child's needs; and (3) the guilt at having instituted life-saving interventions that have contributed to this enigmatic disorder. We look forward to the day when joy and glee predominate and BPD can be prevented.

This small, select series represents the remnants of the most severe cases of BPD. I expanded my vocabulary by adding "twit" spells to the already incomprehensible jargon used at the bedside. Inducing BPD spells while monitoring the airway changes with an endoscope in situ can euphemistically be called novel. I missed seeing a discussion on how easily this went through an institutional review board—if indeed it was reviewed. The findings were striking, and there was unequivocal demonstration of airway collapse and, in effect, a prolonged obstructive apnea provoked by tracheomalacia and dynamic airway collapse during expiration. Airway obstruction and hypoxia in infants with BPD has also been attributed to combinations of bronchospasm, gastroesophageal reflux, mucus plugs, respiratory infections, granulation formation, and extrinsic compression.

These problems with the major airways in BPD have been well documented in the past (1–3). The addendum to the manuscript, however, caught me completely off guard, as I could not make the logical move from documenting airway problems to correcting them with aortopexy, a technique first used by Malone for tracheomalacia and tracheobronchomalacia (4). I couldn't even find aortopexy in the 26th edition of *Dorland's Medical Dictionary.* Nonetheless, aortopexy was carried out in the 5 infants with the most severe BPD spells, and they were successfully extubated. "Aortopexy was a procedure associated with acceptable risks, which appeared to shorten the hospital course substantially." This was a radical, if successful, solution for BPD spells, which perhaps is something to consider when everything else is failing.—A.A. Fanaroff, M.B.B.Ch.

References

1. Bhutani VK, et al: *Am J Dis Child* 140:449, 1986.
2. Sotomayor JL, et al: *Am J Dis Child* 140:367, 1986.
3. McCubbin M, et al: *J Pediatr* 114:304, 1989.
4. Malone PS, Kiely EM: *Arch Dis Child* 65:438, 1990.

The Relationship Between Rhythmic Swallowing and Breathing During Suckle Feeding in Term Neonates

Bamford O, Taciak V, Gewolb IH (Univ of Maryland, Baltimore)
Pediatr Res 31:619–624, 1992 10–10

Background.—Suckle feeding by infants requires efficient coordination for the pharynx to alternate rapidly between functioning as an airway and as a peristaltic pump. The bolus must be totally cleared before the airway reopens to avoid aspiration. Food entering the lung parenchyma can produce inflammation and infection. Delayed swallowing can lead to apnea because breathing is inhibited.

Study Design.—Breathing and swallowing activity were recorded during bottle-feeding in 23 term infants aged 14 to 48 hours. The infants were fitted with a chest strain gauge to monitor chest motion, a nasal thermistor bead assembly to detect air temperature, a pulse oximeter probe, and a vinyl catheter with its tip at the back of the pharynx to record pharyngeal pressure. In addition, the ECG was recorded.

Observations.—A mean of 68% of the swallows were organized into runs, beginning at .6–.8 seconds and slowing to 1–1.3 seconds after

30–40 seconds. Run swallows were more prevalent with advancing age. Swallowing was more regular than breathing. The onset of suckle-feeding decreased both the rate of breathing and the tidal volume, and respiratory air flow became quite irregular. Mild desaturation was frequent but transient; the heart rate did not change. The most frequent sequence was inspiration-swallow-expiration, but swallows could occur in all phases of breathing.

Interpretation.—Newborn infants tend to reduce their breathing drive during suckle feeding. In maturing infants a pattern of coordination that permits ongoing rhythmic breathing probably develops, but how this occurs remains to be learned.

▶ For infants to suckle successfully, there must be coordination between breathing and swallowing. During swallowing, breathing is interrupted, because the pattern of swallowing includes vocal fold adduction and laryngeal compression, stopping airflow while stimulation of pharyngeal receptors inhibits respiration centrally. Thus, during swallowing, breathing stops, and food does not penetrate the airway. Initially, before good coordination occurs, minute ventilation decreases during sucking with a drop in oxygen saturation. Thus, neonates faced with maintaining both ventilation and swallowing reduce respiration; however, with maturation, this is not necessary. It is surprising how quickly such a complex task is mastered by the young neonate.—M.H. Klaus, M.D.

Upper Airway Patency During Apnea of Prematurity
Upton CJ, Milner AD, Stokes GM (City Hosp, Nottingham, England)
Arch Dis Child 67:419–424, 1992 10–11

Background.—Upper airway obstruction is an important factor in apnea in preterm infants, although pure obstructive apnea is rare. It is not clear whether mixed apnea is intrinsically longer than central apnea, or whether these types are part of a spectrum with initially central apnea becoming mixed over time.

Postulate.—It has been postulated that airway closure during central apnea may result in the occurrence of mixed apnea and may be detectable through the absence of cardiac artifact. To analyze this phenomenon in more detail and to determine its importance in the etiology of mixed apnea, a group of preterm infants was studied serially.

Methods.—Twenty-four preterm infants with a gestational age of 32 weeks or less, who were clinically stable in air, had upper airway air flow measured on 83 occasions. A patent airway was confirmed by transmission of a cardiac impulse up the airway.

Observations.—The 309 apneas (of 5 seconds or longer) recorded included 180 central (Fig 10–5), 109 mixed, and 20 obstructive. Airway patency persisted during only 53% of central apneas. The airway was

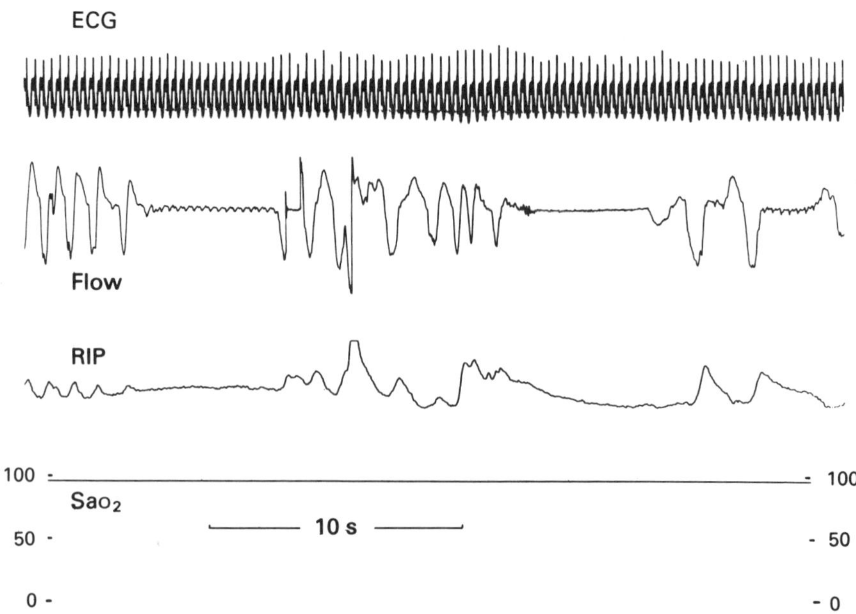

Fig 10–5.—Two short central apneic episodes, first with patent and second with closed upper airway. *Abbreviations: flow,* upper airway flow; *RIP,* abdominal respiratory inductive plethysmography. (Courtesy of Upton CJ, Milner AD, Stokes GM: *Arch Dis Child* 67:419–424, 1992.)

closed throughout in 72% of mixed apneas, including the central element. Mixed apneas were slightly longer than both central and obstructive apneas (table). Airway closure became more frequent as apnea persisted. The duration of apnea correlated closely with the fall in arterial oxygen saturation.

An Hypothesis.—It is proposed that central apnea occurs at end-expiration, often with the airway remaining patent. If airway closure ensues, the initial respiratory effort may overcome obstruction, leading to apparent central apnea. If the first respiratory effort fails to end obstruction, mixed apnea results. The site of airway obstruction remains to be defined.

▶ Richard J. Martin, M.D., Professor of Pediatrics at Case Western Reserve University, and Co-Director of Neonatology at Rainbow Babies and Children's Hospital, a career student of apnea, had the following comments:

▶ The findings of Upton and associates support the concept that upper airway (pharyngeal and/or laryngeal) closure may prolong a short central apnea into a clinically significant episode of mixed apnea, complete with desaturation. Therefore, the author's contention that central and mixed apnea are part of a continuum and are not separate entities seems quite plausible. Periodic breathing may also fit into that continuum, as the ventilatory cycles of

Duration of Apnea (Seconds) With Respect to Apnea Classification and Airway Patency

	Mean (SD)	*Median*	*Range*
Apnoea classification:			
Central (n=180)	6·8 (2·2)	6	5–19
Mixed (n=109)	11·0 (8·3)	8	5–51
Obstructive (n=20)	7·6 (3·4)	6·5	5–20
Airway patency:			
Open (n=102)	6·6 (2·0)	6	5–19
Closed (n=150)	9·7 (7·2)	7	5–51
Open→closed (n=48)	8·2 (4·6)	7	5–33
Closed→open (n=9)	6·0 (0·8)	6	5–7

(Courtesy of Upton CJ, Milner AD, Stokes GM: *Arch Dis Child* 67:419–424, 1992.)

periodic breathing may begin with an obstructed inspiratory effort or high resistance breath (1). It remains to be determined whether passive collapse of the compliant upper airway or failure of active contraction of upper airway dilating muscles (such as the genioglossus) is the major culprit. This model does not neatly explain why some episodes of mixed apnea begin with a series of obstructed inspiratory efforts. Moreover, the authors' rely on superimposition of cardiac artifact on the airflow tracing to indicate upper airway patency, and this is a pretty small amplitude signal whose absence may relate to factors other than airway closure. Regrettably, no one has established a spontaneously breathing neonatal animal model so that underlying mechanisms might be more accessible for study of this widespread clinical problem.—R.J. Martin, M.D.

Reference

1. Miller MJ, et al: *J Appl Physiol* 64:2496, 1988.

Small Preterm Infants (≤ 1500 g) Have Only a Sustained Decrease in Ventilation in Response to Hypoxia

Alvaro R, Alvarez J, Kwiatkowski K, Cates D, Rigatto H (Univ of Manitoba, Winnipeg, Canada)

Pediatr Res 32:403–406, 1992 10–12

Introduction.—The classic "biphasic" ventilatory response of preterm infants to 15% O_2 does not occur in the small (≤ 1,500 g), less-mature infants admitted to intensive care nurseries today. The hypothesis that these infants have a response closer to that of the fetus than that of larger neonates was tested.

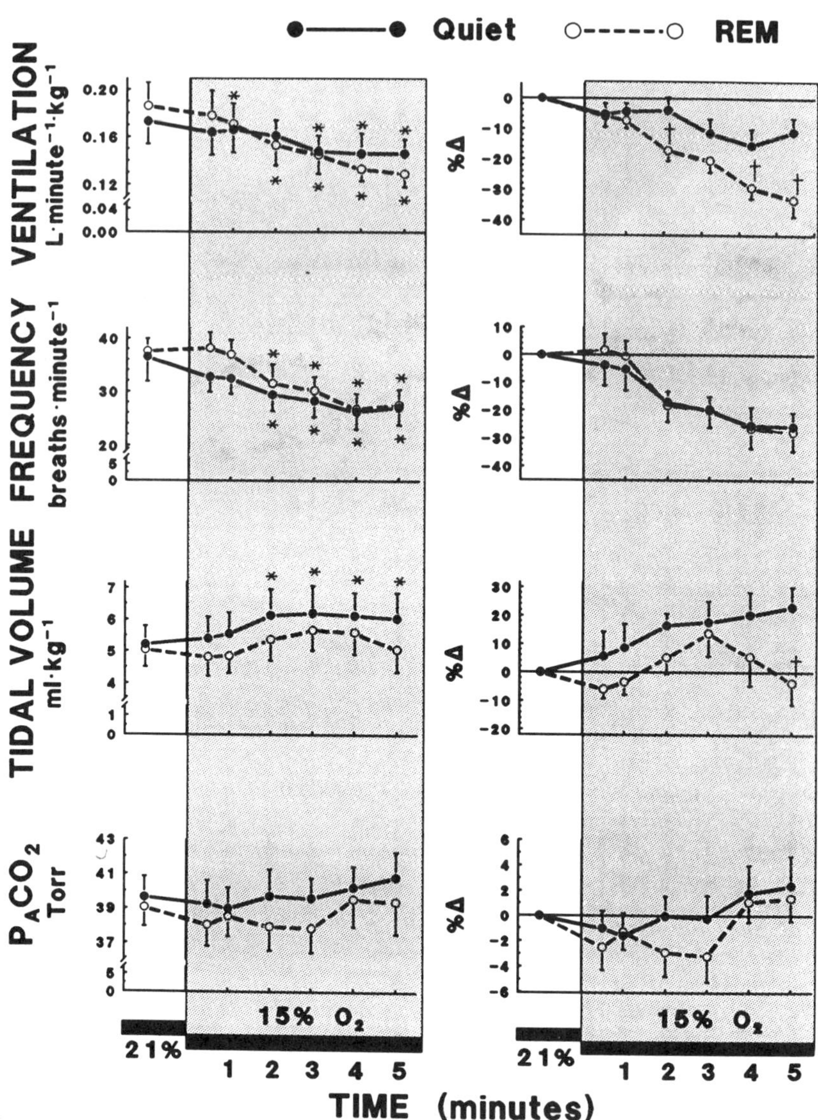

Fig 10–6.—Changes in ventilatory variables in response to 15% O_2. **Left,** sustained decrease in ventilation occurred in both sleep states, mainly because of a decrease in frequency. **Right,** percentages of change show that during REM sleep, ventilation decreased significantly more than in quiet sleep as a result of a lack of increase in tidal volume. Values are mean ± SEM; *asterisk* indicates $P \leq .05$ compared with control; *dagger*, $P \leq .05$ between sleep states. (Courtesy of Alvaro R, Alvarez J, Kwiatkowski K, et al: *Pediatr Res* 32:403–406, 1992.)

Methods.—The study subjects were 14 healthy preterm infants with a mean birth weight of 1,220 g and a mean gestational age of 29 weeks. The infants were studied during rapid eye movement and quiet sleep at a mean postnatal age of 17 days. A nosepiece and a screen flowmeter were used to measure respiratory minute volume and alveolar gases. Sleep states were defined by means of EEG, an electro-oculogram, and body movements.

Results.—The administration of 15% O_2 for 5 minutes resulted in an immediate and sustained decrease in ventilation in both sleep states. These changes in ventilation were primarily related to a decrease in frequency in both sleep states (Fig 10–6). There were negligible changes in tidal volume.

Conclusion.—The classic biphasic response of preterm infants to 15% O_2 consists of an immediate (30 seconds) increase followed by a late (5 minutes) decrease in ventilation. These small preterm infants showed only a sustained decrease in ventilation. The initial increase in ventilation reflecting peripheral chemoreceptor activity was never observed. Thus, the response in smaller preterm infants appears to be closer to that of the fetus, in which low O_2 abolishes breathing.

▶ Infants below a gestational age of 30 weeks appear to respond to hypoxia in a manner similar to the fetus who terminates breathing in low oxygen. The small increase in alveolar PCO_2 with 5 minutes of hypoxia has also been observed in other studies, and it suggests that the central depression is associated with a decrease in metabolism. As noted by the authors, the hypoxemia appears to act by an indirect suprapontine mechanism, because after lesions are placed in either the upper lateral pons or midbrain transaction at the midcollicular level, hypoxemia stimulates respiration without any evidence of depression.—M.H. Klaus, M.D.

Hypoxic Arousal Responses in Normal Infants
Ward SLD, Bautista DB, Keens TG (Childrens Hosp, Los Angeles)
Pediatrics 89:860–864, 1992 10–13

Background.—Failure to respond normally to hypoxia has been proposed as a possible mechanism in sudden infant death syndrome (SIDS), but most victims are not members of a high-risk group. If a disorder of hypoxic arousal is, in fact, important in SIDS, it is important to understand arousal responses to hypoxia in normal infants.

Study Design.—Hypoxic arousal was studied in 18 healthy term infants younger than age 7 months who were not receiving medication. The mean age at evaluation was 12 weeks. The inspired oxygen tension was rapidly lowered to 80 mm Hg for 3 minutes during quiet sleep or until the infant was aroused. A total of 25 challenges were carried out.

Observations.—Failure to arouse from quiet sleep was noted in 68% of challenges. These infants had a mean age of 14 weeks compared with 10 weeks for those who aroused. The mean values for saturation of arterial oxygen (SaO_2) before challenge were similar in those who aroused and those who did not, but the latter infants had significantly lower end-tidal carbon dioxide pressure (PCO_2) values. The lowest SaO_2 and inspired oxygen values during the challenge were not different in the 2 groups. In all cases, the end-tidal PCO_2 values declined during exposure to hypoxia, and the mean decrease was comparable in the 2 groups. Only 2 infants, both of whom failed to arouse, had periodic breathing during the hypoxic challenge, but this was the rule afterward in those who failed to arouse.

Implication.—Most healthy young infants fail to arouse when exposed to relatively mild hypoxia during quiet sleep, despite the apparent presence of a hypoxic ventilatory response. This may contribute to the pathogenesis of SIDS or to other respiratory deaths.

▶ As in other studies, 11% inspired oxygen for a period of 3 minutes failed to arouse the majority of normal infants, although it did result in an increase in ventilation in every infant, which suggests that the peripheral chemoreceptors were activated. Because other respiratory stimuli, such as airway occlusion and hypercapnia, are usually present in a clinical setting where acute hypoxia is observed, the isolated responses to acute hypoxia often are not appreciated. Fewell (1), who performed interesting studies in lambs, noted that the hypoxia arousal response is subject to habituation with repetitive exposure to hypoxia, resulting in progressively lower oxygen saturations to achieve arousal. Hypercapnia facilitated arousal to hypoxia, carotid body denervation significantly reduced the response, and hypoxia produced by airway obstruction played a role in arousal from active sleep but not quiet sleep.—M.H. Klaus, M.D.

Reference

1. Fewell JE, Konduri GG: *Pediatr Res* 24:28, 1988.

Spontaneous Desaturations in Intubated Very Low Birth Weight Infants With Acute and Chronic Lung Disease

Durand M, McEvoy C, MacDonald K (Univ of Southern California, Los Angeles)

Pediatr Pulmonol 13:136–142, 1992 10–14

Purpose.—Patients with chronic lung disease (CLD) have frequent episodes of spontaneous desaturations. Very-low-birth-weight (VLBW) infants frequently have CLD. A study was designed to quantify the frequency and severity of spontaneous desaturation episodes during assisted ventilation in VLBW infants with CLD and to compare the find-

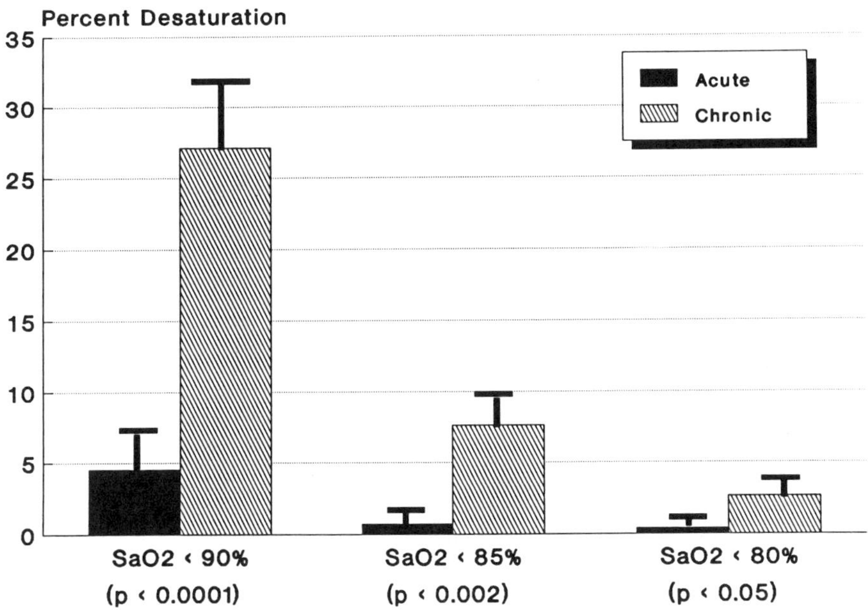

Fig 10–7.—The mean ± 1 SEM values of percent time of spontaneous desaturation below levels of 90% (data include all episodes < 90%), 85% and 80% pulse oximeter oxygen saturation (Sa_{O_2}) in 17 patients with acute disease and 17 infants with chronic lung disease. (Courtesy of Durand M, McEvoy C, MacDonald K: *Pediatr Pulmonol* 13:136–142, 1992.)

ings with those in VLBW infants with acute lung disease (ALD). Computerized pulse oximetry (CPO) was used to document spontaneous desaturation episodes.

Methods.—Four-hour CPO studies were performed in 34 intubated VLBW infants with birth weights ranging from 520 g to 980 g, of whom 17 with a mean postnatal age of 39.4 days had CLD and 17 with a mean postnatal age of 3.1 days had ALD. During the 4-hour study, pulse rate, pulse amplitude, and heart rate were also continuously monitored with the CPO software program. In 12 infants with CLD and 11 infants with ALD, respiratory system mechanics were measured noninvasively at bedside immediately before or immediately after the 4-hour CPO monitoring period via a heated pneumotachograph attached to the patients' endotracheal tubes.

Results.—Spontaneous desaturation to oxygen saturation (SaO_2) below 90% occurred for 4.5% of the time in infants with ALD and for 27.1% of the time in infants with CLD. Spontaneous desaturation to SaO_2 below 85% occurred for .7% of the time in infants with ALD and 7.6% of the time in infants with CLD. For spontaneous desaturation to SaO_2 below 80%, the rates were .4% for ALD and 2.6% for CLD (Fig 10–7). Ventilated infants with CLD had significantly higher respiratory system resistance than did ventilated infants with ALD. In infants with CLD, a higher respiratory system resistance was associated with a higher frequency of spontaneous desaturation. Both groups had comparable respiratory system compliance and inspiratory compliance.

Conclusion.—Very-low-birth-weight infants with CLD who are receiving assisted ventilation have a greater number of spontaneous desaturation episodes than do intubated infants with ALD in the first week of life. The higher frequency of spontaneous desaturation episodes appears to be associated with an increased pulmonary resistance, probably related to airway hyperreactivity or alveolar hypoxia, or both.

▶ Here for all to see is the indisputable evidence that ventilator-dependent preterm infants have frequent periods of spontaneous desaturations. The investigators were able to use all the technological gimmicks and an observer at bedside to exclude motion artifacts and procedure-induced or environmentally related desaturations. Patients with sepsis were excluded; however, an infant subsequently proven to be septic had very frequent episodes of desaturation.

This would have to be classified as a phase I observational study. Although pulmonary resistance, airway hyperreactivity, and alveolar hypoxia were implicated in episodes of desaturation, these parameters were not measured continuously. It is of little consolation to the clinician that the episodes of desaturation can be quantitated. What they desperately desire are the tools to prevent these episodes. Only when the etiology has been clearly delineated will the therapeutic approach become obvious. Until then, rounds in the nursery will recount the number of times an infant "desatted" during the past 24 hours. See also Abstract 10–9.—A.A. Fanaroff, M.B.B.Ch.

Respiratory Complications Associated With Cryotherapy in Premature Infants

Batton DG, Ivery P, Trese M (William Beaumont Hosp, Royal Oak, Mich)
Am J Perinatal 9:296–298, 1992 10–15

Introduction.—Cryotherapy is increasingly accepted as a treatment for retinopathy of prematurity. A 5% rate of respiratory arrest recently was reported with this procedure. Respiratory complications in 14 infants having 17 cryotherapy procedures in a 2-year period were reviewed. Five procedures were done on infants who already were receiving mechanical ventilation.

Findings.—Mechanical ventilatory support had to be augmented in 2 instances because of spontaneously reduced respirations. Three of the other infants had minor respiratory complications; 5 required positive-pressure ventilation because of severe apnea and bradycardia. Infants who required positive-pressure ventilation weighed less than the others, and were younger than those lacking serious respiratory problems (table).

Clinical Data for the 12 Procedures on 11 Patients Who Were Not Already Intubated Before Cryotherapy

	No Major Respiratory Complication (n = 7)	***Apnea and Bradycardia Requiring Positive Pressure Ventilation (n = 5)***
Birthweight (gm)	950 ± 430	719 ± 157
Gestational age (weeks)	26.7 ± 2.0	25.6 ± 1.8
At time of cryotherapy		
Weight (gm)	2610 ± 475[†]	1828 ± 748[†]
Postconceptional age (weeks)	42.0 ± 3.1[†]	36.8 ± 2.4[†]
Age (weeks)	15.3 ± 3.1[†]	11.2 ± 1.2[†]

Note: All data are means ± 1 SD.
[*] $P < .05$ by two-tailed t test.
(Courtesy of Batton DG, Ivery P, Trese M: *Am J Perinatal* 9:296–298, 1992.)

Discussion.—Either cryotherapy or the anesthesia required is associated with a significant risk of respiratory complications, particularly in preterm infants. It is not clear that respiratory complications would be less frequent if general anesthesia were routinely used for cryotherapy in infants treated for retinopathy of prematurity.

▶ Commenting on this article is Richard J. Powers, M.D., Associate Neonatologist, Medical Director, ECMO Program, Children's Hospital, Oakland, California:

▶ In this series, the 42% incidence of respiratory deterioration associated with cryosurgery for ROP is higher than that in previous reports, but the number of patients was small and the population was at higher risk. Others reported a 5% to 10% incidence of similar respiratory changes. Because cryosurgery is commonly performed in tertiary intensive care nurseries, it is important for ophthalmologists and neonatologists to appreciate the risk and understand the mechanisms of associated respiratory deterioration.

Two mechanisms proposed by the authors are narcotic depression of respiratory drive and the vagally mediated oculocardiac reflex. Another mechanism for respiratory deterioration discussed by Brown et al. is general exhaustion and tissue hypoxia resulting from discomfort and struggling when extensive cryotherapy is used in patients with underlying lung disease (1). Mimanish et al. discuss another mechanism, the systemic alpha adrenergic effect of 2.5% phenylephrine administered topically for pupillary dilatation, which leads to bronchospasm in patients with BPD (2).

Endotracheal intubation and general anesthesia may reduce the incidence of complications, but they were used in only 28% of the cases reported in the Multicenter Trial of Cryotherapy for ROP (3). For the majority of cases performed with the patient under local anesthesia in the intensive care nursery, cautious use of narcotics and a lower concentration of phenylephrine (1/2% to 1%) may further reduce complications. Most importantly, the increased awareness of these risks should result in close monitoring and early intervention when changes in respiratory status occur.—R.J. Powers, M.D.

References

1. Brown GC, et al: *Ophthalmology* 97:855, 1990.
2. Miranesh SJ, et al: *J Pediatr* 121:622, 1992.
3. Cryotherapy for Retinopathy of Prematurity Cooperative Group: *Arch Ophthalmol* 108:195, 1990.

Oxygen Desaturation Complicates Feeding in Infants With Bronchopulmonary Dysplasia After Discharge

Singer L, Martin RJ, Hawkins SW, Benson-Szekely LJ, Yamashita TS, Carlo WA (Case Western Reserve Univ, Cleveland, Ohio; Univ Hosps of Cleveland, Ohio; Univ of Alabama,Birmingham)

Pediatrics 90:380–384, 1992 10–16

Introduction.—Very-low-birth-weight (VLBW) infants with bronchopulmonary dysplasia (BPD) are at increased risk for sudden death and poor physical and cognitive outcome. Previous studies have suggested that recurrent, unrecognized episodes of hypoxemia are a cause of morbidity and mortality in these infants. The relationship of feeding methods to desaturation episodes was examined in 46 infants.

Methods.—The study group included 23 full-term healthy infants, 11 infants with BPD, and 12 preterm VLBW infants without BPD. Oxygen saturation (SaO_2) was measured via pulse oximetry before, during the initial 10 minutes of, and immediately after oral feeding. The volume of formula and velocity of intake were also noted. The studies were done at

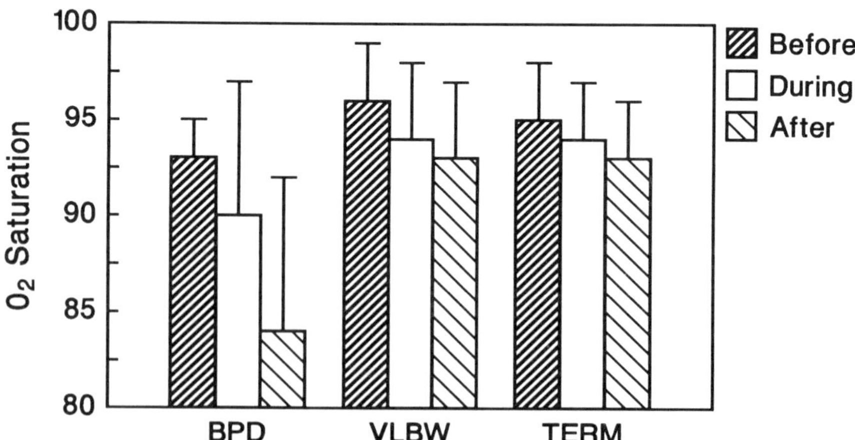

Fig 10–8.—The mean arterial saturation by group before, during, and after feedings. (Courtesy of Singer L, Martin RJ, Hawkins SW, et al: *Pediatrics* 90:380–384, 1992.)

a mean postconceptional age of 43 weeks, while the infants were being fed at home by a parent. Infants with BPD had been discharged home after being weaned from oxygen at the hospital.

Results.—The mean level of Sao_2, the highest level of Sao_2, and periods of desaturation did not differ significantly among groups before feeding. After feeding, infants with BPD had significantly lower mean levels of Sao_2. These infants also spent more time after feeding with an Sao_2 of less than 90% and greater time with an Sao_2 of less than 80% than did term infants or VLBW infants (Fig 10–8). Desaturation in the BPD group was related to both larger volume and faster oral intake during feeding.

Conclusion.—Episodes of desaturation during feeding persist in infants with BPD, even after they are weaned from supplemental oxygen and discharged from the hospital. Alteration of nipple size or frequent pauses may slow down oral feeding and reduce the risk of significant hypoxemia in these infants.

▶ As we search for care procedures to reduce the increased incidence of poor cognitive outcome, stunted growth, cerebral palsy, and mortality in infants with bronchopulmonary dysplasia, closer study of the feeding techniques appears worthwhile. The study infants were discharged home without supplemental oxygen when their average oxygen saturation ranged within or exceeded 88% to 90%. These infants were similar to those studied in hospital by Garg (1), with desaturation both during and especially after feeding. To improve neurologic development, should supplemental oxygen be continued for a longer period during and after feeding as well as smaller volumes administered at a slower pace? Should weaning from oxygen occur based on an assessment of postprandial oxygen saturation?—M.H. Klaus, M.D.

Reference

1. Garg M, et al: *Pediatrics* 81:635, 1988.

A Prospective, Multicenter, Randomized Study of High Versus Low Positive End-Expiratory Pressure During Extracorporeal Membrane Oxygenation

Keszler M, Ryckman FC, McDonald JV Jr, Sweet LD, Moront MG, Boegli MJ, Cox C, Leftridge CA (Georgetown Univ, Washington, DC; Univ of Cincinnati, Ohio; Univ of California, San Diego; et al)

J Pediatr 120:107–113, 1992 10–17

Introduction.—Extracorporeal membrane oxygenation (ECMO) is increasingly being used to allow lung healing in newborn infants with acute respiratory failure, by temporarily replacing the gas exchange function of the lungs. The best way of preventing further deterioration of pulmonary function during ECMO remains uncertain.

Complications Observed During ECMO Therapy

Complication	High PEEP (n = 34)		Low PEEP (n = 40)		
	No.	%	No.	%	*p*
Patent ductus arteriosus	7	20.6	15	37.5	NS
Hypertension	2	5.9	12	30.0	<0.05
Oliguria, renal failure	6	17.6	5	12.5	NS
Seizures	3	8.8	5	12.5	NS
Intracranial hemorrhage, infarction	2	5.9	5	12.5	NS
Air leak	0	0.0	2	5.0	NS
Excessive bleeding	1	2.9	4	10.0	NS
Mechanical problems	3	8.8	4	10.0	NS
Bronchopulmonary dysplasia	0	0.0	2	5.0	NS
Other complications	2	5.9	6	15.0	NS
TOTAL	26*		60		

* Number of complications per patient: .76.
† Number of complications per patient: 1.5.
(Courtesy of Keszler M, Ryckman FC, McDonald JV Jr, et al: *J Pediatr* 120:107–113, 1992.)

Methods.—The value of increased positive end-expiratory pressure (PEEP) was studied by assigning 74 infants with ECMO to receive either high (12–24 cm of water) or low (3–5 cm of water) levels of positive end-expiratory pressure (PEEP). Dynamic lung compliance was measured at 12-hour intervals.

Results.—The 2 study groups were similar in body weight, gestational age, and diagnosis. All 34 infants in the high-PEEP group and 36 of 40 in the low-PEEP group survived. The duration of ECMO averaged 132 hours in the low-PEEP group and 97 hours in the high-PEEP group. Lung compliance in the first 72 hours of ECMO was significantly higher when high PEEP was delivered, and significant radiographic deterioration was less frequent in this group. Complications were half as prevalent in the high-PEEP group (table).

Conclusion.—Delivery of PEEP at 12–24 cm of water helps maintain pulmonary function during ECMO, and it also promotes recovery of the lungs.

▶ Commenting on this article is Richard J. Powers, M.D., Associate Neonatologist, Medical Director, ECMO Program, Children's Hospital, Oakland, California:

▶ In this prospective, multicenter, collaborative trial, the advantages of high PEEP during ECMO are clearly proven. When compared with standard levels of PEEP (3–5 cm of H_2O), the high-PEEP group (12–14 cm of H_2O) had improved lung compliance, less opacification on chest x-ray films and, most importantly, shorter duration of ECMO support. Early decrease in lung compliance and x-ray opacification have been expected for neonates on ECMO. This phase resolves spontaneously in 48–72 hours, as the lungs undergo gradual recovery. As the authors suggest, this process results from multiple factors, including diffused atelectasis, left-to-right ductal shunting, and activation of complement and inflammatory mediators in the lungs by foreign-surface contact of the blood with the ECMO circuit.

This study is especially significant because it proves that this first phase of lung recovery is not necessary and can be avoided by maintaining alveolar volume and the normal distribution of extra vascular lung water. Although total duration of mechanical ventilation and the lenth of hospitalization were not affected, the shorter ECMO duration is still important for several reasons. It means a decreased length of exposure to the known risk of ECMO therapy, chiefly hemorrhage and equipment breakdown. A shorter course of ECMO also means reduced hospital costs. By maintaining improved lung function throughout the course of ECMO, the patient can better tolerate the temporary interruptions of support that intermittently arise from technical problems or the need to change circuit components.

Other strategies for enhancing lung recovery and shortening the ECMO run are reported or are under investigation (1). These include the use of exogenous surfactant, steroids, and liquid ventilation with perfluorocarbon.—R.J. Powers, M.D.

Reference

1. Lotze A, et al: *J Pediatr* 122:261, 1993.

11 The Heart and Blood Vessels

Low-Dose Inhalational Nitric Oxide in Persistent Pulmonary Hypertension of the Newborn

Kinsella JP, Neish SR, Shaffer E, Abman SH (Children's Hosp, Denver; Univ of Colorado, Denver)

Lancet 340:819–820, 1992 11–1

Objective.—The effects of low-dose inhalational nitric oxide (NO) were studied in 9 infants with persistent pulmonary hypertension of the newborn (PPHN) who were candidates for extracorporeal membrane oxygenation (ECMO).

Treatment.—The NO gas, at 10 and 20 ppm, was administered for 15-minute periods through the afferent limb of the ventilator circuit. The first 3 infants were treated with NO for less than 4 hours, and the other 6 were treated with NO for 24 hours.

Outcome.—All infants demonstrated rapid, progressive improvement in oxygenation without a decrease in systemic arterial blood pressure. Six infants treated with low-dose NO (6 ppm) for 24 hours had sustained improvement in oxygenation without the need for ECMO. Those patients were weaned from ventilator and supplemental oxygen therapy within the first month of life, and they showed no evidence of chronic lung disease. None of the patients showed a sustained increase in methemoglobin > 1.5%.

Discussion.—Low-dose inhalational NO improves oxygenation without tachyphylaxis in infants with PPHN. Because the normal decline in pulmonary vascular resistance at birth has been associated with an enhanced activity of the endothelium-derived relaxing factor and NO, a decreased production of endogenous NO may contribute to the failure of postnatal pulmonary vascular adaptation. Inhalational NO causes selective lowering of pulmonary vascular resistance, reducing right-to-left shunting and thus increasing pulmonary blood flow and oxygenation. Furthermore, when administered by inhalation, NO diffuses to vascular smooth muscle and the avid binding of NO by hemoglobin reduces its availability for causing systemic vasodilatation.

Inhaled Nitric Oxide in Persistent Pulmonary Hypertension of the Newborn

Roberts JD, Polaner DM, Lang P, Zapol WM (Massachusetts Gen Hosp, Boston)

Lancet 340:818–819, 1992 11–2

Background.—Inhaled nitric oxide (NO) reduced pulmonary vascular resistance in adults with primary pulmonary hypertension. In hypoxic newborn lambs, inhaled NO rapidly reduces pulmonary artery pressure and increases pulmonary blood flow without reducing systemic vascular resistance. Prompted by these findings, the effects of inhaled NO on systemic oxygenation and blood pressure were examined in infants with persistent pulmonary hypertension of the newborn (PPHN).

Treatment.—Six severely hypoxemic full-term infants with PPHN underwent 7 trials of NO inhalation. The NO gas, at 20, 40, and 80 ppm by volume, was sequentially administered at a fraction of inspired oxygen of .9 for up to 30 minutes via the inspiratory limb of the breathing circuit of a continuous-flow ventilator.

Outcome.—Inhalation of 80 ppm of NO rapidly and significantly increased preductal oxygen saturation (Spo_2) in all infants and increased postductal Spo_2 and oxygen tension in 5. None of the infants had systemic hypotension or increased methemoglobin levels during inhalation of NO.

Conclusion.—Inhaled NO has an important role in the reversal of hypoxemia resulting from PPHN. In PPHN, inadequate endogenous NO production by pulmonary vascular endothelial cells may account for the excessive pulmonary vasoconstriction and pulmonary hypertension and the improved systemic oxygenation with inhaled NO results from pulmonary vasodilation. Nitric oxide can be safely inhaled without causing systemic vasodilation, up to 80 ppm for short periods, in hypoxic infants with PPHN.

▶ Each year, *Science*, the official publication of the American Association for the Advancement of Science, anoints the "molecule of the year." The consensus pick for 1992 was nitric oxide, an incredibly versatile gas (1). "In the atmosphere it is a noxious chemical, but in small controlled doses in the body, it is extraordinarily beneficial. It helps maintain blood pressure by dilating blood vessels, helps kill foreign invaders in the immune response, is a major biochemical mediator of penile erections, and is probably a major biochemical component of long-term memory." In 1992, "the nitric oxide breeze wafting through the scientific world strengthened into gale force winds, stirring up potential drug development and propelling hundreds of heretofore-unrelated scientists together into a new research field" (2).

For neonates with pulmonary hypertension, this potential is being explored, and NO has emerged as the potential messiah. Just imagine that a mere decade ago NO was listed as a biological villain. It was considered an environmental pollutant (categorized with smog and smoke), a destroyer of the ozone layer, a potential carcinogen, and a precursor of acid rain. In the past 5 years, it has been transformed from a rogue into the ultimate messenger molecule, with critical functions as outlined above.

Nitric oxide is now being afforded the attention warranted by its anointment as molecule of the year. Although NO has a lightening-fast life span in vivo, it is long enough to ignite a number of critical reactions. Pulmonary hypertension in the newborn presents a major therapeutic dilemma for the neonatologists who have long groped for an agent that will selectively reduce pulmonary vascular resistance. If the results from the preliminary reports abstracted above can be replicated in the larger multicenter trials, then NO may indeed be that substance.

Lest everyone rush to purchase a NO system, the setup is not that simple. An elaborate system is required to deliver, monitor, and evacuate the gas. The chemiluminescent detectors are expensive, and the administrative setup and exhaust systems are critical, lest there be too early contact with oxygen and the generation of toxic products. The optimal dose must still be established, as Roberts reported success with up to 80 parts per million, whereas Kinsella achieved the desired response with 6–20 parts per million. Furthermore, early experience suggests that NO may not be of benefit to the infant with sepsis and pulmonary hypertension, particularly if cardiac output is compromised. The total clinical experience with NO at this point can only be considered anecdotal. However, the basic research is continuing, and randomized clinical trials in newborns have been launched. The serum optimism thoughout the neonatal community is reaching stratospheric levels. Directors of extracorporeal membrane oxygenation (ECMO) programs are uncertain whether to celebrate or mourn as NO has the potential to significantly reduce the need for ECMO.

The advent of NO heralds a new era in science. The prospects for introducing this powerful new agent into the clinical arena have generated enormous excitement, hope, and enthusiasm. The next few years will determine whether this is, indeed, the magic bullet for the treatment of a wide array of disorders.—A.A. Fanaroff, M.B.B.Ch.

References

1. Koshland D: *Science* December 18, 1992, p 1861.
2. Culotta E, Koshland D: *Science* December 18, 1992, p 1862.

Decreased Serum Insulin-Like Growth Factor-I Associated With Growth Failure in Newborn Lambs With Experimental Cyanotic Heart Disease

Bernstein D, Jasper JR, Rosenfeld RG, Hintz RL (Stanford University, Calif)
J Clin Invest 89:1128–1132, 1992 11–3

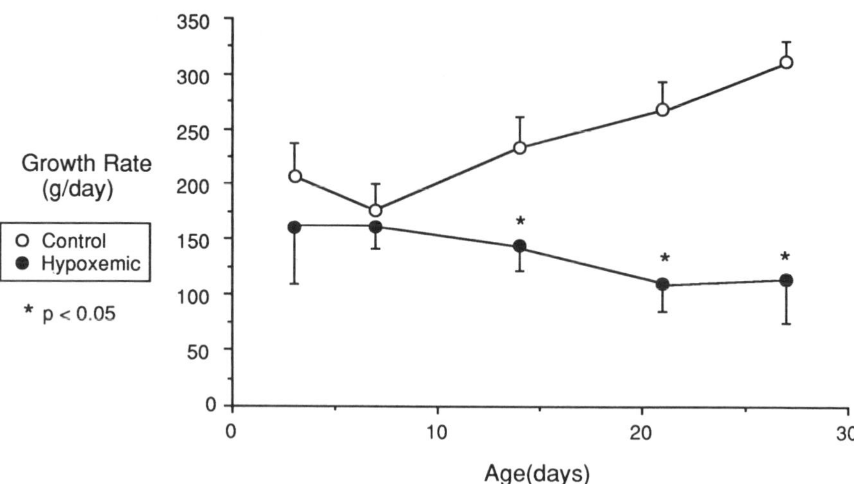

Fig 11–1.—Growth rate compared between chronically hypoxemic and normoxemic control lambs. The *asterisk* indicates $P < .05$ by Student's t test. (Courtesy of Bernstein D, Jasper JR, Rosenfeld RG, et al: *J Clin Invest* 89:1128–1132, 1992.)

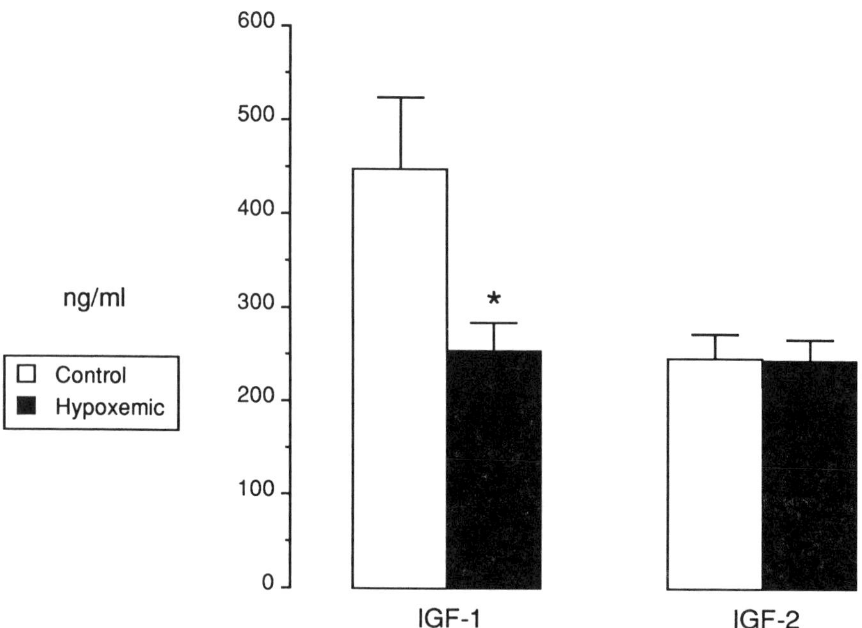

Fig 11–2.—Serum IGF-1 and IGF-2 levels in chronically hypoxemic lambs after 2 weeks of hypoxemia compared with age-matched controls. The *asterisk* indicates $P < .05$ by Student's t test. (Courtesy of Bernstein D, Jasper JR, Rosenfeld RG, et al: *J Clin Invest* 89:1128–1132, 1992.)

Background.—Children with chronic hypoxemia caused by cyanotic congenital heart disease often fail to grow normally. If surgical repair has to be delayed, the effects of hypoxemia on growth can make it difficult to achieve optimal body weight. The exact mechanisms of this growth failure are uncertain.

Methods.—Hormonal measurements were made in newborn lambs with surgically induced pulmonic stenosis and atrial septal defect. Weight gain was 60% of control values during 2 weeks of chronic hypoxemia, when the oxygen saturation ranged from 60% to 74%. Growth hormone and somatomedins, including insulin-like growth factors (IGFs) I and II, were measured along with hepatic growth hormone receptors and circulating IGF-binding proteins.

Findings.—During the time of decreased growth (Fig 11–1), plasma levels of IGF-I (the chief postnatal somatomedin) were reduced by 43% (Fig 11–2). Plasma growth hormone tended to be increased in hypoxemic animals, but not to a significant degree. The plasma levels of IGF-binding proteins were substantially increased, by as much as 154%, in hypoxemic lambs. Growth hormone receptors tended to be decreased, but not significantly.

Interpretation.—In contrast to protein-calorie malnutrition, the reduction in IGF-I associated with cyanotic congenital heart disease is not related to downregulation of hepatic growth hormone receptors. It may be a result of altered signal transduction distal to the growth hormone–receptor binding site. It also is possible that chronic hypoxemia directly alters the transcriptional, translational, or post-translational regulation of IGF-I.

▶ As yet, no explanation for growth failure in congential heart disease fully describes the mechanism; however, this report adds to our knowledge. Although oxygen consumption in cyanotic congential heart disease is not reduced, the increased oxygen consumption secondary to cardiopulmonary problems can be balanced by being less directed toward growth. Reduced peripheral blood flow occurring in chronic hypoxia with cardiac redistribution could result in less flow to the gastrointestinal tract and carcass, leading to less oxygen delivery and decreased absorption. The authors note there is no evidence that hypoxemia alters thyroid function or results in inhibitors to IGF activity. Thus, the changes in this report are probably one aspect of the overall adjustment made during hypoxia, and they help in our understanding of growth failure.—M.H. Klaus, M.D.

Pulmonary and Systemic Arterial Pressure in Hyaline Membrane Disease

Skinner JR, Boys RJ, Hunter S, Hey EN (Princess Mary Maternity Hosp, Newcastle upon Tyne, England; Freeman Hosp, Newcastle upon Tyne, England)

Arch Dis Child 67:366–373, 1992 11–4

Objective.—Serial noninvasive measurements of pulmonary artery pressure can now be acquired using Doppler ultrasound. Accordingly, systolic pulmonary arterial pressure was estimated in the first 10 days of life in 33 infants having hyaline membrane disease. All were ventilator-dependent infants. None received exogenous surfactant. Seventeen healthy premature infants were studied in the first 3 days of life.

Methods.—The peak velocity of pansystolic tricuspid valve regurgitation was measured by Doppler ultrasound, using a blind 1.9-MHz probe. Pressure was derived using the modified Bernoulli equation.

Findings.—The right ventricle-to-right atrial pressure difference, expressed as a ratio of systemic arterial pressure, decreased much more rapidly in the first 3 days in healthy infants than in those who were ill. Ductal patency was prolonged in the latter infants. Pulmonary artery pressure was lower in infants of lesser gestational age. The ratio of pulmonary to systemic arterial pressure declined with age and increased with mean airway pressure and in the presence of pneumothorax. This ratio did not significantly correlate with other signs of the severity of disease.

Conclusion.—There is a range of postnatal circulatory adaptation in infants having hyaline membrane disease. Some maintain a low pulmonary-systemic arterial pressure ratio, even if severe disease occurs. Others have substantial pulmonary hypertension; in some instances, it is related to persistent fetal circulation. In all infants with hyaline membrane disease, circulatory adaptation is delayed.

▶ Martha J. Miller, M.D., Ph.D., Associate Professor of Pediatrics and Reproductive Biology at Case Western Reserve University and Director of Nurseries at MacDonald Hospital for Women, makes the following observation:

▶ Advances in ultrasonographic technology continue to enhance our understanding of the dynamic cardiovascular physiology of premature infants. Doppler ultrasound estimation of pulmonary arterial pressure from tricuspid insufficiency is a valuable new tool for the measurement of pulmonary arterial pressure in the premature infant. At the same time, the results obtained by Skinner and co-workers challenge us with further paradoxes. Multiple regression analysis using age, a: oxygen tension ratio, inspired oxygen fraction, mean airway pressure, $TcPo_2$, PH and $Paco_2$ explained less than 20% of the variability in estimated pulmonary arterial pressure. Furthermore, pulmonary arterial pressure did not consistently correlate with severity of respiratory distress. These new data reveal large gaps in our understanding of the control of pulmonary arterial pressure in the newborn with hyaline membrane disease. The ultrasonographic technique itself, judiciously applied, could be used to answer some of the fundamental questions raised by this study. Such knowledge could in turn lead to design of therapeutic strategies driven by physiologic insight.—M.J. Miller, M.D., Ph.D.

Periodic Variations in Skin Perfusion in Full-Term and Preterm Neonates Using Laser Doppler Technique

Pöschl J, Weiss T, Diehm C, Linderkamp O (Univ of Heidelberg, Germany)
Acta Paediatr Scand 80:999–1007, 1991 11–5

Background.—Recent studies have suggested that infants in the first week of life may be at increased risk of hypothermia because their ability to regulate skin blood flow at the trunk by vasomotion is not fully developed. Thirty-seven neonates were studied to determine skin flowmotion at various skin regions, differences in skin flowmotion between term and preterm infants, and the influence of low skin temperature on the flowmotion pattern in the heel skin.

Methods.—A laser Doppler technique that does not disturb the infant was used to study microvascular skin perfusion and flowmotion. The infants were divided into 5 groups for study purposes. In 10 full-term neonates, skin flow was studied on the back. Flow was examined in the back, thigh, and heel skin in 5 full-term infants. In the third group, flow was studied in the back skin in 7 healthy preterm infants (gestational age, 27–34 weeks). Five preterm infants with respiratory failure were measured in the back, thigh, and heel skin. Finally, blood cell flux and skin and body temperature were measured in 5 preterm and 5 full-term infants at 12–36 hours of age.

Findings.—Three oscillation patterns were distinguished: silent (flow without undulation), arrhythmic (flow with irregular oscillations), and rhythmic (periodic changes of blood flow). All infants showed a similar development of rhythmic oscillations of skin blood flux. Those oscillations were present on the first postnatal day in the heel skin of all full-term and preterm infants, but they were rare in the back and thigh skin. Small changes in skin temperature did not influence the observed flux motion patterns. Rhythmic oscillations became predominant in all body regions on the fourth day of life. At the end of the first postnatal week, oscillation frequencies approached adult values in full-term infants, but they remained at lower levels in preterm infants.

Conclusion.—The delayed maturation of temperature regulation in preterm infants may be attributed, at least in part, to immature skin vasomotion. The oscillation frequency of skin vasomotion increases at a slower rate in these infants than in full-term infants.

▶ When perusing this manuscript, it may be time to dust off the old reprints, but not the concepts. The concepts of capillary blood flow and the relationship to body temperature were all carefully enunciated, studied, and reported beginning more than 3 decades ago, presumably when giants strode the physiology lab (1).

However, as technology advances, physiologic principles are reexamined and our understanding of physiologic and pathologic responses are often enhanced. This study of skin profusion in neonates uses the laser Doppler technique. The terminology (silent, arrhythmic, and rhythmic flow patterns) was new for me. Their technique is noninvasive, and the infants were studied after a 5-minute period of non-REM sleep for 10 minutes. Full-term infants were in incubators, and preterm infants were under radiant warmers. (This fact was overlooked in the discussion.)

The findings that fluctuations in rhythmic flow mature over the first 4 days of life and the oscillation frequency increases at a slower rate in preterm infants were anticipated (2). Low plasma proteins and viscoscity may allow capillary flow without vasomotion.

I would like to have seen the statistical game plan set out a priori, and I still await measurements from a more diverse group of preterm infants as an encore.

If in the last few years you haven't discarded a major opinion or acquired a new one, check your pulse—you may be dead.—Gelett Burgess

A.A. Fanaroff, M.B.B.Ch.

References

1. Brück K, et al: *Biol Neonate* 3:65, 1961.
2. Wu PYK, et al: *Pediatr Res* 14:1374, 1980.

Symptomatic Patent Ductus Arteriosus in Very-Low-Birth-Weight Infants: 1987–1989

Mouzinho AI, Rosenfeld CR, Risser R (Univ of Texas Southwestern Med Ctr, Dallas)

Early Hum Dev 27:65–77, 1991 11–6

Background.—A hemodynamically significant shunt through a patent ductus arteriosus (sPDA) has been reported to occur in 11% to 69% of very-low-birth-weight (VLBW) infants (those weighing 1,500 g or less). The variability of the incidence of sPDA may depend on the differences in diagnostic criteria, population selection, or the use of fluid therapy and volume expanders. An sPDA incidence of 16% in 1979–1980 was

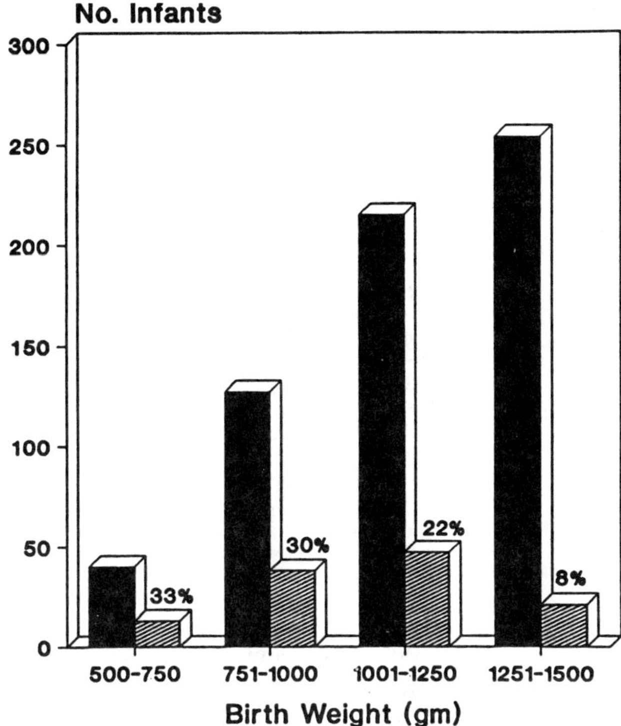

Fig 11–3.—Relationship between birth weight and the incidence of sPDA in infants surviving more than 72 hours. *Solid bars* represent the total number of infants studied and *cross-hatched bars,* infants with sPDA. (Courtesy of Mouzinho Al, Rosenfeld CR, Risser R: *Early Hum Dev* 27:65–77, 1991.)

reported for a totally inborn population of VLBW infants who survived more than 72 hours after birth. Because of numerous changes in the outcomes, weights, fluid management, and colloid administration for VLBW infants since 1980, the incidence and treatment of sPDA from 1987 through 1989 were reviewed.

Methods.—All 119 VLBW infants with sPDA who survived beyond 72 hours after birth were studied. For comparison, control VLBW infants without sPDA were matched to those with sPDA for birth weight and gestational age. The incidence, treatments, outcomes, and possible predictors of sPDA were assessed.

Results.—The incidence of sPDA averaged 19% for the 3 study years. It was inversely proportional to birth weight (Fig 11–3) and to gestational age (Fig 11–4) in all study years. The diagnosis of sPDA was usually made during the second week after birth. Intravenous fluid administration and the use of volume expanders to treat hypotension were similar in control and sPDA infants. Both chronic lung disease and intracranial hemorrhage were associated with the occurrence of sPDA. A multivariate step-wise logistic regression analysis including birth weight,

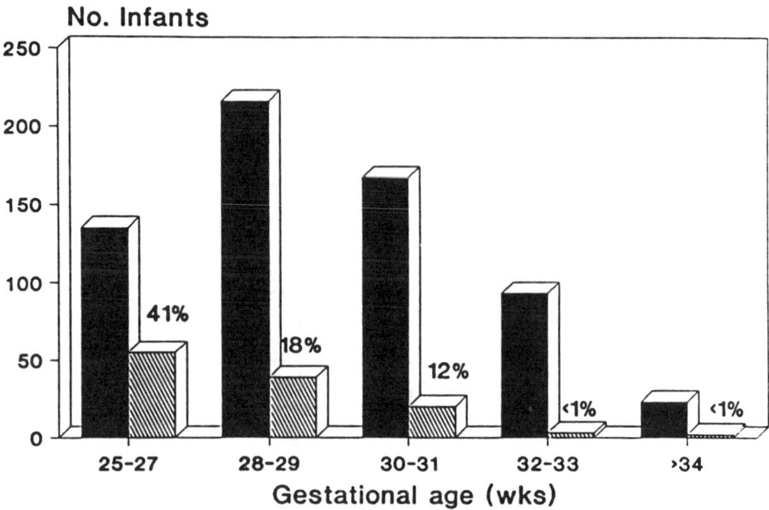

Fig 11–4.—Relationship between gestational age and the incidence of sPDA in infants surviving more than 72 hours. *Solid bars* represent the total number of infants studied and *cross-hatched bars*, infants with sPDA. (Courtesy of Mouzinho AI, Rosenfeld CR, Risser R: *Early Hum Dev* 27:65-77, 1991.)

gestational age, sex, race, fluid management, and use of volume expanders did not result in a model that could predict the occurrence of sPDA. Three quarters of the patients with sPDA initially received medical management consisting of fluid restriction and diuretic therapy, but this therapy was unsuccessful for 66% of these patients. Indomethacin therapy was unsuccessful in 25% of the infants for whom it was used. Forty-three percent of infants with sPDA required surgical ligation.

Conclusion.—During a 10-year period, the survival of VLBW infants increased, and the incidence of sPDA remained low. Conservative fluid management was recommended for VLBW infants, permitting a 12% to 14% fall in birth weight over the first week.

▶ As new therapies are introduced for LBW infants, it becomes an interesting exercise to observe their impact on standard morbidities. Hence, it is intriguing to follow the prevalence of a significant patent ductus arteriosus during the decade preceding the introduction of surfactant. Despite the survival of smaller, less mature infants, the authors claim that their conservative, restrictive fluid policy (designed to lose 12% to 14% during the first week) kept the incidence of patent ductus arteriosus relatively stable. I was struck by the sharp decline in symptomatic PDAs after 31 weeks' gestation (less than 1% compared with 12% at 30–31 weeks). The relationship is not as clearcut when looking at birth weight, although the rate is only 8% for infants with birth weights greater than 1,250 g.

The relationship between the symptomatic PDA and chronic lung disease requires further exploration. Concerns have been expressed that the ductus may reopen with sepsis, is then unresponsive to indomethacin therapy, and contributes significantly to chronic lung disease. Mouzinho reports that, in the present study, infants with a PDA were more prone to have BPD develop, although the relative risk of BPD was similar in the 2 time periods reviewed. We anticipate the next report, which will cover the transition to surfactant therapy; however, with the latent period between study and publication (about 5 years in their first 2 reports), it should not appear much before the next century. See References 1 and 2 for more information on this topic.

Doubt everything at least once, even the sentence "Two times two is four."
—Georg Christoph Lichtenberg

A.A. Fanaroff, M.B.B.Ch.

References

1. Furzan JA, et al: *Early Hum Dev* 12:39, 1985.
2. Gonzalez A, et al: *Pediatr Res* 33:212, 1993.

Randomised Controlled Trial of Colloid Infusions in Hypotensive Preterm Infants

Emery EF, Greenough A, Gamsu HR (King's College Hosp, London)
Arch Dis Child 67:1185–1188, 1992 11–7

Introduction.—Colloid infusions are often used to treat hypotension in preterm infants, but it is not clear whether the improvement in blood pressure is the result of the amount of protein or the volume of colloid infused. The effects were compared of colloid infusions of different volumes and protein content on blood pressure in hypotensive preterm infants.

Systolic Blood Pressure and Colloid Infusions

	Patient group		
	4.5% Albumin	Fresh frozen plasma	20% Albumin
Baseline	31 (22-38)	35 (26-39)	31 (25-39)
One hour after beginning the infusions	38 (25-45)	38 (28-57)	38 (21-44)
One hour after completing the infusions	39 (27-46)	41 (29-51)	37 (25-55)
Four hours after beginning the infusions	39 (19-46)	41 (29-51)	34 (25-42)

Note: Results are given as median (range) values in mm Hg.
(Courtesy of Emery EF, Greenough A, Gamsu HR: *Arch Dis Child* 67:1185–1188, 1992.)

Study Design.—Sixty preterm infants were studied when hypotensive, which was defined as systolic blood pressure < 40 mm Hg for 2 successive hours. In a random fashion, the patients received 5 mL of 20% albumin per kg, 15 mL of fresh frozen plasma per kg, or 15 mL of 4.5% albumin per kg given at a rate of 5 mL/kg/hr in addition to maintenance fluids. Systolic blood pressure was measured from an indwelling arterial catheter or using a Doppler technique.

Results.—Blood pressure before and 1 hour after beginning the infusions did not differ significantly among the 3 groups. However, the increase in blood pressure 1 hour after completing the infusions was significantly greater in infants who received 4.5% albumin or fresh frozen plasma than in those who received 20% albumin. The difference was even more marked at 4 hours after beginning the infusions (table).

Implications.—The volume of fluid, rather than the protein load alone, effectively produces a sustained increase in blood pressure in hypotensive preterm infants. The larger volumes of fluid are given over a longer period, and the prolonged infusion of protein may also have a greater effect by producing a sustained increase in oncotic pressure.

▶ Commenting on this article is Roderic H. Phibbs, M.D., Professor of Pediatrics, University of California, San Francisco:

▶ This paper draws attention to a significant problem that is not yet well understood and also compares some commonly used forms of therapy. First, it is important to point out the types of hypotensive infants that Emery and colleagues studied. The description of the cases indicates that the hypotension studied is not that which appears within minutes after birth and is caused by a massive blood loss during labor and delivery. In that situation, the mechanism of hypotension is clearly hypovolemia, and the appropriate therapy is volume expansion; whole blood seems to be the most effective in improving outcome (1). That condition is relatively uncommon. What Emery and coworkers studied is the much more common problem of hypotension, which develops hours after initial stablization and lasts several days. This is quite common in the very prematurely born infant, and it presents a major therapeutic dilemma, because very little is known about the underlying mechanism. Despite this lack of knowledge, these infants are usually treated with various forms of volume expanders, pressors and, in the more intractable cases, with glucocorticoids. An understanding of the mechanism is not the only thing that is lacking. Although there are some studies that suggest there may be some benefit from correcting this form of hypotension, there are no sufficiently large well-controlled trials that show that any therapy has a beneficial effect on outcome.

The study by Emery et al. is a comparison of some of the various volume expanders commonly given to these infants. However, no data are presented to suggest that the problem is inadequate blood volume. Specifically, there is no information on hematocrit, urinary output, or other signs of adequacy of peripheral perfusion, such as capillary refilling time. In the best of all possible worlds, one would have liked to have data on central venous pressure and mixed venous Po_2—the latter, in particular, because it is probably the best single indicator of adequacy of tissue oxygen delivery.

What Emery and co-workers clearly showed is that if you are going to use a colloid solution for volume expansion therapy in these infants, it is the volume of solution infused and not simply the amount of protein that provides a longer lasting response. This implies that there is not some pool of extravascular fluid that can be easily mobilized simply by producing what was probably a small increase in colloid osmotic pressure (there are no data on the change in plasma albumin concentration before or after therapy, nor are there any data on the change in colloid osmotic pressure). It is possible that a greater infusion of albumin would have had the desired effect.

It is also important to note that this study did not examine some other potentially important volume expanders (there is a practical limit on the number of therapeutic arms you can have in a study like this). The findings of Paxon and co-workers demonstrated the superiority of initial treatment with whole blood rather than initial treatment with albumin, followed later by packed cells. This raises the possibility that whole blood might be an even more effective volume expander than 4.5% albumin or fresh frozen plasma in these infants. The other volume expander to be considered is dextran. Neonatology has almost completely ignored this volume expander, but many authorities on volume expansion consider this to be an excellent volume expander when one does not need red blood cells. Those designing future studies should give serious consideration to dextran.

What is really needed is a series of thorough pathophysiologic studies to define the underlying mechanism(s) in this common problem. These studies would provide (1) a rational choice(s) of therapy, and (2) the design and execution of controlled therapeutic trials that would not only demonstrate which therapy or therapies are most effective in correcting hypotension, but would also demonstrate whether or not such therapy has any beneficial effect on outcome. I hope that the work of Emery and colleagues will prove to be an important start in this direction.—R.H. Phibbs, M.D.

Reference

1. Paxon CL, et al: *Pediatric Res* 10:733A, 1976.

Mortality and Morbidity Rates Among Lower Birth Weight Infants (2000 to 2500 grams) Treated With Extracorporeal Membrane Oxygenation

Revenis ME, Glass P, Short BL (George Washington Univ, Washington, DC)
J Pediatr 121:452–458, 1992 11–8

Background.—Extracorporeal membrane oxygenation (ECMO) is a life-saving treatment for term and near-term newborn infants with a birth weight ≥ 2 kg and acute lung disease with predicted mortality rate

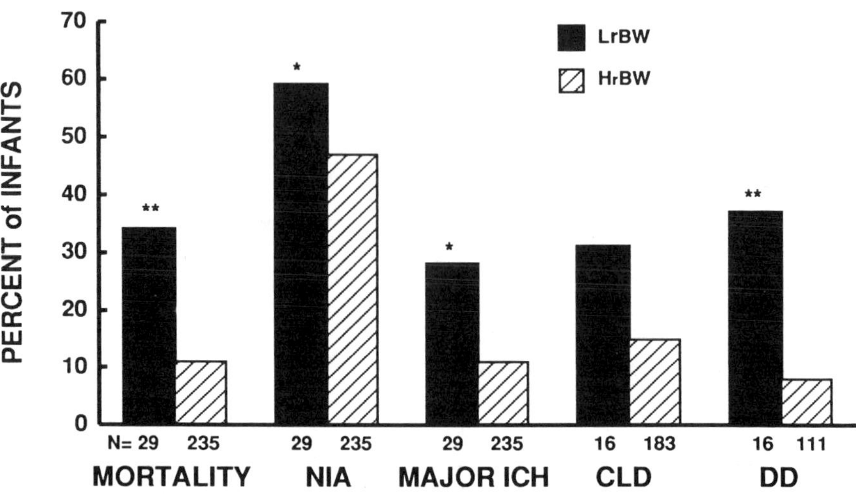

Fig 11–5.—Comparison of mortality and major-morbidity rates among LrBW (*filled bars*) and HrBW (*striped bars*) ECMO-treated neonates. *Abbreviations: NIA*, neuroimaging abnormality; *CLD*, chronic lung disease; *DD*, developmental delay. **P* < .05; ***P* < .01. (Courtesy of Revenis ME, Glass P, Short BL; *J Pediatr* 121:452–458, 1992.)

of 80%, but there is little rationale for the currently accepted lower weight limit of 2 kg.

Study Design.—Between 1984 and 1990, 29 infants with lower birth weight (2–2.5 kg) (LrBW) and 235 with higher birth weight (HrBW) were treated with venoarterial ECMO for respiratory failure, excluding those with congenital diaphragmatic hernia. The relative risk of morbidity and death was compared in both groups. Survivors underwent developmental evaluation at 1–2 years of age.

Outcome.—The mortality rate was 3 times greater for LrBW infants than for HrBW infants, with a relative risk of death of 3.45 for LrBW infants (Fig 11–5). The difference was primarily attributable to the sevenfold increase in deaths among LrBW infants with respiratory distress syndrome. The most frequent cause of death in LrBW infants was intracranial hemorrhage, accounting for 7 of 10 deaths. The overall incidence of any neuroimaging abnormality was significantly greater for LrBW infants, primarily because of the high incidence of major intracranial hemorrhage in those infants. Experience with ECMO did not improve survival rates during the 6-year study. Log linear analysis indicated that outcome was significantly related to birth weight, but not to gestational age. Among survivors, LrBW infants had a significantly higher rate of developmental delay (development quotient < 70 at 1–2 years of age) than HrBW infants.

Implications.—Until further research or new technical advances are conducted, the current lower weight limit of 2 kg for ECMO should not be reduced.

▶ Michele Walsh Sukys, M.D., Assistant Professor of Pediatrics at Case Western Reserve University, and Co-Director of both the Neonatal Intensive Care Unit and ECMO program, expressed the following thoughts regarding this topic:

▶ The authors have continued their tradition of careful consideration of the widely quoted, firmly believed, but largely uninvestigated aspects of the care of patients treated with ECMO. Dr. Short and her group investigate the occurence of intracranial hemorrhage among the smallest neonates treated with ECMO during a 6-year period. Neonates weighing between 2 and 2.5 kg experienced a risk of death 3.45 times greater than that of larger neonates and a 2.5-fold risk of intracranial hemorrhage. This risk was recognized in the 1970s. It was believed to be attributable to the requirement for systemic heparinization, and it contributed to the abandonment for ECMO as a treatment for respiratory distress syndrome. Recently, some ECMO researchers questioned whether this early dismal outcome was pertinent in the '90s, with the increased experience with neonatal ECMO.

Dr. Revenis' data suggest that it is still pertinent. Some argue that patients treated with ECMO are at high risk for mortality without ECMO and, therefore, are at no greater risk as a result of treatment (the so-called "gonna die" selection criteria that are highly sensitive but not specific, and the additional high financial costs incurred despite an ultimate fatal outcome). This study highlights the morbidity of survivors in this high-risk group: relative risk of chronic lung disease, 2.11; significant developmental delay, relative offered to neonates smaller than 2 kg. I would go further and question whether the substantial morbidity of the survivors weighing 2–2.5 kg should not be disclosed as part of an informed consent before ECMO. Finally, the paper reminds us that ECMO is a powerful but risky technology to be reserved for those with a high mortality risk. Perhaps surfactant treatment will reduce the pool of patients and avoid the question altogether.—M.W. Sukys, M.D.

Delayed Repair and Preoperative ECMO Does Not Improve Survival in High-Risk Congenital Diaphragmatic Hernia

Wilson JM, Lund DP, Lillehei CW, O'Rourke PP, Vacanti JP (Children's Hosp, Boston; Harvard Med School, Boston)

J Pediatr Surg 27:368–375, 1992 11–9

Background.—The use of extracorporeal membrane oxygenation (ECMO) has increased survival among high-risk infants with congenital diaphragmatic hernia (CDH) in some institutions but not in others. At some hospitals, deterioration (rather than improvement) often followed emergency repair, and operative delay was therefore advocated. At Children's Hospital in Boston, delayed repair with preoperative stabilization (including ECMO if necessary) was instituted in December 1987. Outcomes with this protocol, as used from 1987 to 1990, were compared

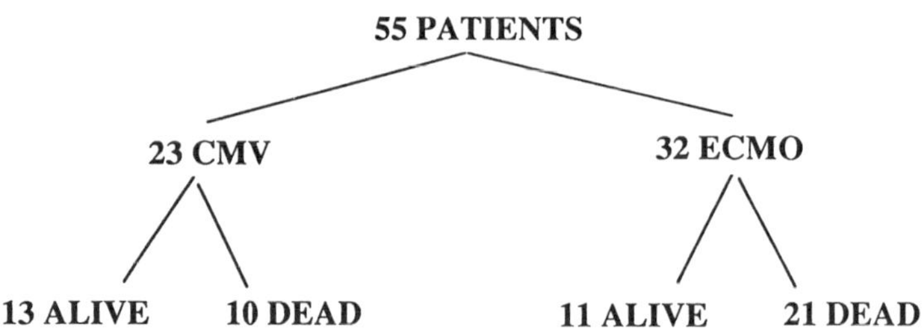

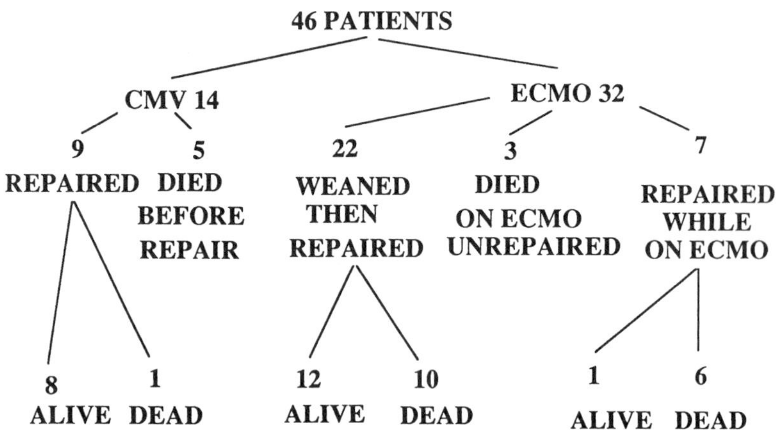

Fig 11–6.—High-risk patients with CDH, 1984–1990. (Courtesy of Wilson JM, Lund DP, Lillehei CW, et al: *J Pediatr Surg* 27:368–375, 1992.)

with outcomes after immediate repair with ECMO if necessary, used for infants with high-risk CDH from 1984 to 1987.

Methods.—One hundred one high-risk infants who were symptomatic within 6 hours of birth, had CDH, and had received ECMO when necessary were studied. Infants born before 1987 were treated with immediate repair, and those born between 1987 and 1990 received operation after 24–36 hours. Contraindications to the use of ECMO were prematurity, intracranial hemorrhage, and other major anomalies.

Results.—Fifty-five infants received immediate operation, and 46 had delayed repair. The 2 groups were similar in gestational age, Apgar score, age at onset of symptoms, best postductal PO_2 ($BPDPO_2$), frequency of antenatal diagnosis, CDH side, requirement for ECMO (Fig

Outcomes With Immediate and Delayed Repair

	Repair		P
	Immediate	Delayed	Value
Series survival	24/55 (43%)	21/46 (45%)	0.9 (NS)
Survival $BPDPO_2 > 100$	21/31 (67%)	20/27 (74%)	0.8 (NS)
Survival $BPDPO_2 < 100$	3/24 (12%)	1/19 (5%)	0.7 (NS)
Survival antenatal diagnosis	6/18 (33%)	9/21 (43%)	0.3 (NS)
ECMO requirement	32/55 (58%)	32/46 (68%)	0.3 (NS)

(Courtesy of Wilson JM, Lund DP, Lillehei CW, et al: *J Pediatr Surg* 27:368–375, 1992.)

11–6; table), and type of repair (primary repair vs. patch). Forty-three percent of patients who received immediate repair survived, and 45% survived after delayed repair (table). Infants in both groups who had a $BPDPO_2$ above 100 had much higher rates of survival than those with a $BPDPO_2$ below 100. Survivors in the delayed repair group received conventional mechanical ventilation and ECMO for a significantly longer period, but they experienced fewer late deaths and fewer pulmonary sequelae than those in the immediate repair group.

Conclusion.—Operative delay with preoperative ECMO did not improve the overall survival of high-risk infants with CDH. Infants who did not respond to aggressive conventional therapy had a poor survival rate despite delayed surgery and preoperative ECMO.

▶ Eileen K. Stork, M.D., Associate Professor of Pediatrics at Case Western Reserve University School of Medicine and Director of the ECMO program made the following observations:

▶ This review constitutes the largest consecutive series of patients with CDH managed in a single center during the ECMO era. Although there was no improvement in mortality among those infants with CDH managed with delayed surgery, the outcome in this cohort was certainly no worse than among those infants repaired emergently. Adding to this the report of fewer late deaths and fewer pulmonary sequelae among the survivors of delayed surgery, one could easily argue that this approach constitutes a more reasonable management strategy for the patient with CDH in the 1990s.

The 1993 ELSO Registry reports only a 59% survival among patients with CDH who were treated with ECMO. This figure compares poorly to other disease categories such as meconium aspiration where survival with ECMO exceeds 90%.

The "take-home" message is that neither ECMO nor delayed surgery has provided the final answer for the high-risk patient with CDH. Even the molecule of the year, nitric oxide (NO), has had a disappointing debut in the CDH arena. At the 10th Annual Childrens National Medical Center ECMO Symposium in March, 1993, investigators in Boston (Fackler, Wilson, et al.) reported no sustained improvement in 4 hypoxic patients with CDH who were treated with NO. This stands in marked contrast to the nearly magical response to NO reported in other disease states complicated by pulmonary hypertension. Stay tuned for more information on this subject. The number of abstracts on NO use in persistent pulmonary hypertension in the newborn submitted to the national meetings this year is staggering.

For more information on the subject of delayed surgery with or without ECMO, see Reference (1).—E.K. Stork, M.D.

Reference

1. Nakayama DK, et al: *J Pediatr* 118:793, 1991.

Neonatal Hypertension: Incidence and Risk Factors

Singh HP, Hurley RM, Myers TF (Loyola Univ of Chicago, Maywood, IL)
Am J Hypertens 5:51–55, 1992 11–10

Introduction.—More and more cases of neonatal hypertension are being diagnosed with the advent of improved methods of blood pressure (BP) monitoring. The incidence and risk factors for neonatal hypertension were studied in 3,179 infants admitted to a neonatal intensive care unit over a 6-year period.

Setting.—The diagnosis of hypertension was based on BP standards suggested by the "Task Force on Blood Pressure Control in Children, 1987" (table). Intra-arterial or intra-aortic and oscillometric techniques were used for BP monitoring.

Results.—Twenty-six infants had hypertension, for an overall incidence of .81%. A significant proportion of these infants had associated thrombocytopenia (35%) and ischemic episodes of the lower extremities (25%). Hypertension was significantly more common among infants

Classification of Hypertension for Term Newborn Infants

Age Group	Significant Hypertension (mm Hg)	Severe Hypertension (mm Hg)
<7 days	SBP ≥96	SBP ≥106
8 to 30 days	SBP ≥104	SBP ≥110

Abbreviation: SBP, systolic blood pressure.
(Courtesy of Singh HP, Hurley RM, Myers TF: *Am J Hypertens* 5:51–55, 1992.)

with an umbilical arterial catheter (UAC) (8.8%) and those affected with bronchopulmonary dysplasia (BPD) (5.9%), patent ductus arteriosus (PDA) (3.07%), and intraventricular hemorrhage (IVH) (2.89%). Common causes of hypertension were renal artery thrombosis in 5 patients, acute renal failure in 5, and central hypertension in 40.

Summary.—An indwelling UAC is the most consistent risk factor for neonatal hypertension. Its presence may predispose the newborn to renal artery thrombosis or aortic thrombosis, or both. Infants with BPD, PDA, and IVH are also at high risk for hypertension. Infants with acute renal failure also need to be observed closely for hypertension.

▶ The monitoring and regulation of blood pressure in the newborn has been rather haphazard. Normative data have accrued slowly, and because of methodologic problems, they have been subjected to harsh criticism, much of it fully justified (1–4). To begin with, the designation of term and preterm infants with indwelling arterial catheters in a normal population surely stretches the definition of normal beyond believable boundaries. Whereas an unattenuated measurement from an intravascular line represents the gold standard with regard to measurement of pressure, infants with these lines have been subjected to therapeutic and pharmacologic interventions that may alter blood pressure. The development of Doppler and oscillometric methods to measure blood pressure have expanded the database, but many more determinations are needed to define the boundaries of normal blood pressure for the full spectrum of newborn infants in the nursery and intensive care unit. A clearer definition of hypotension and hypertension will emerge, which will permit the establishment of more uniform intervention criteria and better comparisons of various therapies.

It is important to note that oscillometric measurements underestimate hypotension in preterm infants, and that blood pressures are different in males and females. There also are significant increases in blood pressure with advancing postnatal age.

This report draws attention to some of the considerations regarding neonatal hypertension. Stringent criteria were used to define hypertension (term, > systolic blood pressure > 96; preterm, systolic blood pressure > 80/50 for 3 days) so that the 26 infants are truly hypertensive. However when contrasted with the adult experience, including thousands of patients, a series of 26 neonates provides minimal insight into the problem. Nevertheless, the usual culprits emerged as significant. We must add corticosteroid therapy, extracorporeal membrane oxygenation, and fluid overload to the list of frequent causes of neonatal hypertension. Renovascular hypertension remains the most common etiology and the debate on catheter position continues. The most recent series again resulted in a tie, therefore, the proponents of high and low catheters can continue to place the catheters where they feel most comfortable.

Nature to be commanded must be obeyed.—Francis Bacon

A.A. Fanaroff, M.B.B.Ch.

References

1. De Sweit M, et al: *Arch Dis Child* 49:734, 1974.
2. Park MK, Menard SM: *Pediatrics* 79:907, 1987.
3. Tan K: *J Pediatr* 112:266, 1988.
4. Hulman S, et al: *J Perinatol* 11:231, 1991.

Mycotic Thromboaneurysmal Disease of the Abdominal Aorta in Preterm Infants: Its Natural History and Its Management

Lobe TE, Richardson CJ, Boulden TF, Swischuk LE, Hayden CK, Oldham KT (Univ of Texas, Galveston; Le Bonheur Children's Med Ctr, Memphis, Tenn)

J Pediatr Surg 27:1054–1060, 1992 11–11

Introduction.—The natural course of myocotic thromboaneurysmal disease of the abdominal aorta, following umbilical artery catheterization, was examined in 5 affected infants by serial abdominal ultrasonography.

Clinical Aspects.—The 1 female and 4 male infants weighed 900–1,200 g at birth. Two catheters were in the abdominal aorta, and the other 3 were above the diaphragm. The infants variably had unexplained anemia, thrombocytopenia, renal failure, hypertension, and emboli to the toes develop. In each case, methicillin-resistant *Staphylococcus aureus* was the infecting organism. Real-time ultrasonography was diagnostic in all instances. Serial studies clearly documented progression to aneurysmal disease in 2 infants. The other 3 infants had aneurysmal changes on initial evaluation.

Course.—Two infants were managed nonoperatively and died of complications of aortic disease. One infant was found at exploration to have necrotic ischemic intestine and died of sepsis when aortic repair was postponed. Another infant lived for 6 months after placement of an interpositional polytetrafluoroethylene graft before dying of pulmonary failure. The remaining infant underwent aneurysm resection and end-to-end anastomosis, along with resection of the left kidney, ureter, and left colon because of gangrene. There is no apparent sequelae as a result of the aortic reconstruction.

Discussion.—The finding of aortic thrombosis after umbilical artery catheterization should promote a careful search for aneurysm formation. Management will depend on the clinical situation and the type of aneurysm that develops. Large amounts of intravenous fluids may be necessary in the early postoperative period.

▶ Commenting on this article is Richard J. Powers, M.D., Associate Neonatologist, Medical Director, ECMO Program, Children's Hospital, Oakland, California:

▶ In this series of 5 cases and additional literature reports of mycotic aortic aneurysm in newborns, the authors present a bleak picture regarding management options and outcome. Although various surgical procedures are discussed for aortic repair, most patients die of either septic or embolic complications. The scenario leading to these complications involves 3 components. The first is an umbilical arterial catheter with its tip in the thoracic aorta (90% of cases involved high umbilical artery catheters). The second component is the development of an intraortic thrombus at the tip of the catheter. The third component is an episode of sepsis, usually coagulase-positive *Staphylococcus* species, which results in bacterial seeding of the thrombus. The authors stress the importance of early identification of an infected thrombus and aggressive management with thrombolytic and antistaphylococcal drugs.

Thrombotic complications are common in the newborn period because of the relative immaturity of the fibrinolytic system. With the recent trend of increasing *staphylococcal* nosocomial infections in intensive care nurseries, infected aortic thrombi and subsequent aneurysms are a persistent risk. As noted by the authors, low umbilical artery catheter placement may be a crucial factor in minimizing this risk. The greater incidence of minor peripheral vascular complications associates with low umbilical artery catheters (1) leads to more timely catheter removal. Conversely, with high umbilical artery catheters, the occult development of an aortic thrombus may be less obvious because of its more proximal location and the absence of external findings.—R.J. Powers, M.D.

Reference

1. Malloy MH, et al: *Pediatrics* 90:881, 1992.

Anomalous Origin of the Left Coronary Artery: A Twenty-Year Review of Surgical Management

Backer CL, Stout MJ, Zales VR, Muster AJ, Weigel TJ, Idriss FS, Mavroudis C
(The Children's Mem Hosp, Chicago)

J Thorac Cardiovasc Surg 103:1049–1058, 1992 11–12

Background.—The surgical management of anomalous origin of the left coronary artery (ALCA) from the pulmonary artery has changed considerably during the past 2 decades. This is a rare congenital anomaly that places the child at risk of myocardial infarction and death. A 20-year review of operative management for this condition was reported.

Patients.—Twenty patients at 2 institutions underwent surgery between 1970 and 1990. There were 14 girls and 6 boys with a mean age of 26 months at operation. Congestive heart failure was seen in 12 patients, cardiogenic shock in 3, and cardiac murmurs in 2. The operation consisted of ligation of the ALCA in 9 patients, anastomosis of the subclavian artery to the ALCA in 5, aortic implantation in 3, anastomosis of the internal mammary artery in 1, intrapulmonary tunnel in 1, and cardiac transplantation in 1.

Outcomes.—Three patients died after ligation, the deaths occurring at 3 weeks, 2 months, and 9 years. None of the deaths occurred after operative establishment of a 2-coronary-artery system or after transplantation. Severe anastomotic stenosis and collateralization was present in 2 patients who had subclavian artery anastomosis.

Conclusion.—Direct aortic implantation at the time of diagnosis was recommended for children with ALCA. If this is not feasible, intrapulmonary tunnel or bypass with the internal mammary artery may be done. Ligation is no longer recommended because of the risk of late death, and patients who have had this procedure and survived it should be considered for establishment of a 2-coronary-artery system.

▶ Anomalous origin of the left coronary artery is usually an isolated lesion, rarely recognized in the newborn period. At birth, the high pulmonary vascular resistance and pulmonary artery pressure results in unsaturated blood flow into the coronary artery. With the reduction in pulmonary artery pressure during the first weeks of life, flow in the left coronary artery reverses and, ultimately, "coronary steel" occurs, resulting in myocardial ischemia. Although angiography has been considered the most sensitive diagnostic imaging technique, pulsed and color-flow Doppler may identify coronary flow into the coronary artery. Surgical intervention is mandatory to establish a 2-coronary-artery system with prograde flow to the left ventricular myocardium. The operative techniques are exquisitely illustrated and detailed in this manuscript. The recuperative potential of the myocardium in the newborn is considerable; nonetheless, early anatomical repair is recommended.

We think in generalities — we live in detail.—Alfred North Whitehead

A.A. Fanaroff, M.B.B.Ch.

12 The Blood

Effect of Hypoxemia on Fetal Hemoglobin Synthesis During Late Gestation

Bard H, Fouron J-C, Prosmanne J, Gagnon J (Univ of Montreal; St Justine's Hosp, Montreal)

Pediatr Res 31:483–485, 1992 12–1

Objective.—The effects of fetal hypoxemia — secondary to acute intermittent maternal hypoxia — on the conversion from fetal to adult type hemoglobin and hemoglobin oxygen affinity in the near-term fetus were determined.

Methods.—Ten fetal lambs ranging in gestational age from 132 to 140 days were studied. After catheterization, half the ewes were exposed to 10% oxygen for 90 min/day on 4 consecutive days. The levels of 2,3-diphosphoglycerate also were determined.

Results.—Fetal arterial oxygen pressure fell from 18.2 to 11.8 mm Hg during hypoxic periods. Fetal hemoglobin synthesis declined in control fetuses, but it did not change significantly in those exposed to hypoxia. Both the level of arterial oxygen pressure at which hemoglobin was 50% saturated and the 2,3-diphosphoglycerate level remained within normal limits.

Conclusion.—Fetal hypoxemia can result in unexpectedly high levels of fetal hemoglobin synthesis at a given stage of gestation. Increased hemoglobin production perinatally suggests fetal hypoxemia.

▶ The intraerythrocytic concentration of 2,3-diphosphoglycerate (DPG) primarily determines blood oxygen affinity. Human fetal blood contains 2 hemoglobins with different affinities for DPG, and the ratio between them is constantly changing. In this simply conceived set of experiments, Bard and colleagues documented that repeated hypoxemia resulted in greater levels of HbF synthesis than would be expected for that period of gestation. The inference is that measuring fetal Hb levels after delivery would provide evidence of intrauterine hypoxemia. Some immediate queries would include when, for what duration, and what was the cause? It is a far cry from the controlled laboratory conditions to the complex intrauterine environment of the human fetus. However, with direct access to the fetus via cordocentesis, the opportunity to test this hypothesis exists.—A.A. Fanaroff, M.B.B.Ch.

Growth of Human Umbilical-Cord Blood in Longterm Haemopoietic Cultures

Hows JM, Bradley BA, Marsh JCW, Luft T, Coutinho L, Testa NG, Dexter TM (Paterson Inst, Manchester, England; Univ of Bristol, England)
Lancet 340:73–76, 1992 12–2

Introduction.—Studies indicate that two thirds of patients with leukemia and other severe bone marrow disorders do not have an HLA-identical sibling marrow donor. These patients must then use volunteer registeries to locate histocompatible donors. It is known that human umbilical cord (HUC) blood contains hemopoietic progenitor cells when measured in standard clonogenic assays for burst-forming units erythroid (BFU-E) and granulocyte-macrophage colony-forming cells (CFU-GM). The results of a comparative investigation of HUC blood and normal adult bone marrow in long-term culture were evaluated to determine whether these materials could be used in marrow reconstitution in clinical transplantation.

Methods.—The HUC blood was collected from umbilical cords after placental delivery. The 132 collections gave a mean volume of 117 mL. The long-term cultures were maintained using the Dexter and co-worker method.

Results.—The total numbers of CFU-mix and megakarocyte colonies in the HUC blood and normal bone marrow were similar. In long-term culture on preformed irradiated marrow stroma, both progenitor cell production and the life span of the cultures were significantly greater in the HUC blood than in normal bone marrow (P = .0007). The 8 experiments in which HUC-blood and normal bone marrow mononuclear cells underwent inoculation into third-party mature irradiated normal bone-marrow cells demonstrated that the plateau phase of CFU-GM growth was significantly higher in the HUC blood cultures.

Conclusion.—These results suggest that cryopreserved HUC blood-derived stem cells offer better quality and quantity than normal bone marrow cells. A single HUC-blood donation appears sufficient for those adults with leukemia or other blood disorders who need cell transplantation to improve their disease status. The banking of HLA-typed HUC blood may facilitate such transplantation, especially in patients without family donors.

► When compared in culture with normal bone marrow, the increased survival of human umbilical cord blood (HUC) is further evidence that the banking of HLA-typed HUC blood for transplantation is possible. Because HUC contains more native T cells than normal adult marrow and has high helper-suppressor activity, the authors suggest it has less potential for inducing graft-vs.-host disease. What other valuable substances are we throwing out in the basket when the placenta is discarded?—M.H. Klaus, M.D.

Decreased Granulocyte-Macrophage Colony-Stimulating Factor Production by Human Neonatal Blood Mononuclear Cells and T Cells

English BK, Hammond WP, Lewis DB, Brown CB, Wilson CB (Univ of Washington, Seattle; Univ of Tennessee, Memphis)

Pediatr Res 31:211–216, 1992 12–3

Introduction.—The increased risk of severe infection in neonates is partly because of their inability to produce adequate numbers of adequately functioning mature neutrophils in response to infection. These deficiencies might be the result of reduced production of colony-stimulating factors (CSF) by neonatal mononuclear cells. The ability of leukocytes from neonates to produce granulocyte-macrophage CFS (GM-CSF) and granulocyte CSF (G-CSF) was assessed.

Methods.—Mononuclear cells (MC) were obtained from umbilical cord blood of healthy term neonates and from peripheral blood of healthy adult donors. Whole MC preparations or purified T-cell or monocyte preparations were assessed for their production of colony stimulating factors, their activity, and their mRNAs in response to various stimuli.

Results.—Neonatal MC produced less than half as much GM-CSF as adult MC. This was because of reduced production of GM-CSF by neonatal T cells, whereas neonatal monocytes produced similar amounts of this factor as adult monocytes. In contrast, neonatal MC produced 4 times as much GM-CSF messenger RNA and more macrophage colony-stimulating activity than adult cells. The T cells did not seem to produce M-CSF or G-CSF.

Conclusion.—Neonatal T cells have modestly reduced the production of GM-CSF. It is unclear whether this deficiency of a factor affecting many neutrophil functions is biologically important.

▶ Readers with an aversion to abbreviations should avoid this article. The glossary of abbreviations reads like an excerpt from the Yellow Pages. The uninitiated and the uninformed (amongst whose ranks I proudly count myself) will constantly be referring to them. However, there will be a sense of accomplishment when you have weaved your way through this polished set of experiments.

The increased risk of severe infection in the neonate has been attributed to a number of factors. These include, but are not limited to, a failure to produce adequate numbers of mature neutrophils in response to infection, plus impaired neutrophil function. This is despite elevated circulating neutrophil precursors in the neonatal bone marrow, perhaps secondary to elevated levels of colony-stimulating activity in neonatal blood (1, 2). Colony-stimulating factors (CSF) regulate the production and function of hematopoietic cells. In addition to causing proliferation and differentiation of hematopoietic precursors, they may also augment the function of mature neutrophils, macrophages, and eosinophils, including possible effects on phagocytosis, tumoricidal activity, and the production of cytokines (3, 4).

This study reaffirms the immaturity of aspects of neonatal T-lymphocyte function. Diminished production of GM-CSF can be added to the impaired production of interferon-γ. The defects are selective because in vitro neonatal T cells produce appropriate amounts of interleukin-2 and lymphotoxin. It is not yet apparent whether the diminished production of GM-CSF by the T lymphocytes is the limiting step in the production of neutrophils in response to infection. As noted by the authors, the finding may be statistically significant but biologically unimportant. However, because GM-CSF also enhances neutrophil locomotion, chemotaxis and oxidative processes in vitro studies are warranted. A better understanding of cytokines may yet reveal the key to adjuvant therapy for neonatal sepsis.—A.A. Fanaroff, M.B.B.Ch.

References

1. Christensen RD, et al: *J Pediatr* 109:1047, 1986.
2. Laver J, et al: *J Pediatr* 116:627, 1990.
3. Clark SC, Kamen R: *Science* 236:1229, 1987.
4. Lopez AF, et al: *J Clin Invest* 78:1220, 1986.

Iron Absorption and Incorporation Into Red Blood Cells by Very Low Birth Weight Infants: Studies With the Stable Isotope ^{58}Fe

Ehrenkranz RA, Gettner PA, Nelli CM, Sherwonit EA, Williams JE, Pearson HA, Ting BTG, Janghorbani M (Yale Univ, New Haven, Conn; Univ of Chicago)

J Pediatr Gastroenterol Nutr 15:270–278, 1992 12–4

Introduction.—The rapidly growing fetus absorbs iron during the third trimester of pregnancy and stores it for use during the first months after birth. This iron storage mechanism does not prevent the iron deficiency sometimes found at about 2 months of age; therefore, mineral supplements are usually recommended at this time. Iron absorption and incorporation into red blood cells was measured in 11 premature neonates at gestational ages between 24 and 33 weeks.

Methods.—Eleven very-low-birth-weight (VLBW) infants participated in the study; they received enteral (nasogastric) feedings at 10 days of age. Nine of these young subjects received a noniron supplemented formula, whereas 2 received a standard, iron-fortified regimen containing .2 mg of iron/dL. The stable isotope ^{58}Fe reference dose study included timed stool and urine collection. Blood samples were drawn before the first iron isotope administration and 2 weeks afterward.

Results.—The iron isotope studies found that gastrointestinal absorption of the ^{58}Fe bolus of 228 micrograms of ^{58}Fe per kg body weight measured 41.6% in the fecal sample, but only 12% of the iron isotope was incorporated into the RBCs by 2 weeks after the initial dose. Both the ^{58}Fe absorption and the ^{58}Fe incorporation into the red blood cells on day 15 significantly correlated with the hemoglobin content and the reticulocyte count of the infants on the first day of the study.

Conclusion.—The use of fecal ^{58}Fe absorption monitoring with red blood cell ^{58}Fe incorporation provides a more complete picture of the outcome of the iron fed to premature infants than either measurement alone. These newborns may have stored most of the absorbed iron for later use in the manufacture of red blood cells.

▶ Commenting on this article is Carolyn Hastings, M.D., Hematologist, Children's Hospital, Oakland, California:

▶ This report on iron absorption and incorporation into the RBCs by VLBW infants using the stable isotope ^{58}Fe is of considerable interest. The authors briefly review the known fate of iron deposition in the infant and note that previous studies of iron absorption and use in growing premature infants have not been performed because of necessary exposure to radioactive iron. Now that a suitable stable isotope is available, digested iron can be traced, and the use for hemoglobin formation can be measured.

In term infants, the hemoglobin concentration begins to decrease soon after birth, reaching a nadir at approximately 6–8 weeks of life; this is known as "physiologic anemia of infancy." Similarly, infants born prematurely experience a decrease (yet begin with a lower hemoglobin concentration) known as "physiologic anemia of prematurity." Red cell survival is known to be shortened, accounting in part for this dramatic decline. Also, there is a striking decrease in hematopoietic activity, as evidenced by a drop in the reticulocyte count and a decrease in bone marrow erythroid precursors. There is some evidence that the newborn may be able to regulate the rate of erythropoiesis in response to various needs. For example, infants who are born anemic do experience a reticulocytosis. Also, an increase in erythropoiesis is seen in small-for-gestational-age infants who have had intrauterine hypoxia. Regulation of erythropoiesis is by erythropoietin, which is produced by the fetal liver and adult kidney in response to hypoxia. Erythropoietin does not cross the placenta and can be detected in the amniotic fluid. Increases in cord blood erythropoietin levels are seen in infants who experience transient hypoxemia immediately before birth. It is interesting to note that in infants born with widely discrepant hemoglobin levels, the nadir achieved is similar, suggesting that the signal for stimulation of erythropoiesis is consistent amongst infants.

During the decline in erythropoiesis in the 6–8 weeks after birth, the hemoglobin level may decrease as rapidly as 1 g per dL per week. Iron from the broken down RBCs is salvaged by the reticuloendothelial system and contributes to neonatal iron stores. After the nadir is achieved at approximately 8 weeks of life, reticulocytosis is evident and heralds the return of active erythropoiesis. Iron obtained in the diet now becomes crucial in the prevention of iron store depletion and the support of ongoing erythropoiesis.

This study monitored the outcome of labeled iron fed to one-week-old premature infants and found that these newborns stored most of the absorbed iron. Based on previous data, it would be expected that the majority of the iron would be absorbed rather than incorporated into RBC production. It would be interesting to repeat the study in infants, both term and preterm, at their physiologic nadirs. Also, a comparative study could be done at that time to look at the contribution of iron supplementation in the diet. Given these limitations, however, this is an important addition to the literature. It supports previous clinical observations and discusses a new method of studying iron incorporation into stores and hemoglobin formation.—C. Hastings, M.D.

Protection Against Immune Haemolytic Disease of Newborn Infants by Maternal Monocyte-Reactive IgG Alloantibodies (anti-HLA-DR)

Dooren MC, Kuijpers RWAM, Joekes EC, Huiskes E, Goldschmeding R, Overbeeke MAM, von dem Borne AEGK, Engelfriet CP, Ouwehand WH (Univ of Amsterdam; Addenbrooke's Hosp, Cambridge, England)

Lancet 339:1067–1070, 1992 12–5

Background.—Hemolytic disease of the newborn infant (HDN) occurs in The Netherlands despite the routine use of anti-Rh(D) immunoprophylaxis in Rh(D)-negative women. An antibody-dependent cell-mediated cytotoxicity (ADCC) assay used to predict the severity of HDN is not entirely accurate, for in some cases HDN is much milder than would be expected from the ADCC value. Maternal ADCC-blocking alloantibodies against paternal antigens on monocytes might protect against severe hemolysis in such cases.

Methods.—The study group included 13 women who produced highly potent anti-D during pregnancy. Although their mean lysis in ADCC was 116% (more than 80% is predictive of severe HDN), their infants showed little or no hemolysis. A control group was made up of 14 women with similar ADCC results whose infants had, as expected, severe HDN. Maternal and paternal serum samples were obtained to determine the nature of the protective antibodies present in some Rh(D)-positive children of severely Rh(D)-alloimmunized women.

Results.—Seven of the women whose infants did not have HDN develop were found to have monocyte-reactive IgG alloantibodies that inhibited lysis by paternal monocytes in the ADCC. In 6 of the samples with monocyte-reactive antibodies, the antibodies had HLA-DR specificity. No such antibodies were found in the women whose infants had severe HDN.

Conclusion.—Non-HLA-class-1 IgG alloantibodies against paternal monocyte blood-group antigens are seen in some severely Rh(D)-alloimmunized women, affording protection from severe HDN to their Rh(D)-positive children. Immunization with paternal monocytes might prove to be a protective measure for future pregnancies in women who are severely Rh(D)-alloimmunized.

▶ "It's not over 'til it's over." The immortal words of Yogi Bera apply to the problem of Rh isoimmunization. Routine anti-RhD administration has reduced the problem to a trickle of cases. The explanation for the residual cases, together with a potential solution, are offered in this manuscript. The importance of careful observation is once again emphasized, as this protocol was triggered by an isolated case amidst an enormous data set.

As hemolytic disease lingers but does not fade into the sunset, the criteria of severity so familiar to the older, or should I say "more experienced" neonatologist, are worth recording. Severity of hemolytic disease in the newborn was based on 8 criteria: "Intrauterine death due to HDN; signs of fetal distress, hepatosplenomegaly or hydrops fetalis; need for intrauterine transfusions; duration of gestation < 37 weeks; induction of delivery, owing to clinical condition of infant with HDN; cord blood hemoglobin concentration below 8.5 mmol/L (13.6 gm/dcl); cord blood bilirubin concentrations above 51 umol/L; and more than 1 exchange transfusion needed. Hemolytic disease in the newborn was defined as 'unexpectedly mild' when at least six of the eight criteria were not satisfied."

The authors conclude that maternal monocyte-reactive IgG alloantibodies provide protection in some newborn infants against hemolytic disease. The distinction and importance of the HLA class I and class II alloantigens are clearly presented in this article. As these antibodies are not present in all infants with mild hemolytic disease, when severe disease would have been indicated, explanations are forthcoming. These include impaired transfer of maternal IgG or impaired fetal phagocytosis of sensitized cells. Hemolytic disease in the newborn remains a fruitful source for learning the immunologic relationship between the mother and her fetus.—A.A. Fanaroff, M.B.B.Ch.

Cytomegalovirus Antibody Detection in Blood Donors and Mothers of Very Low Birth Weight Neonates by Using Three Serologic Methods

Eisenfeld L, McLaughlin JC, Mayo D, Klevjer-Anderson P, Silver H, Krause P, Anderson J, Herson V, Savidakis J, Lazar AM, Rosenkrantz T, DeSilva H, Ryan R, and collaborative group (Hartford Hosp, Conn; St Francis Hosp, Hartford, Conn; Connecticut State Dept of Health, Hartford; et al)

Diagn Microbiol Infect Dis 15:125–128, 1992 12–6

Introduction.—Cytomegalovirus (CMV) infection is difficult to diagnose in low-birth-weight infants without specific laboratory tests. Three serologic methods for CMV antibody detection were compared, and the CMV antibody seroprevalence of blood donors and mothers of very-low-birth-weight neonates was determined.

Methods.—Plasma from the blood of 577 healthy donors and sera from 147 mothers of premature infants were tested for CMV antibody by either an immunofluorescent antibody assay (IFA) or by latex agglutination (LA) at participating hospitals. These samples were then tested by an enzyme-linked immunosorbent assay (ELISA).

Results.—For both plasma or sera, sensitivity and specificity for LA to ELISA were significantly better than for IFA to ELISA. Borderline values explained only 2 of 6 LA-ELISA as well as only 70 of 121 IFA-ELISA discordances. In a random subset of 35 plasma and 13 sera samples tested by all 3 methods, the sensitivity of the LA test was superior to that of the IFA assay. As determined by ELISA, the blood donor group had a CMV seroprevalence rate of 38%; the rate for the maternal population was 53%.

Conclusion.—The LA assay was found to be significantly more sensitive and specific than the IFA assay for CMV screening of both blood donors and maternal populations. In addition, LA is less technically demanding than IFA, has a shorter turnaround time, and is less subjective.

▶ Mary-Lou Kumar, Professor of Pediatrics at Case Western Reserve University and Director of Infectious Disease at Metrohealth–St. Luke, our local expert on cytomegalovirus infections, had the following remarks to add to this abstract:

▶ From my point of view, the institution of policies to routinely provide CMV antibody-negative blood for all infants represents the most significant achievement to date in our effort to control and prevent CMV infections. This study reminds us of the "behind the scenes" efforts by the laboratory required to support blood banks in their efforts to provide neonatal intensive care units and other pediatric facilities with CMV-negative blood. The CMV LA antibody test, which performed well in regards to both sensitivity and specificity in this study, is widely used for screening donor blood. The test's accuracy, simplicity, and low cost have made it the "workhorse" of many blood banks.

One difficulty with provision of CMV-negative blood for all infants in neonatal intensive care units is that blood banks must eliminate the use of blood from all CMV antibody-positive donors. The CMV seropositivity rate noted in the cited study (38%) is fairly typical of that in the volunteer blood donor population. This means that blood from more than one third of donors cannot be used. Although not all CMV antibody-positive blood contains virus, at this point in time no widely applicable technology is available to identify the virus itself. The amount of virus present in CMV-infected blood is far less than with hepatitis B; *viral-coded proteins* (comparable to HBsAg) cannot be detected. Methods to detect *viral genome* by polymerase chain reaction (PCR) DNA amplification, on the other hand, are exquisitely sensitive, and such tests *may* provide a future "CMV screen." Until such time, transfusion-acquired CMV infections can continue to be prevented by use of CMV antibody-negative blood and blood products.—M. Kumar, M.D.

High-Dose Intravenous Immune Globulin Therapy for Hyperbilirubinemia Caused by Rh Hemolytic Disease

Rübo J, Albrecht K, Lasch P, Laufkötter E, Leititis J, Marsan D, Niemeyer B,

Roesler J, Roll C, Roth B, von Stockhausen HB, Widemann B, Wahn V (Children's Hosp of Düsseldorf, Bremen, Mannheim, Bochum, Freiburg, Krefeld, Kleve, Hannover, Essen, Cologne, Würzburg, Germany)
J Pediatr 121:93–97, 1992 12–7

Background.—In Rh hemolytic disease, destruction of antibody-sensitized erythrocytes may be caused by antibody-dependent cellular cytotoxic effects mediated by cells of the reticuloendothelial system. It is hypothesized that high-dose intravenous immunoglobulin (HDivIg) therapy may alter bilirubin production and reduce the rate of exchange transfusions in infants with Rh disease. A pilot study has supported this hypothesis.

Study Design.—In an open, controlled, randomized multicenter trial, 34 patients with Rh incompatibility proved by positive direct Coombs test were treated with conventional treatment, including phototherapy, with or without HDivIg therapy at 500 mg/kg given for 2 hours as soon as diagnosis was established. Exchange transfusions were performed

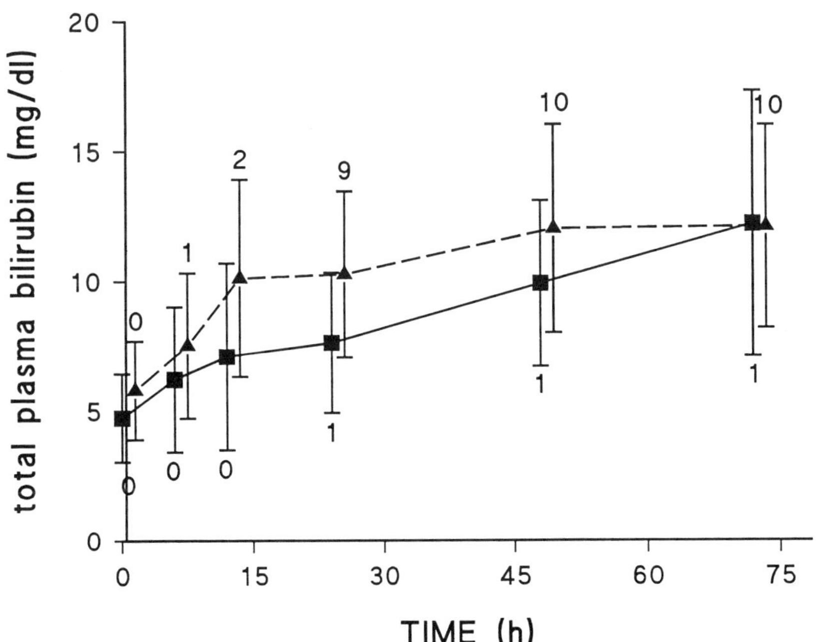

Fig 12–1.—The mean bilirubin concentrations in the treatment group *(solid line)* and the control group *(dashed line)*. *Error bars* indicate standard deviations. Numbers above (below) *bars* indicate the number of exchange transfusions performed until respective time point. Post-exchange-transfusion bilirubin values were included in the calculation of the mean bilirubin levels to document overall treatment efficacy. One patient in the treatment group received exchange transfusion at 80 hours, and 1 patient in the control group at 75 hours. These 2 values are not shown, because documentation of the values in all children according to protocol was scheduled until 72 hours only. (Courtesy of Rübo J, Albrecht K, Lasch P, et al: *J Pediatr* 121:93–97, 1992.)

when bilirubin levels exceeded the modified curves of Polácek by more than 2 mg/dL.

Results.—Of the 32 evaluable infants, 2 (12.5%) of 16 in the HDivIg group and 11 (69%) of 16 children in the control group required exchange transfusions; the difference was statistically significant. Furthermore, bilirubin levels in the HDivIg group were slightly lower despite reduced frequency of exchange transfusion (Fig 12–1). There were no side effects of HDivIg therapy, although 2 infants in the HDivIg group required blood transfusions because of late anemia.

Conclusion.—High-dose intravenous immunoglobulin therapy is a valuable supplement to conventional therapy for RH hemolytic disease. Its mechanism of action, however, remains to be defined. Until more data are available, close monitoring during HDivIg therapy is advisable.

▶ The remarkably low incidence of Rh hemolytic disease in present-day nurseries required 11 units to cooperate in this small trial. The high dose of hyperimmunoglobulin is thought to act by blockade of the Fe receptors in the reticuloendothelial system, preventing hemolysis. Although there were no short-term complications, we lack any long-term follow-up of a large group of infants who received hyperimmunoglobulin. Until we know much more about this treatment, it should remain experimental.—M.H. Klaus, M.D.

13 Endocrine and Metabolic Disorders

Persistence of Impaired Insulin Secretion in Infant Rhesus Monkeys That had Been Hyperinsulinemic *in Utero*

Susa JB, Boylan JM, Sehgal P, Schwartz R (Brown Univ, Providence, RI; New England Regional Primate Research Ctr, Southborough, Mass)

J Clin Endocrinol Metab 75:265–269, 1992 13–1

Background.—The chronically hyperinsulinemic fetal rhesus monkey is similar in many respects to infants of diabetic human mothers. In addition to macrosomia and selective organ enlargement, insulin secretion is altered in the neonatal period. This animal provides a useful model for determining whether the effects of chronic in vitro hyperinsulinemia persist beyond the neonatal period and whether they might contribute to impaired glucose tolerance or diabetes.

Study Plan.—Insulin secretion in early postnatal life was studied in 26 monkeys in which an implanted pump created plasma insulin levels about tenfold greater than baseline. The responses to intravenous glucose and glucagon also were examined starting at age 2 months.

Findings.—Infant monkeys that were hyperinsulinemic in utero had reduced insulin secretion in the first 5 months of life. Plasma insulin and immunoreactive C-peptide responses to intravenous glucose, arginine, and tolbutamide were significantly reduced (by about half) at ages 3–5 months. Repeat testing up to age 3 years showed no differences in insulin or C-peptide secretion.

Conclusion.—Chronic hyperinsulinemia in utero is associated with impaired insulin secretion extending beyond the neonatal period in the rhesus monkey. It is possible that insulin-mediated effects in utero increase the risk that infants of diabetic mothers will have glucose intolerance or diabetes later in life.

▶ This report is part of a series of studies attempting to understand why infants born to mothers with diabetes are at greater risk for glucose intolerance and diabetes developing later in life. These studies were the next step after the observation in a rat model that experimental diabetes or hyperglycemia led to the presence of impaired insulin secretion later in life. The experimental model in this study was used to dissociate fetal hyperinsulinemia from hyperglycemia. Is it possible that although the glucagon and glucose tolerances were normal after 5 months of age, some abnormality has remained that will only reveal itself when the animal is severely stressed?—M.H. Klaus, M.D.

Capillary Recruitment for Preservation of Cerebral Glucose Influx in Hypoglycemic, Preterm Newborns: Evidence for a Glucose Sensor?

Skov L, Pryds O (Univ Hosp, Copenhagen)

Pediatrics 90:193–195, 1992 13–2

Background.—Restriction of the glucose supply can result in brain damage. Preterm neonates, however, are able to tolerate hypoglycemia without signs of impaired brain function. The hypothesis that brain capillaries are recruited in these infants to maintain glucose transport into neurons was examined.

Methods.—Eighteen newborns with an average gestational age of 30 weeks and a mean birth weight of 1,470 g were examined. At a postnatal age of approximately 2 hours, the baseline values of cerebral blood volume (CBV) were recorded, and blood concentration of glucose was measured. The infants then received a bolus infusion of glucose 10% over 2 minutes. By using near-infrared spectroscopy, changes in CBV were measured.

Results.—Treatment with glucose was accompanied by a rapid and significant fall in CBV. Approximately 3 minutes after termination of the glucose infusion, CBV had decreased by a mean of .15 mL/100 g. Thereafter, CBV remained constant (Fig 13–1). Individual reductions were inversely related to the pretreatment blood levels of glucose (Fig 13–2). The amount of deoxygenated hemoglobin in the brain was not

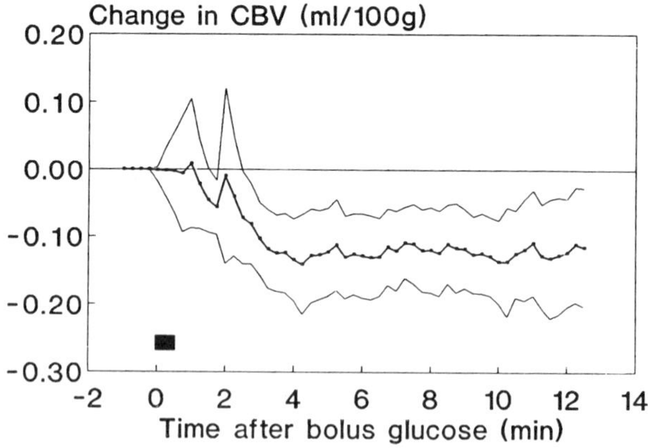

Fig 13–1.—Changes in CBV vs. time after intravenous infusion of glucose. The curve represents the mean value and 95% confidence interval for all 18 newborns. (Courtesy of Skov L, Pryds O: *Pediatrics* 90:193–195, 1992.)

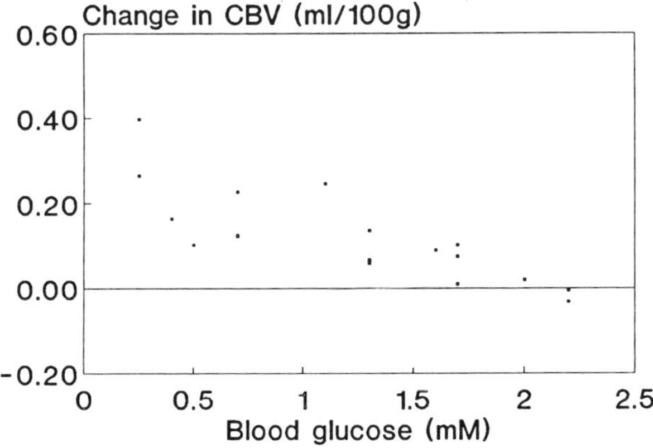

Fig 13–2.—Individual reductions in CBV after intravenous infusion of glucose vs. the pretreatment blood level of glucose ($P < .0001$). (Courtesy of Skov L, Pryds O: *Pediatrics* 90:193–195, 1992.)

affected by treatment with glucose, but changes in CBV paralleled the amount of oxygenated hemoglobin (Fig 13–3). Alterations in blood gas values or in mean arterial pressure were unrelated to changes in CBV.

Conclusion.—The rapidity with which the cerebral vessels in preterm newborns reacted to infusion of glucose may indicate the existence of a cerebral glucose sensor. Capillaries appear to have been recruited in newborns with blood levels of glucose below 2.1 mmol/L, a critical value comparable with those reported in previous studies.

▶ As we continue to learn more about how the neonate functions, it is interesting to note the many adaptations the body makes to maintain a major substrate. Surprisingly, within 3 minutes, the capillaries adjusted to an altered glucose level. The authors suggest that the rapid changes in cerebral blood

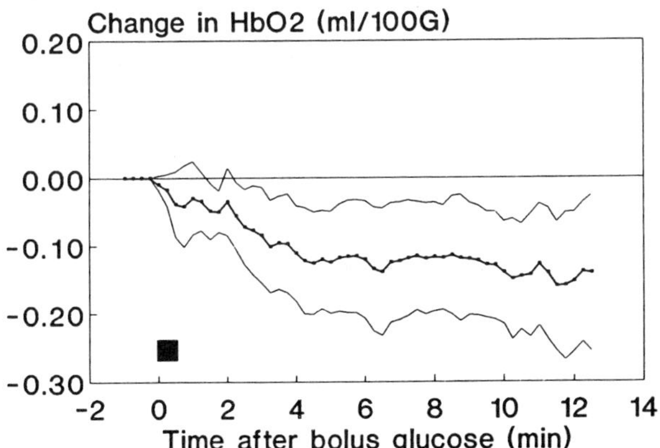

Fig 13–3.—Changes in concentrations of oxygenated hemoglobin (HbO_2) vs. time after intravenous infusion of glucose. The curve represents the mean value and 95% confidence interval for all 18 newborns. (Courtesy of Skov L, Pryds O: *Pediatrics* 90:193–195, 1992.)

volume are mediated by catecholamines, because pretreatment of rats with β-blockers abolished the response.—M.H. Klaus, M.D.

Sodium Restriction Versus Daily Maintenance Replacement in Very Low Birth Weight Premature Neonates: A Randomized, Blind Therapeutic Trial

Costarino AT Jr, Gruskay JA, Corcoran L, Polin RA, Baumgart S (Univ of Pennsylvania, Philadelphia)

J Pediatr 120:99–106, 1992 13–3

Introduction.—The fluid and electrolyte equilibrium of very-low-birth-weight premature neonates is fragile, and hypernatremia associated with hyperosmolality often occurs. The ideal approach to parenteral fluid therapy in critically ill, very-low-birth-weight premature infants is controversial: It is not clear whether large fluid volume and salt replacements should be administered to maintain body water and electrolyte composition, or whether therapy should be limited to avoid fluid overload. To determine whether a sodium-restricted parenteral fluid regimen in the first week of life would prevent hypernatremia, 17 infants with birth weights of less than 1,000 g and gestational ages of 28 weeks or less were randomly divided into a maintenance group that received supplemental sodium, 3–4 mEq/kg per day from days 1–5 of life, and a restriction group that received no sodium supplementation. Parenteral fluid intake was as prescribed by the attending physicians. All urine output was collected, measured, and assayed for sodium and creatinine levels.

Results.—Sodium excretion was similar in the 2 groups, and sodium balance was significantly different between the groups: the daily sodium balance was near 0 in the maintenance group but was consistently negative in the sodium restricted group. Restriction of sodium resulted in a reduction of serum sodium concentration and plasma osmolality. Hyperosmolality and hypernatremia were less likely to develop in the sodium-restricted group. No differences were apparent in the 2 groups as to mortality rate, incidence of patent ductus arteriosus, intraventricular hemorrhage, oliguria, or renal failure. The sodium-restricted group experienced significantly less bronchopulmonary dysplasia than the maintenance group. Neither group had concentrated or dilute urine.

Conclusion.—The fluid management of tiny premature infants may be best accomplished by restricting sodium intake for the first 3–5 days of life. The minimum amount of intravenous water replacement necessary to maintain serum concentrations should be provided. Sodium restriction may prevent hypernatremia and reduce the need for excessive fluid administration.

▶ The transition to extrauterine life imposes a sudden stress on the systems regulating serum osmolality and modulating the various fluid compartments. Consequently, the fluid and electrolyte equilibrium in the very-low-birth-weight infant is precarious during the first week of life. The empiric approach to sodium maintenance therapy is challenged in this well-designed study. Once again, it is necessary to do cost accounting for the alternative approaches to sodium therapy in the first days of life. Restricting sodium intake resulted in a significant daily loss of sodium (equivalent to that provided the sodium-supplemented group) at no apparent increase in morbidity or mortality. On the other hand, those infants receiving maintenance sodium exhibited more hypernatremia and were at increased risk for bronchopulmonary dysplasia. Although only 2 infants in each group were withdrawn from the study because of hypo- or hypernatremia, this represents almost 25% of the study group. Infusions of fluid and electrolytes may contribute to major morbidity, including patent ductus arteriosus, intraventricular hemorrhage, necrotizing enterocolitis, and bronchopulmonary dysplasia.

The survival of even smaller, less mature infants presents challenging fluid and nutritional problems. It is appropriate and timely that the approach to fluid maintenance therapy be critically evaluated. The clinicians are constantly juggling their options as they attempt to establish growth without producing undue morbidity. The almost revolutionary concept of fluid restriction in the early days of life is supported by the data presented.—A.A. Fanaroff, M.B.B.Ch.

Hyperkalemia in Very Low Birth Weight Infants

Shaffer SG, Kilbride HW, Hayen LK, Meade VM, Warady BA (Children's Mercy Hosp, Kansas City, Mo; St Luke's Perinatal Ctr, Kansas City; Univ of Missouri-Kansas, Kansas City)

J Pediatr 121:275–279, 1992 13–4

Objective.—In a prospective study, the incidence and pathogenesis of hyperkalemia during the first 3 postnatal days were examined in infants weighing less than 1,000 g at birth. All had an umbilical or venous catheter inserted for clinical management.

Setting.—Within 12 hours of birth, 31 very-low-birth-weight (VLBW) infants were enrolled in the 72-hour study. Body weight, fluid intake, and urine output were determined every 24 hours; blood samples were obtained every 8 hours; and measurements of the serum levels of aldosterone, plasma levels of renin, and plasma concentrations of atrial natriuretic factor were made at entry and repeated whenever hyperkalemia occurred or at 72 hours.

Results.—Hyperkalemia, defined as a serum level of potassium greater than 6.5 mmol/L, occurred in 16 infants (51.6%), most frequently during the second day of the study. The frequent occurrence of a pH of less than 7.2 in the hyperkalemia group was the only perinatal complication that significantly differentiated those who did or did not have hyperkalemia. During the first 24 hours, the hyperkalemia group had significantly lower creatinine clearance, urine output, and excretion of potassium. Serum concentration of potassium was inversely related to the 24-hour urine output. Estimated extracellular fluid volume, loss in body weight, serum concentration of sodium, fractional excretion of sodium, urine sodium-potassium ratio, and levels of renin, aldosterone, and atrial natriuretic factor did not differ between groups.

Conclusion.—Hyperkalemia occurs frequently in VLBW infants. Infants with low urinary flow rates during the first few hours of life are at greatest risk.

▶ Leonard Kheenmen, Professor of Pediatrics at State University of New York, Stonybrook and Director of Neonatology of the Children's Medical Center at Stonybrook, had these words about this report:

▶ Levels of serum K+ are determined by the balance of input and output of K+ to the extracellular space. Although not clearly stated in the paper by Shaffer et al., it is reasonable to assume that during the first 24 hours, when serum K+ concentrations were rising, exogenous K+ intake was probably negligible. Therefore, extracellular K+ input must have been endogenously derived from the intracellular space. Because serum K+ levels rose in both the normal and hyperkalemic groups of infants during the first 24 hours, renal excretion of K+ was unable to keep up with the intra to extracellular K+ exchange in both groups.

The hyperkalemic group of infants could have achieved higher serum levels of K+ by either having lower renal excretory rates of K+ or higher intra- to extracellular K+ exchange than the normokalemic group. On average, the hyperkalemic infants had a lower renal K+ excretory rate than the normokalemic group; however, we do not know whether there also was a difference in intra- to extracellular K+ exchange between the groups. It would have been relatively easy to calculate the net transfer of K+ from the intra- to the extracellular space for each infant based on changes in plasma K+ concentration, renal K+ excretion, and the volume of the extracellular space. Such information would have clarified the mechanisms of hyperkalemia in a large proportion of extremely-low-birth-weight infants.—L. Kheenmen, M.D.

Catabolic Effect of Dexamethasone in the Preterm Baby

Brownlee KG, Ng PC, Henderson MJ, Smith M, Green JH, Dear PRF (St James's Univ Hosp, Leeds, England)

Arch Dis Child 67:1–4, 1992 13–5

Introduction.—Infants with bronchopulmonary dysplasia are often managed with corticosteroids. However, the risk:benefit ratio of this therapy is not well defined, particularly in less severe cases. Increases in blood urea concentration were investigated to determine whether they were the result of increased protein catabolism.

Methods.—Four groups of infants were examined. Eleven infants had full nitrogen balance studies before and after the start of steroids. The

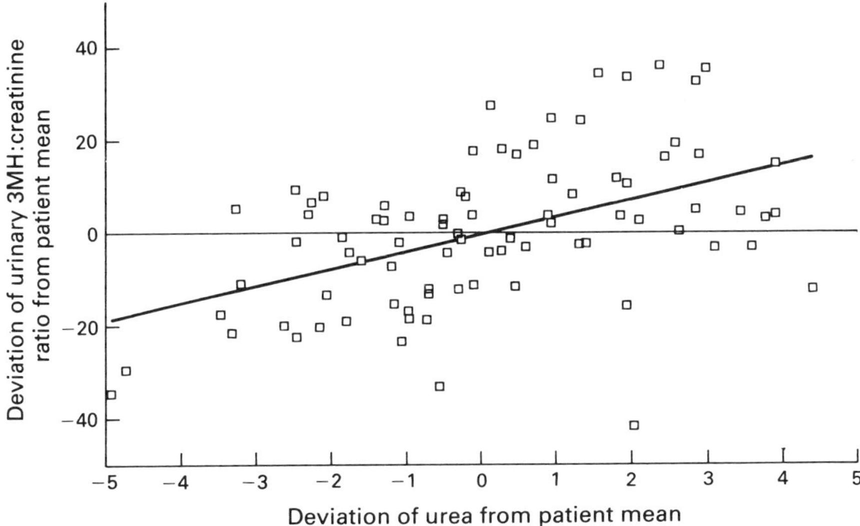

Fig 13–4.—Deviation from patient mean of urine 3MH:creatinine ratio plotted against deviation from patient mean of blood urea concentration. Regression line shown. (Courtesy of Brownlee KG, Ng PC, Henderson MJ, et al: *Arch Dis Child* 67:1–4, 1992.)

day-to-day variations in the 3-methylhistidine (3MH):creatinine ratio was examined in urine studies of 10 healthy preterm infants. The third group, 34 infants who had received a 3-week course of dexamethasone for bronchopulmonary dysplasia, was studied for blood urea and creatinine concentration. Finally, 11 infants were measured before and after dexamethasone therapy for blood urea and creatinine and for urinary 3MH:creatinine ratio.

Results.—The 45 infants in groups 3 and 4 were combined for analysis. Blood urea, a mean of 2.3 mmol/L before the start of dexamethasone, increased to 7.1 mmol/L on the third day of treatment. Concentrations gradually declined to baseline values by the end of the 3-week course. Blood creatinine was falling in these infants before dexamethasone, a trend that continued after the start of the drug. In the fourth group, the mean value for the urinary 3MH:creatinine ratio increased from 46 in the week before steroid treatment to 77 by the end of the first week. This ratio remained elevated in the second week and returned to near-baseline values by the third week of steroid treatment. There was a significant relationship between the urinary 3MH:creatinine ratio deviation from the patient mean and the blood urea deviation from the patient mean after the start of steroid treatment (Fig 13–4). The 11 infants in group 1 were in positive nitrogen balance before steroids and remained so despite treatment; however, they showed a significant reduction in nitrogen retention.

Conclusion.—These findings suggest a loss of muscle tissue with dexamethasone treatment, for 3MH emanates almost entirely from the breakdown of actin in skeletal muscle cells. The increase of protein catabolism observed with steroid adds to the risk side of the risk:benefit equation. Physicians are cautioned against the use of dexamethasone in less severe cases of bronchopulmonary dysplasia.

▶ Commenting on this article is Cynthia Bearer, M.D., Ph.D., Director of Neonatology and Pediatric Environmental Health, Tod Childrens Hospital, Youngstown, Ohio, and Associate Professor of Pediatrics, Northeastern Ohio University College of Medicine, Kent, Ohio:

▶ This paper confirms the clinical observation that no matter how many calories per kg of body weight an infant given steroids receives daily, the growth of that infant is poor. That the mechanism of poor weight gain is the result of increased protein breakdown is well demonstrated in this paper. The authors point out that this effect is one factor on the risk side of the risk:benefit ratio. Unfortunately, the risk:benefit ratio is poorly defined for steroid use, and firm criteria for its use have not been established. Perhaps future collaborative research in this area will be directed toward a clearer definition of the criteria for initiation of systemic steroid therapy.—C. Bearer, M.D., Ph.D.

Elevated Growth Hormone Secretory Rate in Premature Infants: Deconvolution Analysis of Pulsatile Growth Hormone Secretion in the Neonate

Wright NM, Northington FJ, Miller JD, Veldhuis JD, Rogol AD (Univ of Virginia, Charlottesville, Va; Univ of California, Irvine)

Pediatr Res 32:286–290, 1992 13–6

Background.—Growth hormone (GH) can be detected in the human fetal pituitary by the ninth week of gestation. Previous studies have noted higher GH concentrations in fetuses and in premature infants than in term infants. It is uncertain whether the increase in premature infants is secondary to increased secretion of GH or is a result of decreased GH clearance. Researchers sampled neonates at 15-minute intervals and performed deconvolutional analysis of the resultant plasma GH values to estimate GH secretory and clearance parameters.

Methods.—The study group included 5 premature infants ranging in gestational age from 24–34 weeks and 6 term infants born at 38 to 42 weeks' gestation. All had indwelling catheters and were sampled every 15 minutes for 6 hours. Growth hormone was measured by a modification of a double-antibody radio immunoassay. Deconvolutional modeling separated secretory and clearance function in each subject.

Results.—Premature infants had higher secretory burst amplitudes than term infants (mean, 2.2 vs. 1.4 μg/L/min). Higher production rates and a higher mass of GH per secretory burst were also observed in the

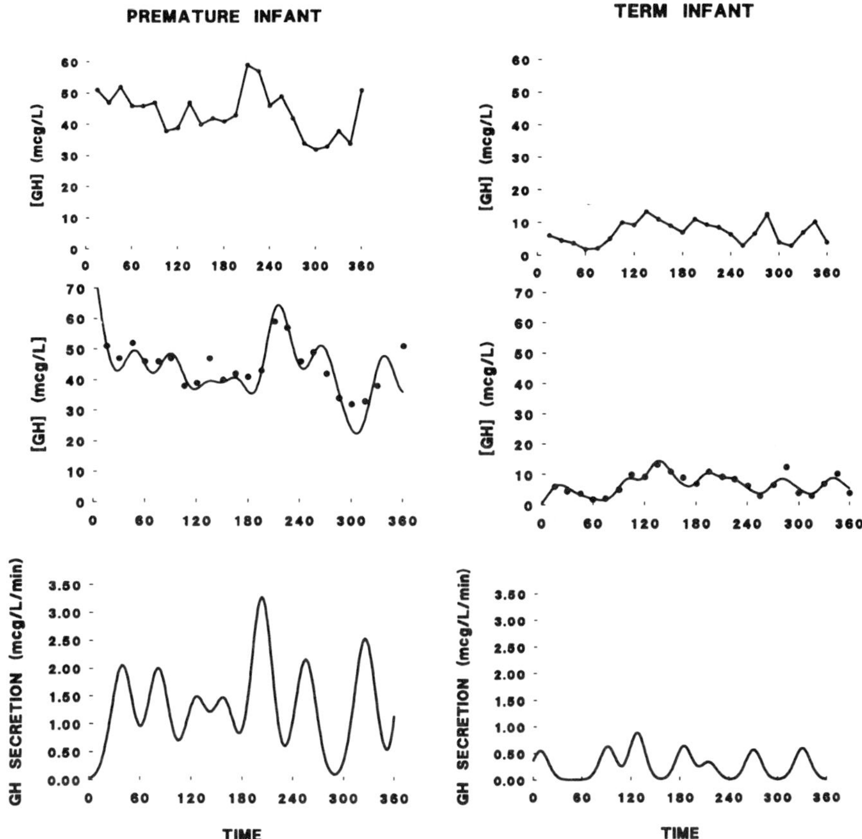

Fig 13–5.—Growth hormone secretory profiles of 2 representative subjects (a 25-week gestation premature infant on the **left** and a 38-week term male infant on the **right**). **Top panel** depicts observed plasma GH concentrations (μg/L) over time (minutes), plotted using CLUSTER. **Middle panel** shows discrete GH concentrations as above, in addition to reconvolved fit of these data predicted by deconvolution analysis shown by the *continuous line*. **Bottom panel** represents deconvolved secretory bursts over time, which account for observed GH concentrations (secretory rate, μg/L/min vs. time). (Courtesy of Wright NM, Northington FJ, Miller JD, et al: *Pediatr Res* 32:286–290, 1992.)

preterm group. The GH secretory burst frequency, half-duration of burst, and mean interval between peaks did not differ significantly between the 2 groups, but the integrated plasma GH concentration showed a strong trend toward higher values in preterm infants.

Conclusion.—The application of deconvolutional modeling revealed that the elevated circulating GH concentrations found in premature infants result from increased pulsatile GH secretion, with a greater mass of GH secreted per burst, rather than from decreased GH clearance (Fig

13–5). This finding is in agreement with the estimated GH $t^{1/2}$, similar for the 2 groups of infants.

▶ Commenting on this article is Julian Irias, M.D., Director, Division of Endocrinology, Children's Hospital, Oakland, California:

▶ Reliable detection of pituitary insufficiency in preterm infants would be facilitated by fuller characterization of pituitary function in "normal" and sick infants. This question is problematic, most obviously so with regard to the pituitary-adrenal axis. Ill and well preterm infants have similar cortisol levels, although the former "should" have higher levels. Hanna et al. (1) found that very small, stressed premature infants had pituitary-adrenal responses to corticotropin-releasing hormone (CRH) like those of older children, and they suggest that very premature brains may not recognize stress or that their CRH secretion may be insufficient. If so, some premature infants might benefit from treatment with hydrocortisone—if we could identify them, decide when treatment should start and stop, and deal with the likely adrenal suppression.

Turning to GH secretion, it is of interest not only for its own sake but also as a possible "handle" on changes in other pituitary hormones. Because newborns normally have higher growth hormone levels than older infants, a low level could, for instance, be an early marker for a lesion causing multiple deficiencies. However, GH dynamics in prematures remain incompletely characterized. This report provides strong evidence that the premature infants studied secreted more GH during each pulse than did the term newborns. In contrast, Lanes et al. (2) studied a larger number of infants but sampled them less frequently, found higher growth hormone levels in the term infants than in the preterm infants, and found no response to growth-hormone releasing hormone in either group. Difficult as these studies are, it would seem that more are needed.—J. Irias, M.D.

References

1. Hanna, et al: *J Clin Endocr Metab* 76:384, 1993.
2. Lanes R, et al: *Biol Neonate* 56:252, 1989.

Maternal-Child Blood Group Incompatibility and Other Perinatal Events Increase the Risk for Early-Onset Type 1 (Insulin-Dependent) Diabetes Mellitus

Dahlquist G, Källén B (Univ of Umeå, Sweden; Univ of Lund, Sweden)
Diabetologia 35:671–675, 1992 13–7

Introduction.—There is considerable evidence that nongenetic risk factors play an important etiologic role in type 1 (insulin-dependent) diabetes. In the fetal period, rubella embryopathy and exposure to nitrosamine compounds have been linked to an increased risk of the disease.

Results of Study of Medical Records for Children With Type 1 (Insulin-Dependent) Diabetes and Controls With a Diagnosis of Maternal-Child Blood Group Incompatibility

Variable	Type diabetic cases	Control children	Odds ratio	95% confidence interval
Total number	21	40		
ABO incompatibility	12	20	1.57	1.18–2.08
Rh incompatibility	7	15	1.29	0.36–4.84
Blood transfusion	10	11	2.29	0.71–7.52
Phototherapy	16	21	3.23	0.82–16.3
Phototherapy or transfusion	18	23	8.34	1.25–197
Transfusion and phototherapy	8	8	2.50	0.52–15.4
Phototherapy or transfusion, stratified for year of birth and ABO vs Rh			17.8	2.69–424
Phototherapy stratified for year of birth, ABO vs Rh, transfusion			8.16	1.87–58.9
Transfusion stratified for year of birth, ABO vs Rh, phototherapy			2.26	0.54–11.9

(Courtesy of Dahlquist G, Källén B: *Diabetologia* 35:671–675, 1992.)

The relationship of perinatal events to type 1 diabetes was examined in a case-control study.

Methods.—The nationwide Swedish Childhood Diabetes Registry and the Swedish Medical Birth Registry identified 2,757 infants who had a diagnosis of diabetes during the period 1978–1988. Three age-matched control children were randomly selected for each case infant. A number of variables were analyzed for cases and controls, including maternal age, parity, diagnoses during pregnancy, smoking habits, maternal weight gain, birth weight, and neonatal diagnoses.

Results.—Maternal age 35 years and older was a risk factor for type 1 diabetes in children, with an odds ratio (OR) of 1.36. Short duration of gestation was a weak but significant risk factor. Other statistically significant risk factors were maternal diabetes (OR, 3.90), maternal nonsmoking (OR, 1.54), preeclamptic toxemia (OR, 1.9), cesarean section (OR, 1.32), and maternal-child blood group incompatibility (OR, 1.61). Most odds ratios were increased in children with disease onset before the age of 5 years. In the case of maternal-child blood group incompatibility, the OR was 4.13 at an age of onset below 5 years. The odds ratios remained significantly increased when each risk factor was analyzed after standardization for all other risk factors.

Conclusion.—Perinatal events are related to an increased risk for childhood type 1 diabetes. The most striking finding was the effect of maternal-child blood group incompatibility (table). The more severe cases needing phototherapy and/or blood transfusion were found to have a greater risk than milder cases.

▶ By linking the Swedish birth and childhood diabetic registries, the authors were able to evaluate perinatal risk factors that could relate to childhood type I diabetes (insulin-dependent). This study gives no clue why maternal-infant blood group incompatibility and type I diabetes are strongly associated. The authors suggest that the hypoglycemia, hyperinsulinemia, and hyperplasia of the islet cells of Langerhans known to occur with blood group incompatibility might be evidence that circulating immune complexes are altering and possibly permanently damaging the beta cells in the early days of life. This study not only reveals the potential of computerized national medical records, but also reports an interesting clue for detectives tracking the etiology of diabetes.—M.H. Klaus, M.D.

The Relation of Fetal Growth to Plasma Glucose in Young Men

Robinson S, Walton RJ, Clark PM, Barker DJP, Hales CN, Osmond C (Southampton Gen Hosp, England; Shirley Health Ctr, Southampton, England; Addenbrookes Hosp, Cambridge, England)

Diabetologia 35:444–446, 1992 13–8

Background.—Limited growth in fetal life and early infancy correlates with increased mortality from cardiovascular disease in adult life. Non-insulin-dependent diabetes, which is associated with ischemic heart disease, evidently is programmed in utero and in early infancy. It is possible that reduced growth in early life indicates an adverse environment.

Study Design.—Glucose tolerance was investigated in 42 men aged 18–25 years for whom data on birth weight, placental weight, and head circumference were available. A standard 75-g oral glucose load was administered.

Findings.—Lower birth weight correlated with higher 30-minute plasma glucose levels, independently of gestational age, current body mass, height, and social class. Neither plasma insulin levels nor proinsulin levels were related to birth or placental weight or head circumference. Systolic blood pressure increased with the plasma glucose after adjusting for body mass index.

Implication.—These findings are consistent with the suggestion that nutritional and other influences that retard early pancreatic growth may cause impaired glucose tolerance and diabetes in adult life.

▶ These investigations have been stimulated by long-term follow-up (50–70 years) studies that observed that infants with the lowest weights at birth and at 1 year had the highest death rates from ischemic heart disease. These investigations also noted that the plasma glucose levels at 30 minutes and 2 hours were inversely related to the weights at birth and 1 year. The data in this report support previous long-term studies and expand a new area of exploration: how the environment of the infant is related to adult disease. Conceptually, workers in this area believe that the long-term associations of retarded growth result from adverse influences occurring at critical periods of fetal development that irrevocably alter the structure and function of the organism during its entire life. These observations have focused internists on the concept of critical periods of development.—M.H. Klaus, M.D.

Association Between Magnesium, Calcium, Phosphorus, Copper, and Zinc in Umbilical Cord Plasma and Erythrocytes, and the Gestational Age and Growth Variables of Full-Term Newborns

Speich M, Bousquet B, Auget J-L, Gelot S, Laborde O (Faculté de Pharmacie, Nantes, France; Hôpital Femme-Enfant, Nantes, France)

Clin Chem 38:141–143, 1992 13–9

Background.—Mineral element disorders may lead to fetal death or to various abnormalities in the fetus, infant, or adult. Limited data are available, however, on mineral values in newborns. This study determined reference values in umbilical cord plasma and erythrocytes for magnesium, total calcium, phosphorus, copper, and zinc, and searched for pos-

Mean (SD) Reference Values for Minerals in Umbilical Cord Plasma and Erythrocytes of Male and Female Newborns

	n	Pl-Mg	Erc-Mg	Pl-Ca	Pl-P	Pl-Cu	Erc-Cu	Pl-Zn	Erc-Zn
		mmol/L				µmol/L			
Males	35	0.86	1.77	2.46	1.52	5.45	12.7	16.4	43.2
		(0.09)	(0.14)	(0.24)	(0.24)	(2.17)	(2.75)	(3.60)	(13.0)
Females	31	0.84	1.74	2.50	1.63	5.73	13.1	15.6	37.2
		(0.08)	(0.16)	(0.19)	(0.25)	(2.13)	(3.29)	(2.21)	(13.7)
Total	66	0.85	1.76	2.48	1.57	5.58	12.9	16.0	40.4
		(0.08)	(0.15)	(0.22)	(0.25)	(2.14)	(3.00)	(3.02)	(13.6)

(Courtesy of Speich M, Bousquet B, Auget J-L, et al: *Clin Chem* 38:141–143, 1992.)

sible relationships between gestational age and growth variables and the concentrations of these minerals.

Methods.—The study subjects were white full-term infants (35 boys and 31 girls) who were delivered vaginally after uncomplicated pregnancies. No infant had a congenital malformation. Cord blood specimens were drawn within 5 minutes of delivery. Because no statistically significant sex-related differences were apparent at birth for the variables studied, the results for boys and girls were pooled (table).

Results.—Positive correlations were observed for the number of weeks of gestation and erythrocyte zinc and for plasma calcium and erythrocyte copper. Plasma copper was the most significant variable in the stepwise-regression equation for birth height as the dependent variable. Erythrocyte zinc, followed by plasma zinc, were the most significant regressors accounting for birth weight.

Conclusion.—Umbilical cord blood provides a sufficient amount for the assays performed and corresponds well to infant blood. The neonatal reference values obtained here will be of use in future comparative studies of newborns with various pathologies or whose mothers have a history of disease.

▶ A thimbleful of knowledge is added to the meager database regarding trace minerals in the cord blood. They may serve as reference values for comparison with sick term newborns or the offspring of a complicated pregnancy. However, as there are often gradients from maternal to fetal blood, would the purist not demand cord arterial blood to develop "reference values"? Although a considerable segment of the discussion was devoted to the gestational age relationship, these deductions are restricted to the narrow range of gestational age (37–42 weeks) from which the data were gathered. Assuredly, with the measurement techniques perfected, a similar data set from preterm infants should be forthcoming. Further investigation may also quantify the mutagenic or teratogenic effects of disturbances in trace mineral nutrition and metabolism, together with a role in intrauterine growth. By the way, my beret goes off to the French infants, all of whom had Apgar scores of 10 at 1 and 5 minutes—or should I compliment those assigning the scores? I really do accept that those were healthy, term, appropriately grown infants—but all 66 had Apgars of 10 at 1 and 5 minutes?—A.A. Fanaroff, M.B.B.Ch.

Thyroid Dyshormonogenesis: Severe Hypothyroidism After Normal Neonatal Thyroid Stimulating Hormone Screening

de Zegher F, Vanderschueren-Lodeweyckx M, Heinrichs C, Van Vliet G, Malvaux P (Univ of Leuven, Belgium; Univ of Brussels, Belgium; Univ of Louvain, Belgium)

Acta Paediatr 81:274–276, 1992 13–10

Background.—Although neonatal thyroid stimulating hormone (TSH) screening programs are remarkably successful in diagnosing congenital hypothyroidism, the disease may still be found later. This may be attributed to false negative results on neonatal screening or to the acquisition of hypothyroidism after the screening. The latter possibility occurs in children with a hypoplastic thyroid gland "decompensating" later in infancy and in a few athyroid infants of monochorionic twin pairs who received euthyroid blood from the unaffected twin until birth. After normal results on neonatal TSH screening, 4 patients had severe hypothyroidism caused by thyroid dyshormonogenesis.

Patients.—All 4 children had normal neonatal thyroid function. All had normal growth velocity and normal plasma levels of TSH, thyroid hormone, or both in the neonatal period. Two children had a family history of goiter. Seen between 12 weeks and 5 years of age, all children had severe primary hypothyroidism with declines in height velocity. In all 4 children, thyroid dyshormonogenesis was diagnosed, based in part on the presence of a goiter, the absence of an iodine-deficient diet, and the lack of evidence of thyroid antibodies. Two children had elevated plasma thyroglobulin levels and a positive perchlorate discharge test, suggesting an organification defect. All children received thyroid hormone replacement therapy and achieved catch-up growth.

Conclusion.—Physicians treating children, especially those from families with a history of thyroid dyshormonogenesis, should be aware that a normal neonatal thyroid screening result does not exclude the possibility that severe hypothyroidism may develop later in infancy or childhood. Identification of these children is based on a decline in height velocity and an increase in thyroid volume, thyroid function studies being necessary for final diagnosis. The 4 children described may have experienced a gradual decrease in thyroid hormone secretion because of delayed expression of an inborn error of thyroid hormone metabolism.

► Neonatal screening for thyroid disorders has achieved phenomenal success. The programs have been cost effective, and many infants in whom the diagnosis would have been delayed because of lack of obvious symptoms have been the beneficiaries of early thyroid replacement therapy. It is not surprising to learn that there are some gaps in the screen. The 4 infants reported in this study slipped through the screen. However, in evaluating these screen failures, it becomes apparent that the underlying disorder, "thyroid dyshormonogenesis," for a multitude of reasons masquerades as euthyroid on the initial screens. It is the primary-care providers who must back up the screening process. They were equal to the task as the delayed growth in length served to push the warning buttons and set in motion the necessary physical and biochemical tests to determine the cause. Thyroid dyshormonogenesis is a diabolical term for an apparent inborn error of thyroid hormone metabolism that is characterized by a gradual decrease in thyroid secretion for unknown reasons.

Vulsma (1) noted that there is considerable transfer of T4 from the mother to the fetus in late gestation, at least when the infant has severe congenital hypothyroidism. This was not believed to be the mechanism for the normal thyroid screens in de Zeghers series above. See also References 2 and 3.—A.A. Fanaroff, M.B.B.Ch.

References

1. 1991 YEAR BOOK OF NEONATAL AND PERINATAL MEDICINE, pp 248–249.
2. 1992 YEAR BOOK OF NEONATAL AND PERINATAL MEDICINE, pp 274–275.
3. 1992 YEAR BOOK OF NEONATAL AND PERINATAL MEDICINE, pp 276–277.

Delayed Diagnosis of Infants With Abnormal Neonatal Screens
Listernick R, Frisone L, Silverman BL (Northwestern Univ, Chicago)
JAMA 267:1095–1099, 1992 13–11

Background.—During the past several decades, advances in assay techniques have enabled a variety of disorders to be identified through mass screening of newborn infants. However, some affected infants slip through the screening process and fail to receive timely medical attention. The effectiveness of 1 neonatal screening program was reviewed.

Methods.—Since May 1991, Illinois has required neonatal screening for phenylketonuria, hypothyroidism, galactosemia, biotinidase deficiency, 21-hydroxylase deficiency, and hemoglobinopathies. A single laboratory in Chicago performs the tests and notifies state health authorities of abnormal results. Physicians are notified immediately by telephone in urgent cases and by mail of borderline or mildly abnormal results. The state's Genetic Disease Program staff is responsible for follow-up.

Results.—During the period from January 1989 through March 1991, 10 children with abnormal test results had received inadequate care. In each case, the physician of record had received prompt telephone communication of the findings. Seven children had a hemoglobinopathy, and 3 had 21-hydroxylase deficiency. The mean patient age at clinical diagnosis was 215 days for children with sickle cell anemia and 32 days for infants with 21-hydroxylase deficiency. There were no deaths, but 6 children had potentially life-threatening complications. In some cases, parents had not scheduled medical follow-up or had changed their address or telephone number between birth and the time of diagnosis. However, it was also apparent that physicians were not diligent in providing follow-up and were at times unaware of the implications of genetic screening.

Conclusion.—Screening programs are worthless without the means to ensure proper follow-up. Improvements must be made in each step of the process, beginning with the mechanics of the state screening program itself. Parents as well as physicians should be notified and hospital personnel educated on the importance of the tests and the need to verify parents' addresses and telephone numbers. There is a clear ethical and legal mandate that infants identified through screening programs receive prompt medical attention.

▶ Although neonatal screening programs have been especially helpful in identifying rare diseases, they have also often failed to notify some patients. In one study, 16% of all missed cases were the results of inadequate follow-up of screening results (1). While in Georgia, a program to screen for hemoglobinopathies without any built-in system of follow-up revealed that 31% of infants with sickle cell disease died with infection or splenic sequestration (2). Sadly, in this study, 27% of the patients with sickle cell disease on screening were never informed of the disease until their children became symptomatic. In examining each delay in diagnosis, inadequate education of the physician was a frequent problem. To reduce a delay in diagnosis to a minimum, it is imperative that every physician and family be notified of the possibility of the disease and essential information about the problem. Increasing the counseling time will be necessary because of a high false positive rate in some conditions.—M.H. Klaus, M.D.

References

1. Holtzman C, Slazyk WE: *Pediatrics* 78:553, 1986.
2. Weatherall DJ, Clegg JB: *The Thalassemia Syndromes*, ed 3. Oxford, England, Blackwell Scientific Publications, 1981.

14 Developmental Pharmacology and Toxicology

Effect of Morphine and Pancuronium on the Stress Response in Ventilated Preterm Infants

Quinn MW, Otoo F, Rushforth JA, Dean HG, Puntis JWL, Wild J, Levene MI (Gen Infirmary, Leeds, England)

Early Hum Dev 30:241–248, 1992 14–1

Background.—Pain and the stress response associated with it may be important in infants receiving intensive care. Little is known about the stress of mechanical ventilation in premature infants. The effect of sedation of ventilated infants on stress response was assessed in a group of ill premature infants.

Methods.—Ninety-five premature infants who had hyaline membrane disease and were struggling against the ventilator were studied. The newborns were assigned randomly to 1 of 3 treatment groups: morphine (M), pancuronium (P), or morphine with pancuronium (M+P). The morphine dose was 50 μg/kg/hr, which was increased to 100 μg/kg/hr in group M infants if they continued to struggle. Pancuronium, 100 μg/kg, was administered as needed to inhibit spontaneous respiration. Plasma catecholamine concentrations were assessed on entry and at 24 hours. Blood pressure and ventilatory requirements were noted on entry and at 6 hours.

Findings.—The 29 infants in group M had a significant decrease in noradrenaline levels. However, 7 of those infants had to be withdrawn because of failure to settle. The 28 infants in group P and 38 in group M+P had no significant changes in noradrenaline levels. Group comparisons indicated that group M infants had a significant noradrenaline decrease compared with those in group P. The immediate effects of treatment on blood pressure and ventilatory needs were comparable in the 3 groups. The clinical outcomes did not differ for any parameter measured.

Conclusion.—In infants who are adequately sedated with morphine, there is a significant decline in noradrenaline levels. Therefore, morphine may reduce the stress of neonatal intensive care.

▶ Commenting on this article is Linda Franck, R.N., M.S., Ph.D. Candidate, Director of Critical Care Nursing, Children's Hospital, Oakland, California:

▶ This study is significant in that it reflects a major shift in thinking about neonatal pain and stress. Sufficient evidence exists to indicate that neonates have the capacity to mount stress responses and experience pain. We must now focus our attention on evaluating our interventions to reduce the stress of neonatal care. However, several crucial issues remain unresolved. First, neuroendocrine, physiologic, and behavioral measures that are valid, reliable, and feasible in daily clinical care are still needed. Second, we must recognize that there is great individual variability in neonatal stress responses, requiring that pharmacologic treatment be individualized. Finally, methods for weaning opiates to minimize withdrawal symptoms must be explored so as not to further stress the infant when pharmacologic support is discontinued.

This study contributes to our knowledge about neonatal responses to sedation and paralysis, but it leaves us with more questions than answers. For example, are adrenaline and noradrenaline the best measures of stress response in neonates? Is 24 hours an appropriate interval to detect changes in stress levels? How do physiologic parameters relate to the neuroendocrine markers? What factors contributed to the need for increased morphine in some infants?

However, the most compelling questions raised by this study concern the use of mechanical ventilation. Why was such a large number of infants perceived as "fighting the ventilator" to the degree that sedation or paralysis was required? Could sedation and paralysis have been avoided by the use of alternative ventilation techniques to achieve better synchrony with the infant's own respiratory effort? Unfortunately, the authors do not report what strategies were attempted before the decision was made to sedate or paralyze. We must be vigilant that our increased awareness of the importance of symptom management does not obscure our diagnosis and treatment of the root problem. Even in today's health-care economy, an ounce of prevention is still worth a pound of cure.—L. Franck, R.N.

Pharmacokinetic-Pharmacodynamic Relationships of Morphine in Neonates

Chay PCW, Duffy BJ, Walker JS (Prince of Wales Children's Hosp, Randwick, Australia; St Vincent's Hosp, Darlinghurst, Australia)

Clin Pharmacol Ther 51:334–342, 1992 14–2

Background.—Morphine administered by infusion is used widely for analgesia and sedation in neonates but less frequently for postoperative pain. Reports that newborn infants are more susceptible to the respira-

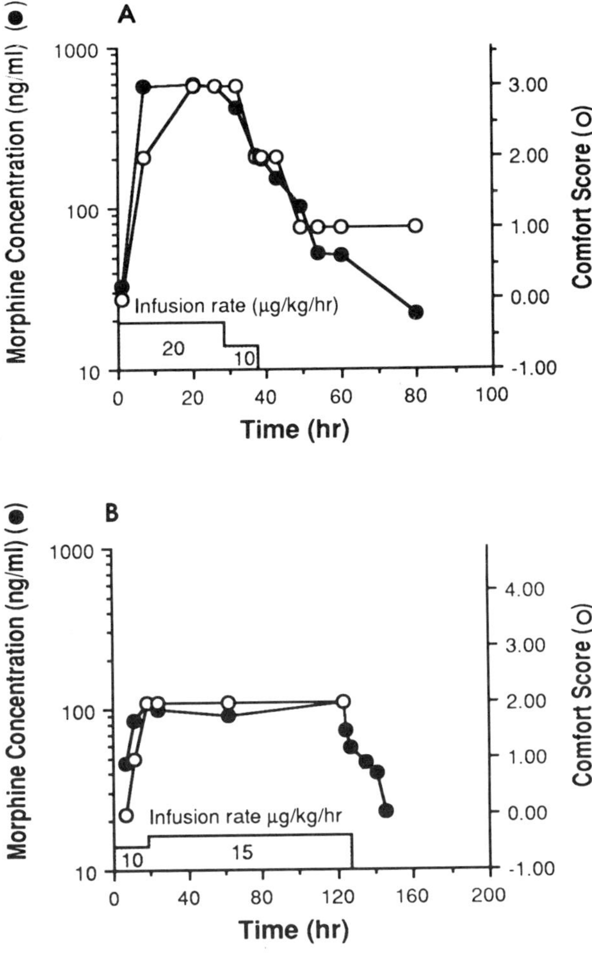

Fig 14–1.—Plasma concentration-time profiles and concurrent comfort scores during and after an intravenous infusion of morphine. **A,** profile in a typical patient in whom adverse effects attributable to high plasma morphine were noted; **B,** similar data in a patient with no adverse effects. *Closed circles* indicate measured plasma concentrations; *open circles,* corresponding comfort scores. (Courtesy of Chay PCW, Duffy BJ, Walker JS: *Clin Pharmacol Ther* 51:334–342, 1992.)

tory depressant effects of morphine than adults are have contributed to the reluctance to use morphine in neonates for pain management. The relationship between analgesic effects and serum concentrations of morphine and its glucuronide metabolites during continuous infusion was examined in term and preterm neonates.

Method.—Nineteen mechanically ventilated infants were receiving morphine for pain relief, sedation, or other clinical indications. The infants were divided into a preterm group and a term group. A 4-point scale was used to assess the adequacy of pain relief and sedation. Elimination half-life, total plasma clearance, and volume of distribution were monitored.

Findings.—The elimination half-life was 9.6 ± 3 hours, total plasma clearance was 2.55 ± 1.65 mL/min/kg by area analysis or 2.09 ± 1.19 mL/min/kg by steady-state data, and the volume of distribution was 2.05 ± 1.05 L/kg. These values were not significantly different in preterm and term neonates. The plasma clearance was twofold lower and the volume of distribution was significantly lower in neonates with adverse reactions to morphine (Fig 14–1); however, the half-life was not different. The mean morphine concentration required to produce adequate sedation in 50% of the patients was 125 ng/mL, but concentrations above 300 ng/mL were potentially associated with adverse effects. Morphine-6-glucuronide was not detected in the plasma of any neonate. This may explain why neonates require high plasma concentrations of unchanged morphine for sedation.

Conclusion.—The high incidence of adverse effects from morphine administration in neonates may be attributed to high plasma concentrations of morphine because of diminished clearance. Plasma morphine concentrations of approximately 125 ng/mL were required for adequate sedation and analgesia in neonates maintained on ventilation, but adverse effects occurred at concentrations greater than 300 ng/mL.

▶ Celeste M. Marx, Pharm.D., Assistant Professor of Pediatrics, Case Western Reserve University School of Medicine, makes the following insightful comments on this important topic:

▶ This has been a tremendous year for growth in our understanding of the metabolism of morphine in infancy. These authors present a careful analysis of the pharmacokinetics of morphine and 2 of its metabolites in 19 mechanically ventilated newborns with dosage titrated to clinical response. Several observations are quite interesting. Morphine-6-glucuronide (M6G), a potently analgesic metabolite of morphine, was not measured in the plasma of the 6 infants tested for it, despite the use of an assay more sensitive than that used in prior reports noting its absence (1). However, shortly after the publication of this report, Choonara described the detection of M6G in the plasma of 10 of 12 infants tested (2). Bhat et al. also examined the plasma and urine of sick preterm infants who were given morphine, and they were able to demonstrate the presence of M6G in plasma 24 hours, but not 4 hours, after single-dose administration (3). Part of these differences may relate to the well-established interpatient variability in this population. However, preterm and neonatal metabolism is not so immature that this potent and long-acting metabolite cannot be formed in detectable quantities.

The second observation of interest is that when patients were grouped by presence of excessive opiate effect (bradycardia, carbon dioxide retention, and urinary retention), the mean morphine steady state plasma concentration was much higher (with mean volume of distribution being much lower) in those infants with adverse effects compared with those without them; this occurred despite a similar rate of elimination for both groups. Variability in toxic response to morphine may have a pharmacokinetic basis. Nevertheless, a complete understanding of the reasons for age-based differences in response to morphine requires careful attention to the measurement of effects relative to plasma concentration. This study was an attempt to define the relationship between dose and plasma concentration and analgesic/sedative response in these infants. Analgesia and sedation responses were not distinguished, and they were described only by a coarse 4-point descriptive scale. It is unfortunate that their tool was not validated as a measure of either analgesia or sedation (distinct effects) in newborns before its application. The author's "comfort score" should not be confused with the COMFORT Scale, which is a valid and reliable measure of behavioral and physiologic distress in mechanically ventilated children, including term newborns (4). At present, there is no valid measure of the distinct behavioral responses of distressed premature infants. Although it was not clear whether any of the newborns had conditions that were likely to be painful, analgesic effect was not assessed by any neonatal pain scale, such as that developed for postoperative infants (5). The limited pharmacodynamic methodology of Chay and colleagues does not stand alone, as a recent evaluation of the pharmacokinetics and pharmacodynamics of meperidine in a similar neonatal population used simple assessment of vital signs and ventilation parameters to define drug effect (6). Although side effects are important safety considerations, they are not the primary effect for which the drug is given. Because of the limitations of pharmacodynamic observations, derived "therapeutic" plasma concentrations for morphine remain to be defined.—C.M. Marx, Pharm.D.

References

1. Choonara IA, et al: *Br J Clin Pharmacol* 28:599, 1989.
2. Choonara IA, et al: *Br J Clin Pharmacol* 34:434, 1992.
3. Bhat R, et al: *J Pediatr* 120:795, 1992.
4. Ambuel B, et al: *J Pediatr Psychol* 17:95, 1992.
5. Barrier G, et al: *Intensive Care Med* 15:S37, 1989.
6. Pokela M, et al: *Clin Pharmacol Ther* 52:342, 1992.

Maternal and Umbilical Cord Concentrations of Fentanyl After Epidural Analgesia for Cesarean Section

Desprats R, Dumas J-C, Giroux M, Campistron G, Faure F, Teixeira MG, Grandjean H, Houin G, Pontonnier G (Hôpital LaGrave, Paul Sabatier Univ, Toulouse, France)

Eur J Obstet Gynecol Reprod Biol 42:89–94, 1991 14–3

Introduction.—Fentanyl is frequently used in epidural analgesia for cesarean section. The drug appears to have no important maternal side effects, but little is known about the transplacental transfer of fentanyl. A highly sensitive radioimmunoassay method was used to measure maternal and umbilical concentrations of fentanyl in 16 women scheduled for cesarean section.

Methods.—The 16 women were all at term and were to be surgically delivered because of a narrow pelvis. All received a single epidural injection of 85 mg of bupivacaine .5%, 60 mg of etidocaine 1%, and 100 μg of fentanyl with epinephrine 1:200,000. Maternal blood samples were obtained at 5, 15, 30, and 60 minutes after the injection and at the time of birth. Blood samples were taken from the umbilical cord at birth.

Results.—The mothers showed no clinical evidence of sedation or respiratory depression. All of the infants were in good health and showed normal progress during the first 6 days. Fentanyl appeared rapidly in the maternal circulation, with peak concentrations at 15 or 30 minutes. In all but 1 patient, concentrations decreased rapidly between 30 and 60 minutes. The infants were born at an average of 27 minutes after the epidural injections. The average umbilical concentration represented 43% of the maternal concentration at birth, with a range of 17% to 95%. The mean fentanyl concentrations in neonates were .13 ng/mL for the umbilical vein and .06 ng/mL for the artery.

Conclusion.—With the form of analgesia used in this patient group, fentanyl levels reaching the fetus after cesarean section were low and did not affect the neonatal condition. Nevertheless, the likelihood of fentanyl uptake by fetal tissues recommends caution when the drug is used repeatedly during spontaneous or induced labor.

▶ The pharmacokinetic exposure and response of the fetus are accumulating in dribs and drabs. The above series expands the information concerning the use of fentanyl as part of the epidural analgesic cocktail. The development of the microassay for fentanyl (1) paved the way for this data set. The rapid transfer to and accumulation of fentanyl by the fetus was impressive, even if no adverse effects could be documented. The authors' warning concerning the use of repeated doses of fentanyl to the mother should not go unheeded, and the resuscitation team needs to be aware of all the constituents in the epidural analgesia, not merely that the nature of the anesthesia was via the epidural route. In this way, if a neonate is depressed, apneic, or hypotensive secondary to maternal fentanyl administration, the cause will be quickly recognized and remedied.

As fentanyl is used more frequently in the neonatal intensive care unit, its pharmacokinetic characteristics need to be better understood. Arnold (1) noted that infants receiving extracorporeal membrane oxygenation required increasing plasma concentrations to maintain satisfactory sedation, suggesting rapid tolerance to the sedative effects of fentanyl.—A.A. Fanaroff, M.B.B.Ch.

Reference

1. Arnold JH: *J Pediatrics* 119:639, 1991.

Drug Screening of Newborns by Meconium Analysis: A Large-Scale, Prospective, Epidemiologic Study

Ostrea EM Jr, Brady M, Gause S, Raymundo AL, Stevens M (Wayne State Univ, Detroit)

Pediatrics 89:107–113, 1992 14–4

Introduction.—A method to identify drugs and their metabolites in the meconium of newborns was shown to be easy, specific, and sensitive. A previous study using this method found drug abuse during pregnancy in 73% of patients based on maternal interview, in 73% based on drug analysis of meconium, and in 75% based on maternal hair analysis. This method was used in a large-scale, prospective screening of neonates to determine the prevalence and epidemiologic characteristics of drug use in a high-risk, urban population.

Methods.—The meconium of 3,010 neonates was analyzed for the presence of metabolites of cocaine, morphine, and cannabinoids. The neonates were delivered at a tertiary perinatal center in Detroit in 1988–1989. Demographic, clinical and laboratory data on the mothers and infants were compiled and analyzed.

Results.—Of the screened infants, 44% were positive for drugs, 31% were positive for cocaine, 20.5% were positive for morphine, and 11.5% were positive for cannabinoid. In contrast, only 11% of mothers gave self-reports of illicit drug use during pregnancy. Maternal drug users were significantly more likely to be service patients, single, multigravid (more than 3), with little or no prenatal care, and to have had meconium-stained amniotic fluid. Cocaine users had significantly shorter duration of labor than did other women. In 32% of all positive test results, the presence of more than 1 drug was demonstrated. Among neonates, positive screens were associated with significantly higher incidences of prematurity, low birth weight, smaller length and head circumference, and an Apgar score of less than 6 at 1 minute. Meconium screens were positive in 88 of the infants whose mothers admitted drug use during pregnancy compared with only 52% with positive urine screens; however, 12% of these newborns had negative meconium screens.

Conclusion.—The presence of drug metabolites was detected in 44% of specimens of neonatal meconium, 4 times more than the 11% rate of drug usage obtained from maternal self-report. This discrepancy may be based in part on the use of self-report during routine maternal history taken by the physician, although other methods can provide more accurate information on maternal drug use. Because many infants exposed to drugs in utero may appear normal at birth and may have mothers who deny drug use, drug screening and a high index of suspicion may be necessary to detect infants at risk.

▶ It is a sad reflection on our society when there is evidence of drug abuse in 44% of women delivering at an urban tertiary center. Abuse of multiple drugs was noted in 32% of all positive meconium tests. This report reaffirms the value of meconium as a screening medium for drug use during pregnancy and confirms the unreliability of maternal history with regard to the use of illicit drugs (1). Meconium now offers an easy, rapid, and sensitive method to detect intrauterine exposure of the fetus to drugs. It remains to be proven that the method is also cost-effective. The appallingly high prevalence of drug usage casts a deep shadow of doubt on those who believe that the drug epidemic is abating.

Drug use in pregnancy has emerged as a major public health problem. It results in untold fetal wastage and drastically increases the perinatal morbidity. Many of the drugs may not produce immediate or recognizable effects on the neonate. Cocaine use is associated with an increased incidence of prematurity, intrauterine growth retardation, microcephaly, cerebral infarction and, possibly, other teratogenic effects resulting from disorders of neuronal migration or differentiation (2). Long-term consequences may include delays in physical and mental developmental and learning disabilities. The full expanse of this drug epidemic will not be available for many years. The early devastation is becoming more apparent, and the time is more than ripe to find a solution to this tragedy. Establishing the magnitude of the problem, as noted above, may gain the attention of legislators and public health officials so that the problem can really be tackled in earnest.

The greatest right in the world is the right to be wrong.—Harry Weinberger

A.A. Fanaroff, M.B.B.Ch

References

1. Ostrea EM, et al: *J Pediatr* 115:474, 1989.
2. Volpe JJ, et al: N *Engl J Med* 327:399, 1992.

Enhanced Prevalence of Ankyloglossia With Maternal Cocaine Use

Harris EF, Friend GW, Tolley EA (Univ of Tennessee, Memphis)

Cleft Palate Craniofac J 29:72–76, 1992 14–5

Background.—Partial ankyloglossia results from the persistent midline attachment of the tongue to the floor of the mouth. The association between maternal cocaine use and ankyloglossia in newborns was investigated.

Methods.—The study sample included 500 term neonates examined on a case-control basis. Drug use was determined by testing the mother and newborn for the major metabolite of cocaine, benzoylecgonine. Each infant was assessed for ankyloglossia (Fig 14–2) and several other oral conditions; birth weight and crown-heel length were also recorded, together with a number of maternal characteristics.

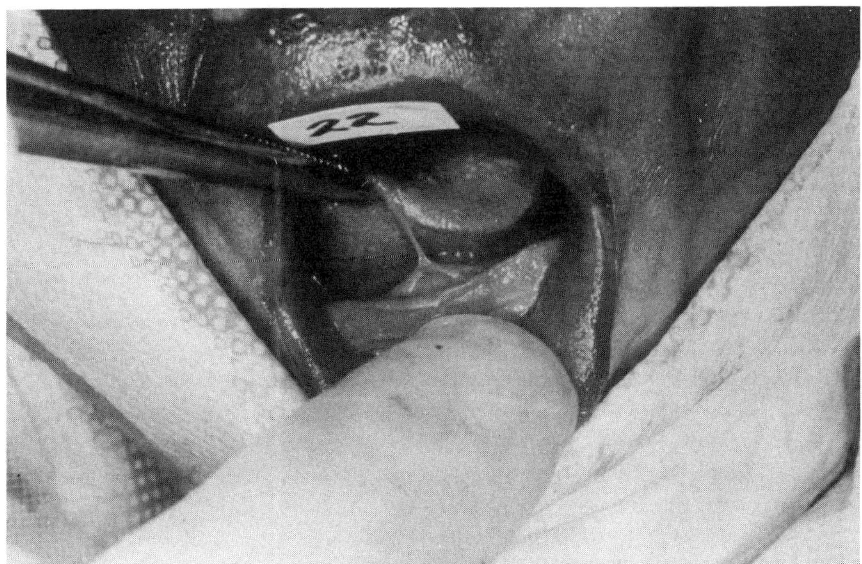

Fig 14–2.—An example of ankyloglossia with shortened, thickened frenulum restraining tongue mobility. (Courtesy of Harris EF, Friend GW, Tolley EA: *Cleft Palate Craniofac J* 29:72–76, 1992.)

Results.—Sixty-eight infants tested positive for maternal cocaine use. These infants had an increased likelihood of short length (2.4 times) and lower birth weight (1.8 times). Ankyloglossia was present in 4.4% of the 500 newborns and was more common in boys (6%) than in girls (2.3%). Both black and white infants exhibited an incidence of 4% to 5%. The incidence of ankyloglossia was 10.4% in infants born to cocaine users vs. 3.5% in infants born to nonusers. The other maternal factors examined were not associated with ankyloglossia.

Conclusion.—Maternal cocaine use was the primary determinant of partial ankyloglossia in these infants. The higher frequency of the condition in male infants may reflect their slower maturation. Recent studies have suggested that cocaine-induced defects occur during the embryonic period of gestation. Ankyloglossia may be a nonspecific consequence of maternal cocaine abuse and the multiple interactive risk factors characteristic of the life-style of these women.

▶ Not only does cocaine affect brain growth, but in some infants it also results in a shortened frenulum or tongue-tie. I disagree, however, with the authors' belief that this single problem can either delay speech or retard the development of a mature swallowing pattern.—M.H. Klaus, M.D.

Pharmacokinetics of Midazolam During Continuous Infusion in Critically Ill Neonates

Jacqz-Aigrain E, Daoud P, Burtin P, Maherzi S, Beaufils E (Hôpital Robert Debré, Paris)

Eur J Clin Pharmacol 42:329–332, 1992 14–6

Objective.—Midazolam is a short-acting, water-soluble benzodiazepine that may be useful for sedation of critically ill neonates. The pharmacokinetics of midazolam during continuous infusion in critically ill neonates of various gestational ages were examined.

Treatment.—Midazolam, .2 mg/kg given as an intravenous bolus followed immediately by a continuous infusion of .06 mg/kg/hr, was administered to 15 critically ill neonates who were undergoing mechanical ventilation for respiratory distress syndrome. The mean gestational age was 32.8 weeks (range, 29–41 weeks).

Outcome.—Hypotension occurred in 4 neonates, 3 of whom were also given fentanyl. Hypotension occurred immediately after the bolus dose of midazolam in 3 patients. Plasma clearance of midazolam was 1.7 mL/kg/min, and the elimination half-life was 12 hours; both parameters correlated significantly with gestational age (Fig 14–3). The clearance

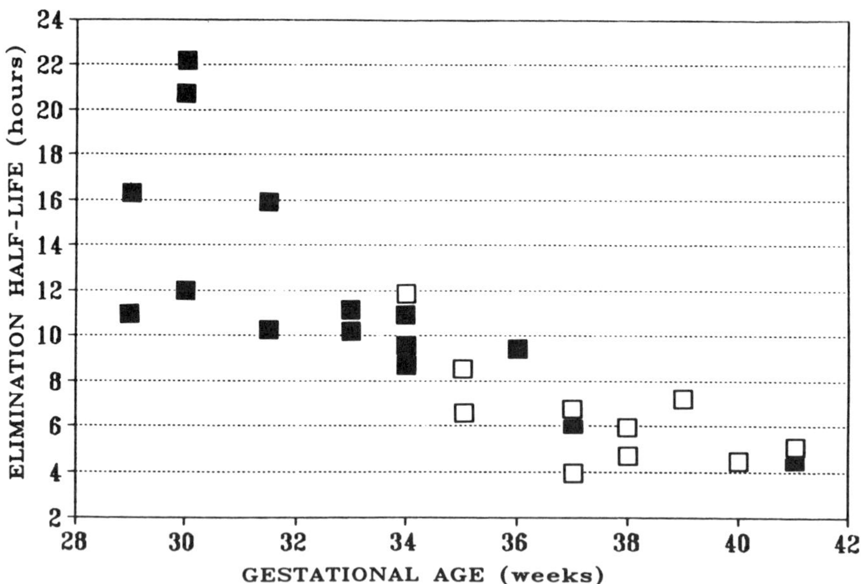

Fig 14–3.—Linear regression between elimination half-life of midazolam and gestational age: $Y = -1.07 \times + 47.1$; $r = .82$, $P < .001$. Elimination half-life was calculated after bolus administration (*open squares*) and at the end of continuous infusion (*filled squares*). (Data obtained after intravenous bolus were presented previously.) (Courtesy of Jacqz-Aigrain, Daoud P, Burtin P, et al: *Eur J Clin Pharmacol* 42:329–332, 1992.)

rate was reduced and the elimination half-life was prolonged when compared with those of young adults and children.

Conclusion.—Midazolam may be used to achieve rapid brief sedation during the neonatal period. However, it should be administered cautiously, particularly in premature infants or when fentanyl is also given. Intravenous bolus doses of midazolam should be avoided.

▶ Celeste M. Marx, Pharm.D., Assistant Professor of Pediatrics, Case Western Reserve University School of Medicine, comments:

▶ This study extended the first author's previous work with the single-dose pharmacokinetics of midazolam in the first week of life (1) to assess a more gestationally diverse population that was given the agent by an initial loading bolus followed by a continuous infusion. When data from both studies are combined, elimination half-life of midazolam correlates well with gestational age ($r = .82$) in the first week of life. The active metabolite, 1-OH midazolam, was measurable in infants in this recent study. The longer half-lives and metabolite presence, like the single-dose data (1), should not be misconstrued to imply that midazolam is "not really short-acting in preterm neonates" (2). This study was not designed to determine the efficacy or duration of action of midazolam for newborn sedation. It may be inferred that the efficacy of midazolam was not optimal, because nearly one half of the infants received fentanyl concomitantly. Unfortunately, it was not established that the infants actually needed sedation by any defined criteria, either initially or later. Although use of fentanyl does not interfere with the measurement of midazolam plasma concentration, it does complicate evaluation of midazolam efficacy and safety. The risk of hemodynamic instability in the presence of fentanyl may be very different from that when using midazolam as a sole agent. The optimal dose of fentanyl as a supplemental analgesic during infusion of midazolam is not known.

The authors' choice of initial midazolam bolus (loading) dose and continuous infusion doses are important factors relating to their adverse safety experience. It is unclear how the infusion dose was selected. The initial study did not examine any correlation of efficacy and plasma concentration to allow a specific plasma concentration to be targeted. A relatively large bolus dose of midazolam (standardized for weight) was given to all infants. No adjustment was made for an infant's individual response or tolerance of side effect. It does not appear that midazolam infusion administration was discontinued in the face of protracted hypotension refractory to albumin infusion. It is possible that neither the pharmacokinetics nor the safety data are clinically relevant to midazolam safety with proper use, i.e., the same as those that would be seen after administration of a minimum effective dosage of midazolam alone. Because of that element, these data are not an adequate argument for avoiding "bolus" administration of midazolam; they only call for avoiding the use of the large initial dose chosen in this investigation, particularly in combination with fentanyl. Midazolam is a useful sedative that should undergo additional study in newborns.

Until more complete data are available, each therapeutic use of either sedative in a neonate should be treated as an individual experiment to define the minimum effective dose without unacceptable side effects. That is, *small* incremental boluses of a single agent should be given, titrated to adequate effect without unacceptable cardiovascular side effects. Once the effective dose is established, it is given as often as necessary or is continuously infused if doses are required too frequently to be practical. Neonatal research with objective observations of sedation onset and recovery after the dose effective for newborns of various maturities will indicate whether intermittent dosage or continuous infusion is best for this population.

As an additional safety concern, the authors do not state whether the midazolam product administered contains benzyl alcohol. The dose of benzyl alcohol administered should be monitored during the use of midazolam in immature newborns.—C.M. Marx, Pharm.D.

References

1. Jacqz-Aigrain E, et al: *Eur J Clin Pharmacol* 39:191, 1990.
2. Van den Anker JN, Sauer PJJ: *Eur J Clin Pharmacol* 5:152, 1992.

The Effect of Benzodiazepines on the Fetus and the Newborn

Laegreid L, Hagberg G, Lundberg A (Gothenburg Univ, Sweden)

Neuropediatrics 23:18–23, 1992 14–7

Introduction.—Benzodiazepines (BZD) are frequently used in pregnancy. The potential impact of maternal use of BZD on the fetus and the newborn infant was evaluated in a prospective longitudinal study.

Setting.—Seventeen children born to 16 mothers who used BZD only throughout pregnancy (BZD group) were studied. For comparison, 21 newborns who were exposed to psychotropic drugs other than BZD during pregnancy (drug group) and 29 newborns with no known fetal exposure to drugs (reference group) were also studied. The pregnancy and perinatal periods were evaluated, and a neurologic examination, consisting of 38 items subgrouped in terms of reflexes/reactions, tonus, and other symptoms and signs, was performed on the second day of life.

Results.—Infants in the BZD group had lower birth weight relative to birth length when compared with both drug and reference groups. Infants in the BZD group had significantly more perinatal complications, such as intrauterine asphyxia, instrumental delivery, respiratory disturbances, and infection work out than those in the reference group. Furthermore, BZD-exposed infants differed significantly from the reference group in half of the 38 neurologic and behavioral items, ranging from depression of the CNS to hyperirritability. Infants of 2 mothers with the highest consumption of BZD showed clear intoxication or withdrawal symptoms.

Conclusion.—Maternal use of BZD is associated with impaired intrauterine growth, increased frequency of perinatal complications, and significantly deviating neurobehavior.

▶ Because BZDs are frequently used in pregnancy in Sweden, it is appropriate that prospective longitudinal studies be undertaken to determine their effects on the fetus. This report represents the first results of these studies. Although somewhat limited in scope, it further documents the importance of the chemical milieu of the fetus on subsequent physical and mental development. The adverse effects of alcohol, tobacco, narcotics, and cocaine have all been substantiated (1). We learn that in women who take benzodiazepines, there are more perinatal problems, the fetal growth is impaired, and the neurobehavioural responses soon after delivery can be differentiated from those in neonates not exposed to other chemical compounds. The features selected were more characteristic of drug abstinence or intoxication. None of the infants showed the athetoid posture or tremor and dystonia that were characteristic of BZD withdrawal, and no major malformations were documented to support the teratogenicity of BZD. It remains to be seen whether these findings are transient or will translate into permanent problems. Because there was a reduction in head circumference, it is probable that permanent sequelae will occur, particularly as the home environment is unlikely to be optimal and will not compensate for the poor perinatal environment. The women who were taking benzodiazepines smoked more, lived less frequently in stable pair relationships, and had more pregnancies and abortions than did the reference group. The same boring message emerges: drugs taken by the mother can harm the fetus and should be avoided. See also Abstract 2–6.

I have learned to use the word impossible with the greatest caution.—Werner von Braun

A.A. Fanaroff, M.B.B.Ch.

Reference

1. Volpe JJ, et al: *N Engl J Med* 327:399, 1992.

Population Pharmacokinetics of Gentamicin in Neonates Using a Nonlinear, Mixed-Effects Model

Jensen PD, Edgren BE, Brundage RC (Children's Hosp of St Paul, Minn; Med Univ of South Carolina, Charleston)

Pharmacotherapy 12:178–182, 1992 14–8

Background.—Pharmacokinetic studies of neonates are usually hampered by the limited availability of serum samples. A new statistical program using a nonlinear, mixed-effects model (NONMEM) may prove particularly useful in these patients. A NONMEM program was used to assess the pharmacokinetics of gentamicin in neonates, and these results were compared with those obtained in a separate study.

Methods.—A total of 443 serum samples taken from 150 neonates receiving gentamicin were evaluated. A NONMEM computer program run on a VAX 11/785 computer performed data analysis.

Results.—Regression analysis indicated that gentamicin clearance rates could be computed from: Clearance (L/hr) = $.120 \times (\text{weight}/2.4)^{1.36}$. Equations for volume of distribution were also obtained: Volume (L) = $.429 \times$ (weight). Interindividual variation was 26.2% for clearance and 15.9% for volume of distribution. Intraindividual variation, accounting for all other sources of residual error, was 11%. These results compared favorably with those in a group of neonates analyzed by standard 2-stage population analysis.

Conclusion.—Although NONMEM is still experimental, these results are in close agreement with other NONMEM and conventional analyses. The modest covariance correlation coefficient of .53, found between clearance rate and volume of distribution, supports clinical experience.

▶ Commenting on this article is Michael Reed, Pharm.D., Associate Professor of Pediatrics, Case Western Reserve University, and Director, Pediatric Clinical Pharmacology and Toxicology, Rainbow Babies and Children's Hospital, Oakland, California:

▶ The pharmacokinetics of gentamicin in a group of neonates were determined using population-based statistical methods. Serum gentamicin concentrations were obtained from 150 neonates who were receiving the drug for suspected or documented infection. All infants were younger than 7 days' postnatal age, between 25 and 43 weeks (mean, 35 weeks) of gestation, and they weighed between .62 and 4.9 kg (mean, 2.4 kg). Each infant received 2.5 mg of gentamicin per kg of body weight, which was infused intravenously over 30 minutes; documented infusion times ranged from 10 to 120 minutes. After the first gentamicin dose, blood samples were obtained for the determination of the gentamicin concentration in serum. A total of 443 heel stick samples were obtained as routine clinical data, usually at 1, 7, and 11 hours after infusion of gentamicin, and they were analyzed in the clinical laboratory by radioimmunoassay. The measured serum gentamicin concentration-time data were entered into a nonlinear, mixed-effects model (NONMEM) computer program to generate gentamicin pharmacokinetic parameter estimates. The accuracy of the NONMEM-derived regression model to predict serum gentamicin concentrations was assessed in another group of 30 infants with similar clinical characteristics who were receiving gentamicin.

Various regression models were tested relative to their ability to describe the important gentamicin pharmacokinetic parameters: body clearance (Cl) and volume of distribution (Vd). A knowledge of these values allows accurate prediction of resultant serum drug concentrations after any size dose administered. The final regression model described by the authors for the "typical value of clearance (TVCL)" for the population was TVCL = .12* (wt / 2.4)$^{1.36}$ L/hr and, for the "typical value of volume of distribution (TVVD)" for the population, TVVD = (wt) L* .429, where wt is patient body weight. Comparison of the 2 pharmacokinetic methods to predict serum peak and trough gentamicin concentrations, i.e., applying population-derived regression relationships or standard individual pharmacokinetic methods revealed small, nonstatistically (or clinically) significant differences.

The results of this study confirm those from previously published reports describing the accuracy of population-based pharmacokinetic methods in predicting resultant gentamicin serum concentrations during the neonatal period. These population-based pharmacokinetic techniques may be useful in those clinical settings where the available number of blood samples is severely restricted and/or sample acquisition is many times less than optimal for calculation of a patient's individual gentamicin pharmacokinetics.

Gentamicin is the most common antibiotic administered to neonates. A member of the aminoglycoside class of antibiotics, the use of gentamicin may be associated with serious adverse effects, including oto- and nephrotoxicity. Recognition that the occurrence of these adverse effects may be related to the serum aminoglycoside (gentamicin) concentration has fostered the near-universal use of serum drug concentration monitoring to guide aminoglycoside dosing. Knowledge of a drug's pharmacokinetic characteristics allows initial dose selection, which achieves predetermined target serum drug concentrations with the least number of dose adjustments. Traditional strategies to define a drug's pharmacokinetic behavior involve obtaining detailed disposition data from individual patients; this can be extremely difficult in seriously ill neonates. This method of pharmacokinetic analysis for gentamicin requires a minimum of 2–3 blood samples obtained at specific time points. Moreover, this approach requires a knowledge of the exact time a blood sample is obtained relative to gentamicin administration, an extremely important but often overlooked and undocumented piece of information at the bedside. One attempt to overcome these limitations and enhance the clinical usefulness of suboptimal or incomplete data is to perform population-based, rather than patient-specific, pharmacokinetic evaluations.

Population-based strategies to describe the pharmacokinetics of a number of different drugs have expanded during the past decade (1). This method of pharmacokinetic analysis provides pharmacokinetic information for a specific drug relative to the patient population of interest rather than the individual patient. In addition, this analytic method accepts all data points (including those that may have been obtained incorrectly or at suboptimal times) that provide limited information about an individual's specific pharmacokinetic values but can be pooled to provide information about the population. Based on these criteria, it is understandable that neonates are a primary target patient population frequently used to assess the validity of these techniques and to refine methodology.

The data derived from this study describe a similar regression relationship to estimate gentamicin pharmacokinetics in neonates, confirming the findings of previous reports (2, 3). These regression formulas can be used to estimate a neonate's gentamicin body clearance (TVCL) and volume of distribution (TVVD) rapidly for calculation of the initial gentamicin dose for a particular infant. Regardless of how the initial dose is selected, the accuracy of dose selection should be confirmed in each patient. Does this approach allow a more accurate means to calculate initial gentamicin dose requirements for seriously ill neonates as compared with our current dose estimates based on gestational and postconceptional age? Probably not. These pharmacokinetic methods *do* expand the depth and sophistication of our understanding of a drug's disposition profile in a patient population that poses many challenges in the conduct of clinical research.—M. Reed, Pharm.D.

References

1. Thompson AH, Whiting B: *Clin Pharmacokinet* 22:447, 1992.
2. Grasela TH, et al: *Clin Pharmacol Ther* 37:199, 1985.
3. Thompson AH, et al: *Dev Pharmacol Ther* 11:173, 1988.

15 The Genitourinary Tract

The Accuracy of Antenatal Ultrasonography in Identifying Renal Abnormalities

Johnson CE, Elder JS, Judge NE, Adeeb FN, Grisoni ER, Fattlar DC (Case Western Univ, Cleveland, Ohio)

Am J Dis Child 146:1181–1184, 1992 15–1

Purpose.—Most fetuses with mild renal pelvic dilation diagnosed antenatally by ultrasound ultimately prove to be normal. Although there have been many retrospective studies of the epidemiology of fetal renal abnormalities, reliable incidence figures for the general population are lacking. The accuracy of using ultrasonographic measurement of the antenatal renal pelvic diameter for the prediction of renal abnormalities was investigated.

Patients and Methods.—During a 3-year period, more than 7,500 pregnant women underwent ultrasonography at a teaching hospital that provides primary and tertiary obstetric care. Sixty percent of the patients were non-Hispanic whites, 30% were black, and 9% were Hispanic. Fifty-six fetuses were identified as having suspected fetal hydronephrosis or cystic lesions; all had measurement of the renal pelvic diameter in the anteroposterior dimension. After the third day of life, the neonates underwent ultrasonography again, and those with abnormal results had a cystogram and renal diuretic scan.

Results.—Nineteen subjects had a pelvic diameter of 9 mm or less, 28 had a pelvic diameter of more than 9 mm, and 9 had hypoplasia, renal agenesis, or cystic malformations. There were no cases of obstruction in the 50 kidneys with an anteroposterior pelvic diameter of 15 mm or less. Eleven of the 14 kidncys with a pelvic diameter of larger than 15 mm had obstruction or vesicoureteral reflux. Five of the 12 kidneys believed to be multicystic antenatally proved to be hydronephrotic.

Conclusion.—Although most fetuses with antenatally suspected hydronephrosis prove to be normal after birth (Fig 15–1), fetuses with a renal pelvic diameter of greater than 15 mm are likely to have hydronephrosis. The incidence of renal and bladder abnormalities was about 2.8 in 1,000 pregnancies studied by antenatal ultrasound.

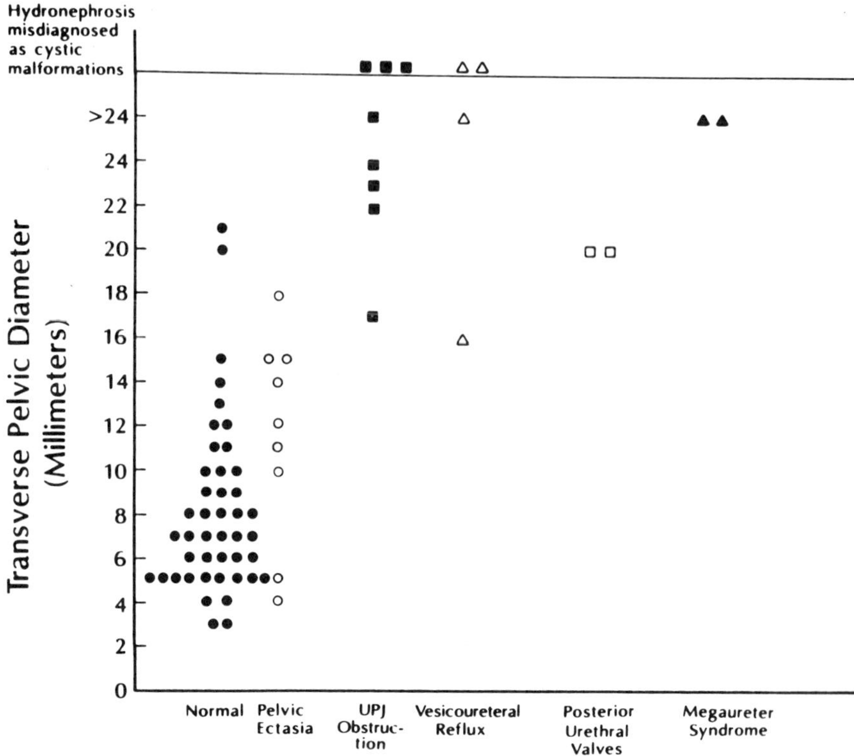

Fig 15–1.—Transverse anteroposterior pelvic diameter on antenatal ultrasonogram classified by final diagnosis. Each point represents 1 renal unit. *Abbreviation: UPJ,* ureteropelvic junction. The area above the dotted line indicates hydronephrosis misdiagnosed as cystic malformations. Different symbols represent various diagnoses. (Courtesy of Johnson CE, Elder JS, Judge NE, et al: *Am J Dis Child* 146:1181–1184, 1992.)

Ultrasound Screening of Newborn Urinary Tract

Scott JES, Lee REJ, Hunter EW, Coulthard MG, Matthews JNS (Univ of Newcastle Upon Tyne, England; Royal Victoria Infirmary, Newcastle Upon Tyne, England)

Lancet 338:1571–1573, 1991 15–2

Objective.—It has been hypothesized that a noninvasive method of screening newborns for ureteric reflux may allow appropriate action to prevent reflux nephropathy. To test this hypothesis, ultrasound screening was undertaken among infants born at 1 hospital during 1986.

Study Design.—Ultrasound was performed on 1,086 unselected newborn infants, and the findings were recorded on videotape. Infants with dilated renal collecting systems underwent further investigations, including micturating cystourethrography, intravenous urography, or radioisotope study. A postal follow-up survey was conducted when the children were age 3 years, and 657 families (62%) responded. A search for nonresponders who subsequently had renal radioisotope studies revealed 5 nonresponders.

Findings.—Ureteric reflux was diagnosed in 6 children (.6%). However, the diagnosis was suspected at the neonatal scan in only 3 infants (.3%). Diagnosis was made at follow-up in the other 3 children. In 2 infants, the renal collecting system was too small to be measured on the neonatal scan, and in 1, the reflux was not apparent at the neonatal scanning. Five infants had hydronephrosis on the neonatal scan, including 3 (.3%) with nonrefluxing hydronephrosis. More than half of the children with hydronephrosis or ureteric reflux had only slight dilatation (less than 5 mm) on the neonatal scan. Review of the original videotapes showed no difference in internal dimensions between the right and left kidneys. The internal dimension was 5 mm or less in both kidneys in 96.3% of infants and 4 mm or less in 93.3%. Other renal abnormalities were noted on neonatal scans of 4 infants.

Conclusion.—Routine renal ultrasound scanning of newborns appears to have no value in detecting those who may have ureteric reflux. Further studies are needed in a large cohort of healthy infants to define the sensitivity and specificity of ultrasound screening in predicting reflux.

Nonoperative Management of Unilateral Neonatal Hydronephrosis

Koff SA, Campbell K (Ohio State Univ, Columbus)

J Urol 148:525–531, 1992 15–3

Introduction.—The use of maternal ultrasound has led to detection of fetal hydronephrosis in numerous asymptomatic infants. Surgical intervention for suspected obstruction has become a popular, though controversial, management approach. Forty-five infants were analyzed to define the natural history of unilateral neonatal hydronephrosis and to determine the accuracy of diagnostic studies for assessing obstruction.

Methods.—The infants were to be followed nonoperatively, with surgical intervention reserved for proven deterioration of renal function in the affected kidney. A combination of ultrasound, diuretic renography, and cystography was used to evaluate the condition. Prophylactic antibiotics were given during the first year of life or until improvement of hydronephrosis.

Results.—Thirty of the infants had mild hydronephrosis, showed no renal deterioration, and did not require surgical repair. Severe hydronephrosis was seen in the remaining 15 cases. These infants had marked pelviocaliceal dilatation and parenchymal thinning, as well as significantly decreased renal function. During follow-up, hydronephrosis completely disappeared in 2 infants, showed mild-to-marked improvement in 5, and was unchanged in 8. In all patients, percentage and absolute renal function rapidly increased; none had contralateral compensatory hypertrophy develop. None of the 15 infants with initially impaired renal function has required surgical intervention.

Conclusion.—Despite initial decreases in renal function, many kidneys of newborns with severe hydronephrosis are not biologically obstructed. Nevertheless, standard diagnostic tests suggested or diagnosed obstruction in these infants. Sequential ultrasonographic and radionuclide studies should identify evidence of obstructive injury before surgery is undertaken. Improvement in renal function that occurs after surgery may actually reflect normal maturation of the kidney.

▶ Commenting on this article is Sumner Marshall, M.D., Clinical Professor of Urology, University of California, San Francisco, and Director, Division of Pediatric Urology, Children's Hospital, Oakland, California:

▶ One principal theme that emerges from these 3 papers (Abstracts 15–1, 15–2, and 15–3) is that the physician should be aware of the limitations of ante- and neonatal ultrasonography. It often may be difficult to differentiate between multicystic and hydronephrotic kidneys, as well as to identify which children might need interventional therapy.

The physician is faced with the dilemma of deciding just how extensive a workup should be initiated when an anatomical abnormality is reported on ante- or neonatal ultrasonography. Despite the fact that a large proportion of these abnormalities are of no clinical significance and very possibly need no or only minimal follow-up, once the family has been informed of the abnormal finding, their level of concern usually rises rapidly. Therefore, it is incumbent on the physician to handle this parental anxiety by providing either reassurance that nothing further need be done or by appropriate guidance for more complete evaluation. For example, if only mild-to-moderate dilation of the collecting system (hydronephrosis) is noted, follow-up sonograms alone are quite adequate. When dealing with more severe hydronephrosis, it is critical that some type of functional evaluation be done. A large number of these kidneys are not anatomically obstructed and will not require surgical intervention. A diuretic renogram should help differentiate the surgical from the nonsurgical cases.

In the majority of cases of renal abnormalities identified on ante- or neonatal ultrasonography, no interventional therapy is necessary. All too often, we treat the x-ray film rather than the patient. Surgical intervention is fraught with measurable risks, and it should not be performed unless there is evidence of potential damage to the kidney secondary to a true anatomical obstruction.—S. Marshall, M.D.

Outpatient Inguinal Herniorrhaphy in Premature Infants: Is It Safe?

Melone JH, Schwartz MZ, Tyson KRT, Marr CC, Greenholz SK, Taub JE (Univ

of Calif, Davis; Sutter Surgery Cent, Sacramento, Calif)
J Pediatr Surg 27:203–208, 1992 15–4

Introduction.—In infants, inguinal herniorrhaphy is usually performed as an outpatient procedure. However, in premature infants, it is usually performed as an inpatient procedure because of the increased incidence of apnea and bradycardia subsequent to administration of general anesthesia.

Patients and Methods.—Data were reviewed on 1,294 outpatient inguinal herniorrhaphies performed over a 5-year period. Of the infants, 124 were premature, with a gestational age of 24–36 weeks, a postnatal age of 3–24 weeks, and a postconceptional age of 34–59 weeks. Ventilatory support had been required in 22 infants, apnea/bradycardia occurred in 11, and bronchopulmonary dysplasia occurred in 9. General anesthesia was used in all infants and endotracheal intubation was used in 75%. The average time in the operating room was 40 minutes, and the average time in the recovery room was 94 minutes.

There were no perioperative deaths. One patient became apneic with extubation, but no further episodes were noted. Another patient had a brief apneic period at home that was relieved by gentle stimulation. Bradycardia of 80 beats per minute was noted in 2 patients in the recovery room and resolved spontaneously. With extubation, laryngospasm occurred in 2 patients; in 1, it resolved spontaneously, and brief reintubation was necessary in the other. Postoperative ventilation was necessary in 2 patients. There was 1 postdischarge emergency room visit. None of the infants required readmission after discharge from the outpatient surgical center.

Conclusion.—In these infants, the previously reported high incidence of apnea and bradycardia did not occur. This was true even among those infants with a previous history of apnea and bradycardia. Although the reasons for this are not known, it is possible that the fact that preoperative and postoperative narcotics were not used and that muscle relaxants were used sparingly may have been contributory factors. Routine inpatient inguinal herniorrhaphy is not necessary in premature infants.

► Each year, the number of extremely-low-birth-weight infants discharged from the hospital increases. Many of them are scheduled to return in the near future for repair of an inguinal hernia or two. The surgical/anesthesia/nursing team has some far reaching decisions to make regarding inpatient vs. outpatient surgery, type of anesthesia/analgesia, and type and duration of monitoring. A few recent studies have provided revealing information pointing the team in the right direction.

I found the title to Melone et al.'s study to be amusing. In the form of a rhetoric question, it explores the safety of outpatient surgery. However the study was retrospective and no inpatients were used for comparison; therefore, we must deduce that the results justified the preconceived notion of the team. If they didn't believe that it was safe, they would not have started doing ambulatory surgery in the first place. Not surprisingly, they conclude that it is indeed safe, a conclusion that has been reached by other investigators (1, 2)

The infants did not receive continuous pneumography nor oxygen saturation monitoring; thus, the true incidence of apnea is unknown. Kurth (2) had documented a significant occurrence of apnea and desaturation, suggesting that all infants should be monitored with pulse oximetry postoperatively. Veverka (1) had reported the safety of spinal anesthesia for outpatient herniorrhaphy, suggesting that it reduced the incidence of postoperative apnea in preterm infants. It would appear that the use of inhalational anesthesia by experienced personnel who avoided muscle relaxants and narcotics pre and intraoperatively worked equally well for Melone. Thus, there is a choice concerning the anesthetic technique.

In sum, the repair of an inguinal hernia can be carried out on former premature infants in an outpatient setting. An experienced surgical team is mandatory, and if Kurth's guidelines are followed, "infants younger than 60 postconceptional weeks should be monitored continuously for at least 12 hours postoperatively." Although I am confident that this 12-hour period will be whittled down, I believe that the concept of continuous monitoring should not be compromised.—A.A. Fanaroff, M.B.B.Ch.

References

1. 1992 Year Book of Neonatal and Perinatal Medicine, pp 162–163.
2. 1992 Year Book of Neonatal and Perinatal Medicine, pp 166–168.

The Urinary System in Down Syndrome: A Study of 124 Autopsy Cases

Ariel I, Wells TR, Landing BH, Singer DB (Women and Infants' Hosp, Providence, RI; Children's Hosp of Los Angeles, Calif)
Pediatr Pathol 11:879–888, 1991 15–5

Introduction.—Although malformations of the kidney and urinary tract are described in several chromosomal aberrations, they generally have received little attention in cases of Down syndrome. In a study of 124 autopsy cases of Down syndrome there were 18 fetuses of 16–22 weeks' gestation, which were aborted after Down syndrome was diagnosed by amniocentesis; 9 stillborn fetuses and newborn infants who died on the first day of life, all but 1 of them at more than 30 weeks' gestation; and 97 patients up to 25 years of age.

Findings.—Renal weight was reduced by 14% on average, and renal hypoplasia was evident in 21% of the cases. Glomerular microcysts were found in nearly one fourth of the patient series, chiefly in the subcapsular region. Focal tubular dilatation was found in 10 kidneys and simple cysts were found in 7. Obstructive uropathy was present in 8 cases. Two of 9 fetuses and newborn infants had bladder neck stenosis with hydroureters and bilateral cystic dysplasia. All cases of renal cystic dysplasia were associated with obstructive lesions of the urinary tract.

Conclusion.—These findings suggest that obstructive uropathy is associated with Down syndrome and that, when severe, it can lead to early perinatal death. Chromosomal analysis is appropriate whenever obstructive uropathy is identified in a fetus or newborn infant.

▶ Descriptive reports do not make for exciting reading, yet they represent an important step in the process of elucidating the pathophysiology of various disorders. The association between obstructive uropathy and Down syndrome appears significant in the fetus and early newborn period. This series, which originates from autopsy findings, is a select group that does not reflect the true incidence of obstructive uropathy in trisomy 21. An obstructive uropathy with oligohydramnios sequence may distort the facial features to the extent that the observer misses the classical features of trisomy 21. The recommendation for chromosomal analysis in all fetuses and newborns with obstructive uropathy therefore may not be that far fetched.

In a prospective study, Rosendahl (1) noted abnormalities of the genitourinary tract in 27 of 4,586 fetuses at 18 weeks and in 19 fetuses at 34 weeks' gestation. Screening failed to detect abnormalities in only 4 infants. Whereas the screening process can work well, little progress has been made with regard to intervening on the fetus with obstructive uropathy. Reuss and associates (2) reported that 31 of 43 infants with an obstructive uropathy diagnosed but not treated in utero died soon after birth. The vast majority of these infants (89%) had multiple malformations, chromosomal abnormalities, or lesions incompatible with life; therefore, in utero attempts at correction would indeed have proven futile. Arnold (3) reported on the prenatal experience with 56 infants who had the prenatal diagnosis of pelviureteric obstruction. Diagnosis was confirmed after delivery in only 45 of these infants, and a conservative approach to surgery was recommended if renal function was adequate. This contrasts with the more aggressive approach recommended on this side of the Atlantic.

The recurrent theme has been to adopt a conservative approach to urogenital anomalies identified in the fetus. See also Abstract 4–18.

Nothing is so firmly believed as what is least known.—Michel Eyquem de Montaigne

A.A. Fanaroff, M.B.B.Ch.

References

1. 1992 YEAR BOOK OF NEONATAL AND PERINATAL MEDICINE, pp 71–72.
2. Reuss A, et al: *Lancet* 2:950, 1988.
3. 1991 YEAR BOOK OF NEONATAL AND PERINATAL MEDICINE, pp 260–261.

Cryptorchidism: A Prospective Study of 7500 Consecutive Male Births, 1984–8

Chilvers CED, for the John Radcliffe Hospital Cryptorchidism Study Group (Univ of Nottingham, England)

Arch Dis Child 67:892–899, 1992 15–6

Introduction.—Cryptorchidism is an important congenital defect associated with infertility and testicular cancer. A research group in England examined a 4-year cohort of infant boys born between 1984 and 1988 to

TABLE 1.—Results of Screening for Neonatal Undescended Testis: Boys Examined in the John Radcliffe Hospital, November 1984 to October 1988

Birth weight (g)	*No examined at birth*	*Cryptorchid**			
		At birth		*At 3 months*	
		No	*Rate* (%)	*No*	*Rate* (%)
(a) Excluding boys with severe congenital abnormalities noted at birth:					
<2000	130	59	45·4	10	7·7†
2000–2499	238	32	13·4	6	2·5
≥2500	7032	270	3·8	99	1·41‡
Total	7400	361	4·9	115	1·55
(b) Including boys with severe congenital abnormalities noted at birth:					
<2000	134	63	47·0	10	7·5§
2000–2499	246	37	15·0	8	3·3‖
≥2500	7061	276	3·9	100	1·42¶
Total	7441	376	5·1	118	1·59

* Cryptorchid by position: cryptorchidism seen at 3 months decided at special pediatric surgical outpatient clinic.

† Two boys declared by their general practitioner as having descended testes assumed to have descended testes by the author's criteria.

‡ One boy who left the area assumed to have descended testes and 4 boys declared by their general practitioner as having descended testes assumed to have descended testes by the author's criteria.

§ Two boys declared by their general practitioner as having descended testes and 3 boys with severe congenital abnormalities assumed to have descended testes by the author's criteria.

‖ Two boys with severe congenital abnormalities assumed to have descended testes by the author's criteria.

¶ One boy who left the area assumed to have descended testes, 4 boys declared by their general practitioner as having descended testes, and 1 boy with a severe congenital abnormality assumed to have descended testes by the author's criteria.

(Courtesy of Chilvers CED, for the John Radcliffe Hospital Cryptorchidism Study Group: *Arch Dis Child* 67:892–899, 1992.)

TABLE 2.—Relationship Between Cryptorchidism and Other Characteristics Recorded at Birth: Boys Examined at John Radcliffe Hospital, Results Are Number (%)

	Descended	*Undescended*	
	(n=7039)	*At birth only (n=246)*	*At 3 months (n=115)*
Hernia	2 (0·03)	0 (0)	4†§ (3·5)
Hydrocoele	599 (8·5)	35‡ (14·2)	7† (6·1)
Hypospadias	110 (1·56)	6 (2·4)	6§ (5·2)
Small scrotum	251 (3·6)	106‡ (43·1)	64†§ (55·7)
Poor scrotal rugation	10 (0·14)	14‡ (5·7)	10§ (8·7)

Note: Excluding boys with severe congenital abnormalities at birth.
† Two sided $P < .05$ for difference between those undescended at birth only compared with those undescended at 3 months.
‡ Two sided $P < .05$ for difference between those descended at birth compared with those undescended at birth only.
§ Two sided $P < .05$ for difference between those descended at birth compared with those undescended at 3 months.
(Courtesy of Chilvers CED, for the John Radcliffe Hospital Cryptorchidism Study Group: *Arch Dis Child* 67:892–899, 1992.)

determine the incidence of undescended testis and risk factors for this condition.

Methods.—The 7,441 boys, almost all (98.2%) of whom were born at John Radcliffe Hospital, were examined for cryptorchidism during the first 24 hours of life. Those with severe congenital malformations were excluded from the study. All except testes well down in the scrotum were classified as undescended. The boys were examined again at home 3 months after birth. If a testis was still undescended, the child was referred to a pediatric surgical outpatient clinic for final assessment.

Results.—At birth, unilateral cryptorchidism was seen in 3% of the boys, and bilateral cryptorchidism had occurred in 1.92%. At 3 months, the rate of cryptorchidism was 7.7% in infants less than 2,000 g, 2.5% in those between 2,000 and 2,499 g, and 1.41% in those weighing ≥2,500 g. These rates were considerably higher than previously reported (Table 1). Boys with undescended testes at 3 months were more likely to have hypospadias, a small scrotum, and poor scrotal rugation compared with boys having normally descended testes at birth (Table 2). Descent at 3 months in infants cryptorchid at birth was more likely the lower the testis was along the normal pathway of descent and in infants with low birth weight, bilateral cryptorchidism, and normal scrotal size. The rate of orchidopexy at 3 years was 1.24%, substantially lower than in other series.

Conclusion.—Of the 115 infants with cryptorchidism confirmed at 3 months, 9.6% had normally descended testes at follow-up, 16.5% were borderline, and 73.9% had an orchidopexy. Of the 92 infants known to have had an orchidopexy, 85 were cryptorchid at 3 months, 3 were late descenders, and 4 were judged normal at birth.

► Neonatologists do not usually let their minds wander to the realms of testicular cancer and infertility, the well-established long-term sequelae of cryptorchidism. They have, however, long been aware that an undescended testis is present in 2% to 3% of full-term infants and as many as 30% of preterm infants, and that the condition is bilateral approximately 25% of the time. This large prospective study sheds some further light on the factors associated with cryptorchidism, including seasonality. I was somewhat startled to be introduced to the concept of the "ascending testis," which helps explain why there are apparently more orchidopexies than cases of cryptorchidism.

Cryptorchidism is associated with a number of minor malformations, including a small scrotum with poor scrotal rugation, hydrocele, inguinal hernia, and hypospadias. To this list should be added the increased number of epididymal malformations. These include separation of the testis and epididymis, angulation, atresia and a long mesorchium (1). Parrott (2) reported that the undescended testis demonstrates significant histologic abnormalities that are present at birth. This, together with congenital ductal lesions in the vas deferens and epididymis, accounts for the high incidence of infertility. Hence, an undescended testis should not be considered as a single entity but, rather, as part of a wider spectrum of embryopathy.

Smyth (3) reported that the incidence of cryptorchidism is higher in infants with cerebral palsy and attributed the condition to spasticity of the cremaster muscle. File this fact in the "Believe-It-or-Not" section.—A.A. Fanaroff, M.B.B.Ch.

References

1. Koff WJ, Scaletscky R: *J Urol* 143:340, 1990.
2. Parrott TS, et al: *Pediatrics* 83:591, 1989.
3. Smyth JA, et al: *J Pediatr Surg* 24:1303, 1989.

Prenatal Testicular Torsion: Principles of Management

Brandt MT, Sheldon CA, Wacksman J, Matthews P (Children's Hosp Med Ctr, Cincinnati, Ohio)

J Urol 147:670–672, 1992 15–7

Background.—Testicular torsion in the perinatal period is a rare condition that includes 2 separate entities, prenatal or in utero torsion and postnatal torsion. Researchers retrospectively studied all newborns at the study institution who had neonatal testicular torsion between 1976 and 1990.

Methods.—Data were collected for 23 infants (25 torsed testes). All underwent immediate exploration when medically stable. Excluded were those infants with a normal scrotal examination at birth who had torsion later. Long-term follow-up was available for 20 patients.

Results.—Emergency exploration revealed no viable testes, and no testes were salvaged. Seventeen testes were removed and confirmed to have complete necrosis. Six testes were replaced in the scrotum; all showed severe atrophy at follow-up. Torsion was predominantly on the left side (60%). All neonates but 1 were term deliveries, and 60% of the infants were above the 90th percentile in birth weight. The mean maternal parity was 3. Twelve of 13 patients who underwent orchiopexy returned for follow-up; all had normal testicular development. Results were also normal in 6 of the 8 patients undergoing neither contralateral exploration nor orchiopexy who were available for follow-up.

Conclusion.—Prenatal and postnatal torsion of the spermatic cord represent distinct clinical and pathologic entities. Prenatal torsion is almost exclusively extravaginal. Prompt exploration is an important step in the management of this condition. Evaluation and protection of the remaining gonad may be best accomplished by elective early inguinal exploration with orchiectomy and contralateral scrotal orchiopexy.

▶ Commenting on this article is Sumner Marshall, M.D., Clinical Professor of Urology, University of California, San Francisco, and Director, Division of Pediatric Urology, Children's Hospital, Oakland, California:

▶ Testicular torsion is one of the few real surgical emergencies of pediatric urology. Unless the compromised vascular supply to the torsed testis is reversed within a few hours, the testis becomes infarcted and nonviable. However, when testicular torsion is seen at birth, the actual "insult" to the testis has usually occurred in utero; by the time of birth, this testis is most likely already nonviable. In the neonate, the torsion usually involves the entire spermatic cord with surrounding tunica vaginalis, (extra vaginal torsion) as opposed to that occurring in the older boys, that of intravaginal torsion. The usual presentation is a swelling of the intrascrotal contents; over the subsequent few weeks, the swelling generally subsides, with progressive atrophy of the involved testis. There is little controversy regarding pexing of the contralateral testis in cases of postnatal torsion, given the high probability of an underlying anatomical abnormality of inadequate attachments of the contralateral testis. In cases of prenatal torsion, subsequent torsion of the contralateral testis is less likely, although certainly possible. Although extravaginal torsion is the usual presentation in this age group, intravaginal torsion has also been reported. I have seen such a case myself.

The status of the involved testis should be evaluated preoperatively with either a Doppler ultrasound study or an isotope testicular scan; it should be realized that the results could be misleading if there has been secondary inflammatory reaction, which could be misinterpreted as normal or even increased blood flow. Surgical exploration should be done as an elective procedure rather than as an emergency. At the time of surgery, if an incision into this testicle results in no bleeding, the testis is likely completely infarcted and, therefore, nonviable. Given the potential torsion of the contralateral testicle, combined with the relatively low risk of damage to this testicle by fixation, I agree with the authors' suggestion to proceed with orchiopexy at the time of removal of its nonviable mate.—S. Marshall, M.D.

16 Miscellaneous Topics

Temperature, Metabolic Adaptation and Crying in Healthy Full-Term Newborns Cared for Skin-to-Skin or in a Cot

Christensson K, Siles C, Moreno L, Belaustequi A, De La Fuente P, Lagercrantz H, Puyol P, Winberg J (Karolinska Hosp, Stockholm; Hosp Doce de Octubre, Madrid)

Acta Pædiatr 81:488–493, 1992 16–1

Background.—The human infant has a low or moderate capacity for nonshivering thermogenesis. Among mammals whose offspring are in this category, mothers arrange a nest and use their own body as a heat source. The human mother behaves in a similar way by holding her baby skin-to-skin. The effects of skin-to-skin care and cot care were compared in reference to temperature control, metabolic adaptation, and crying behavior.

Methods.—Included in this study were 50 vaginally delivered, healthy, full-term infants. Twenty-five were randomized to be kept skin-to-skin with the mother for 90 minutes after birth and 25 to be kept in a cot for

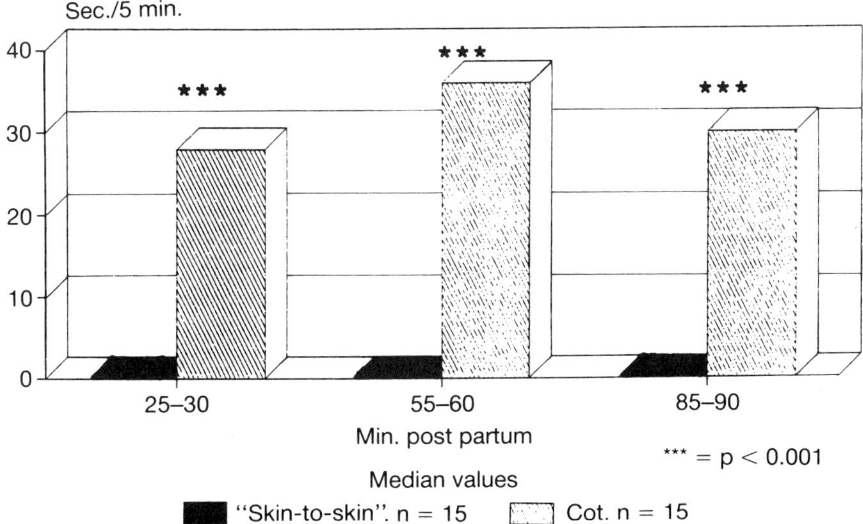

Fig 16–1.—The medians for crying time during 3 5-minute observation periods in healthy, full-term newborn infants kept skin-to-skin with the mother or in a cot. (Courtesy of Christensson K, Siles C, Moreno L, et al: *Acta Paediatr* 81:488–493, 1992.)

the same period of time. The mean room temperatures did not differ significantly between the groups.

Results.—There were significant differences in mean skin and axillar temperatures between the groups, particularly towards the end of the 90-minute observation period. Except at the intercapsular measurement point 30 minutes after birth, the skin-to-skin group was always warmer. There were 41 crying episodes registered among cot infants, but only 4 among skin-to-skin infants. Cot infants had significantly longer crying times during all 3 observation periods (Fig 16–1). The cot group also had a lower glucose level and slower normalization of the base deficit than the skin-to-skin group.

Conclusion.—Human mothers can be an important heat source for the newborn. This finding should be of special interest in developing countries, where neonatal hypothermia is associated with increased morbidity and mortality.

▶ The healthy newborn certainly seems happier on the warm skin of his mother than wrapped in a cot. At the same time, as we learn more about neonatal physiology and behavior, it appears that neonates' metabolic responses are also normalized more quickly when the neonates are managed with their mothers. Is this how the whole system was planned?—M.H. Klaus, M.D.

Design and Performance of Blanket Heat Shields for Neonates

Walterspiel JN (Univ of South Alabama, Mobile)

Acta Paediatr Scand 80:993–998, 1991 16–2

Introduction.—Various types of blanket shields are used to diminish heat loss in premature infants under radiant warmers. The influences were quantified of the different design features on the effectiveness of the shields.

Methods.—In 2 separate studies, 2 sets of shield designs were tested on groups of 14 infants. The effectiveness of the shield was determined by the amount of power consumption required by servo-controlled radiant warmers set to maintain a skin temperature of 36.6°C. Each type of shield was tested on every infant. Under control situations, no shield was used. One shield consisted of a thin, plasticized PVC food wrap stretched over the side rails of the bassinet. Another was a single-layer plastic blanket leaving the head uncovered. This same plastic blanket was also used without a cutout for the head and as a double layer with the head uncovered. After the first study, the most efficient shield (full body cover) was modified by adding a cut to slip around the endotracheal tube.

Results.—Power consumption was significantly affected by infant weight, with the lower-weight infants requiring more energy to maintain

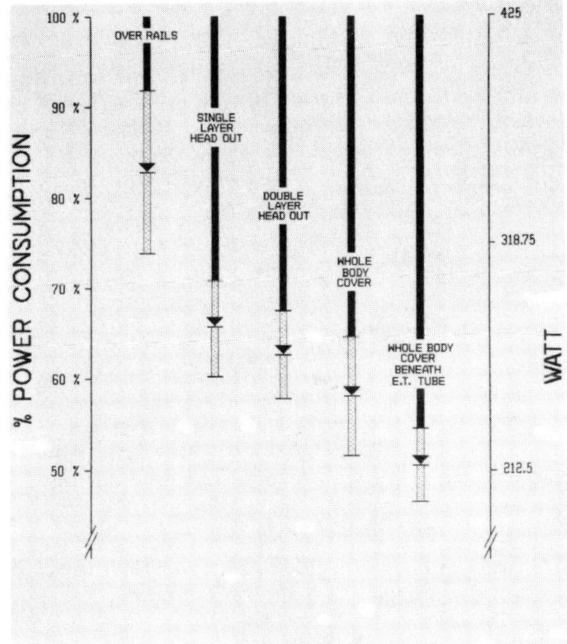

Fig 16–2.—Decreases in power consumption when infants were housed under the different shields. *Arrows* point to means; *shaded areas* cover 95% confidence intervals. The absolute values shown on the right are the ones measured for no shield in the first study (425 Watt) and under the whole-body cover that was tucked under the connecting tubes to the ventilator in the second study (212.5 Watt), (Courtesy of Walterspiel JN: *Acta Paediatr Scand* 80:993–998, 1991.)

skin temperature. The type of radiant warmer also had an influence; to achieve the same results, a newer model consumed less electrical power than an older one. The most efficient heat shield was the single layer covering the whole infant (Fig 16–2). This design reduced power consumption even more when the blanket was tucked under the connecting tubes to the ventilator. All variations of the plastic blanket shield were at least twice as effective as plastic wrap over the side rails.

Conclusion.—The most popular shield proved least efficient. A plastic blanket that covers the whole infant as close to the skin as possible appears to be the optimal design. A soft anchor around the endotracheal tube lessened the risk of displacement.

▶ Thermal regulation served as the foundation from which the fledgling subspecialty of neonatology emerged. Lamentably, it is frequently necessary to remind those now practicing or supervising this well-established profession to return to the their roots. It has mistakenly been taken for granted that the thermal needs of the infant are always being appropriately attented to and that the neutral thermal environment has been realized. Resarch output on thermal regulation has dwindled to a trickle as seemingly more glamorous—and certainly better funded—topics are tackled. This abstract serves to focus on this important matter and, in the process, it proves that practice does not always make perfect. The most popular heat shield, plastic wrap stretched over the rails, proved to be the least efficient, whereas a cover that was close to the body but did not necessarily include the head was twice as effective. It is important to recognize that the results were expressed as the relative reduction in power consumption between the shields, as seen in Figure 16–2. The starting point was the 100% power consumption without a shield or 0% reduction. The reader should note that, of the 14 infants, 5 had no studies without a shield, because the institutional review board permitted exchange of, but not removal of, shields. Furthermore, as commented in passing by the author, "displacement of the shield by an active infant was a common problem. The shields were pulled down toward the feet with the endotracheal tube sliding out of the incision."

Transparent plastic blankets diminish convection and evaporation, dampen the fluctuation of radiant energy, and may reduce oxygen consumption in addition to diminishing any infrared radiation to the infant (1, 2). Applying the blanket in the correct manner facilitates the attainment of the neutral thermal environment and may improve outcome for the infant. My understanding is that the computer-controlled incubators in Cincinnati continue to enhance survival of the smallest, least mature infants (3).

Imagination is more important than knowledge.—Albert Einstein

A.A. Fanaroff, M.B.B.Ch.

References

1. Baumgart S: *Pediatrics* 74:1022, 1984.
2. Chessex P, et al: *J Pediatr* 113:373, 1988.
3. Perlstein PH, et al: *Pediatrics* 57:494, 1976.

Interferon Alfa-2a Therapy for Life-Threatening Hemangiomas of Infancy

Ezekowitz RAV, Mulliken JB, Folkman J (Children's Hosp, Boston)
N Engl J Med 326:1456–1463, 1992 16–3

Introduction.—Infants with hemangiomas experience an excessive growth of the capillary endothelium and accompanying complications. The most common tumor in infancy, hemangioma, affects 10% to 12% of white infants and as many as 22% of preterm infants weighing less than 1,000 g. Although most are small and benign, some hemangiomas can cause serious consequences. Interferon alfa-2a, developed as an antiviral agent, has been reported to improve Kaposi's sarcoma (a vascular tumor) in patients with AIDS. Twenty very young patients with life-threatening or vision-threatening hemangiomas, who had not responded to corticosteroid therapy, were treated with interferon alfa-2a.

Methods.—Twenty infants and children with severe hemangiomas, including lesions that had invaded or blocked vital organs or tissues, participated in the trial. The recombinant human interferon alfa-2a given had a specific activity of 3 million units per .5 mL. Each patient received up to 3 million units per square meter of body surface area by subcutaneous injection every day.

Results.—Eighteen of the 20 neonates, infants, and young children who were treated with interferon alfa-2a for life-threatening hemangiomas experienced a 50% or more tumor regression. These results occurred after an average of 7.8 months of treatment. Two infants generally improved overall after the stabilization of the tumor. Only 1 patient had an adverse reaction to treatment—superficial sloughing of the skin on the cheek, which later healed. Other side effects that resolved included transient neutropenia and fever.

Conclusion.—These results indicate that treatment with interferon alfa-2a can lead to the early regression of lethal tumors such as corticosteroid-resistant hemangiomas in infants. Because no long-term adverse effects occurred with interferon alfa-2a, further clinical study with this medication and a longer follow-up of the children successfully treated in this clinical trial are recommended.

▶ Commenting on this article is James Feusner, M.D., Oncologist and Hematologist, Children's Hospital, Oakland, California:

▶ This report of the use of interferon-alfa-2a in the treatment of 20 patients with hemangiomas is of considerable interest. The authors have tackled what is a very problematic area of treatment as a result of the variable natural history of hemangiomas of infancy. The vast majority of these lesions tend to regress spontaneously but at a variable rate (cessation of growth may occur as early as 2 months and as late as 48 months after diagnosis). However, some can be life-threatening because of the location or association complications of congestive heart failure or thrombocytopenic hemorrhage. Current treatment is not very satisfactory: only 30% respond to steroids. This report follows 2 previous reports of response to interferon alfa-2 in hemangioma or hemangiomatosis in children (1, 2). The report would be more impressive if coagulation data were included on patients 3 and 4 and earlier follow-up pictures and/or scans were presented on patients 4 and 6. It would be important to know whether any of these patients were still receiving prednisone, either at a full dose or tapering dose, to address the possibility of there being synergistic effects of interferon alfa and predisone on these vascular lesions. Also, more details regarding initial dosing and follow-up escalation of dosing in each of the responding patients would be important to others attempting to treat patients similarly.

Given these limitations, however, this is an important addition to the literature, and it supports the previous clinical observations and the growing laboratory observations of the ability of interferons to interfere with new capillary blood vessel development.

References

1. White CW, et al: *J Pediatr* 118:59, 1991.
2. Orchard PJ, et al: *Lancet* 2:565, 1989.

17 Postnatal Growth and Development

The Relation of Fetal Length, Ponderal Index and Head Circumference to Blood Pressure and the Risk of Hypertension in Adult Life

Barker DJP, Godfrey KM, Osmond C, Bull A (Univ of Southampton, England; Yorkshire Regional Health Authority, Harrogate, England)

Paediatr Perinat Epidemiol 6:35–44, 1992 17–1

Introduction.—Low birth weight (as related to placental weight) correlates with hypertension in later life. The highest blood pressures have occurred in individuals with heavy placentas and birth weights that were lower than expected from placental weight. The factors underlying the relationship between low birth weight and adult hypertension are uncertain.

Study Plan.—Blood pressures in 327 individuals aged 46–54 years were related to birth weight, placental weight, length at birth, ponderal index, and head circumference. All had been born after 38 weeks' gestation.

Observations.—Higher blood pressure in adult life correlated with both lower birth weight and greater placental weight. The latter association was statistically stronger. Among subjects whose placental weight was 1.25 lb or less, mean blood pressure increased as the ponderal index at birth declined. In those with greater placental weights, the mean blood pressure and the risk of hypertension increased as body length decreased, and also as the ratio of head circumference to length increased.

Implications.—The strength of these associations and their occurrence in men and women of all social classes, as well as in the first- and later-born children, suggest that they will be confirmed in other groups of adults. If this is the case, research can focus on those maternal influences that determine hypertension in the next generation.

Relation of Fetal and Infant Growth to Plasma Fibrinogen and Factor VII Concentrations in Adult Life

Barker DJP, Meade TW, Fall CHD, Lee A, Osmond C, Phipps K, Stirling Y (Univ of Southampton, England; Northwick Park Hosp, Harrow, Middlesex, England)

BMJ 304:148–152, 1992 17–2

Background.—Several recent studies have suggested that retarded growth in utero and during infancy correlates with cardiovascular disease in adult life. High plasma levels of both fibrinogen and factor VII are independently associated with increased rates of ischemic heart disease, and they may predispose to thrombosis and atheromatous disease.

Study Design.—Plasma levels of fibrinogen and factor VII were measured in 597 men born in Hertfordshire in 1920–1930 who still lived there, and whose weights at birth and at age 1 year had been recorded. For 148 men in Preston, born in 1935–1943, birth size had been measured in detail.

Findings.—The plasma fibrinogen and factor VII levels in the larger group of men decreased with increasing weight at age 1 year, independently of smoking status, alcohol consumption, body mass index, and social class. The levels did not correlate with birth weight. In the younger group, fibrinogen levels fell progressively as the ratio of placental weight to birth weight decreased.

Conclusion.—Reduced growth in fetal life and early infancy closely correlates with higher plasma levels of hemostatic factors. Along with recent reports indicating that early growth relates to blood pressure and glucose tolerance in adult life, these findings support the importance of early developmental events in the development of cardiovascular disease.

▶ Commenting on this article is Thomas B. Newman, M.D., M.P.H., Associate Professor of Laboratory Medicine, Pediatrics, Epidemiology, and Biostatistics, University of California, San Francisco:

▶ These 2 studies (Abstracts 17–1 and 17–2) both correlate anthropometric measurements made in the first year after birth with findings 50 or more years later. The investigators found several highly statistically significant associations. What should a practicing clinician make of these findings?

It is hard to know whether the observed associations were casual. Even if they were casual, it is not at all clear whether they still apply to infants born in the 1990s. Also, even if, for example, today's low-birth-weight infants will be more likely to be hypertensive or have high factor VII levels 50 years from now, would it matter? There are much better reasons to try to prevent low birth weight. Thus, these findings will be of interest primarily to developmental biologists or physiologists, rather than to clinicians.—T.B. Newman, M.D., M.P.H.

Hyperbilirubinemia in Low Birth Weight Infants and Outcome at 5 Years of Age

van de Bor M, Ens-Dokkum M, Schreuder AM, Veen S, Brand R, Verloove-Vanhorick SP (Univ Hosp Leiden, The Netherlands)

Pediatrics 89:359–364, 1992 17–3

Background.—Bilirubin can cause cerebral damage, but the neurotoxicity of moderate hyperbilirubinemia in preterm infants has not been established. A national survey in The Netherlands found that a dose-response relationship exists between the maximal serum total bilirubin concentration and the risk of adverse neurodevelopmental outcome at 2 years of age. Because the status at 2 years of age may not indicate the long-term outcome of low-birth-weight infants, the relationship between the maximal serum total bilirubin concentration in the neonatal period and the outcome at 5 years of age was studied.

Methods.—Of 1,338 infants enrolled in 1983, 814 children were evaluable at the age of 5 years. Their neurodevelopmental status was blindly assessed by 3 specially trained pediatricians with the aid of standardized tests. Cross-tabulation and logistic regression analysis were used to test the association of maximal neonatal serum total bilirubin and neurodevelopmental outcome at age 5 years.

Odds Ratios in Children With and Without Intracranial Hemorrhage (ICH) After Correction for Possible Confounding Factors

Maximal Serum Bilirubin Concentration		Odds Ratio (n)	
μmol/L	mg/dL	No ICH (n = 684)	ICH (n = 130)
≤150	≤8.7	1.0 (189)	1.0 (21)
151–200	8.8–11.6	0.8 (323)	1.9 (66)
201–250	11.7–14.6	1.0 (136)	3.3 (29)
251–300	14.7–17.5	0.8 (31)	5.6 (13)
>300	>17.5	1.3 (5)	>>> (1)
Overall†		1.0 [0.8, 1.38]‡	1.8* [1.1, 3.2]‡

* $P = .04$; no ICH vs ICH (likelihood ratio test).
† Bilirubin as a linear term in the logistic model.
‡ 95% confidence interval.
(Courtesy of van de Bor M, Ens-Dokkum M, Schreuder AM, et al: *Pediatrics* 89:359–364, 1992.)

Results.—Handicaps were observed in 13.4% of the children at 5 years of age. No significant differences were seen in the maximal total serum bilirubin concentrations of neonates who did and did not have a handicap at 5 years of age. This lack of a significant relationship was maintained in spite of logistic regression analysis correcting for gestational age, birth weight, intracranial hemorrhage, ventriculomegaly, seizures, bronchopulmonary dysplasia, and socioeconomic status. However, children who had an intracranial hemorrhage as neonates had a significantly higher risk of a handicap for each 50-μmol/L increase in maximal bilirubin concentration than children without an intracranial hemorrhage. After correction for confounding factors, a relationship between maximal bilirubin concentration and risk of a handicap was seen among children with an intracranial hemorrhage (table). No such relationship was seen in children without an intracranial hemorrhage.

Conclusion.—The significant relationship found between neurodevelopmental outcome at 2 years of age and maximal serum total bilirubin concentration in the neonatal period of preterm infants was not significant at 5 years of age. A dose-response relationship was seen, however, among 5-year-old children who had experienced intracranial hemorrhage as neonates.

► M. Jeffreys Maisels, M.D., Director of Pediatrics at William Beaumont Hospital, Royal Oak, Michigan, and Clinical Professor of Pediatrics at Wayne State University and University of Michigan Medical Center, one of the advocates of a kinder, gentler approach to hyperbilirubinemia, is always eager to express an opinion on anything related to bilirubin.

► Dr. van de Bor and her colleagues once again provide us with outcome data in a large cohort of low-birth-weight infants. When their earlier paper was published (1) the ability to achieve 100% follow-up in surviving children at age 2 years elicited expressions of wonderment. A 98% follow-up at age 5 years almost strains our credulity! The data confirm previous observations that periventricular-intraventricular hemorrhage (PV-IVH) has little or no effect on maximum serum bilirubin levels. Thus, it is unlikely that PV-IVH acts here as a confounder—a variable that affects both the risk factor (bilirubin) and the outcome variable (handicap).

For reasons that are not clear, the authors chose to use odds ratios rather than risk ratios in their tables. Most of us understand the concept of *risk* far better than we understand *odds*. The risk ratios (calculated from Table 5 in the original article) change minimally over the range of bilirubin levels from 101 to 300 μmol/L (5.9–17.5 mg/dL). The risk of a handicap when the serum bilirubin level was ≤ 5.8 mg/dL was 9.5%, and between 5.9 and 8.7 mg/dL it was 14.8% (relative risk, 1.6). However, at levels of 14.7 to 17.5 mg/dL, the risk had only increased to 15.9% (relative risk, 1.7). When an intracranial hemorrhage was present, however, the risk of handicap increased substantially with increasing bilirubin levels.

What does this mean? The authors speculate that their failure to find as strong a relationship (between rising bilirubin levels and handicap in the absence of PV-IVH) at 5 yeasr as was found at 2 years, may be a result of abnormalities of motor development improving with time. An alternative explanation is that the earlier associations occurred by chance. When tested in a controlled trial (albeit in premature infants of higher birth weight and gestation), early phototherapy reduced the risk of exchange transfusion but had no effect on mental or motor development (2).

On the other hand, is the issue worth quibbling about? Compared with the noxious interventions inflicted on small infants in our neonatal intensive care units, phototherapy must certainly rank among the more benign. Thus, if there is even a small risk of increasing handicap with rising serum bilirubin levels, it seems reasonable to use phototherapy quite early in this population and particularly if PV-IVH is present. The use of fiberoptic phototherapy in conjunction with conventional phototherapy more or less doubles the efficiency of the treatment and has made it much easier to control serum bilirubin levels in these infants (3). Exchange transfusions are rapidly going the way of clysis!—M.J. Maisels, M.D.

References

1. Van de Bor M, et al: *Pediatrics* 83:915, 1989.
2. Scheidt PC, et al: *Pediatrics* 85:455, 1990.
3. Holtrop PC, et al: *Pediatrics* 90:674, 1992.

Effects of Intraventricular Hemorrhage and Socioeconomic Status on Perceptual, Cognitive, and Neurologic Status of Low Birth Weight Infants at 5 Years of Age

Vohr B, Coll CG, Flanagan P, Oh W (Brown Univ, Providence, RI)

J Pediatr 121:280–285, 1992 17–4

Background.—It has previously been suggested that visual evoked response (VER) might assist in identifying children who were at increased risk for long-term perceptual and visual-motor abnormalities. The impact of socioeconomic status and the severity of intraventricular hemorrhage (IVH) on the overall cognitive performance of 5-year-olds were compared. The correlation of scores of eye-hand and visual function (observed at ages 1 and 2 years) with perceptual scores at age 5 years was also investigated.

Methods.—The participants of this prospective longitudinal study were divided into 3 groups as preterm neonates; there also was a control group. The groupings were based on their IVH status (no IVH, grade I–II IVH, and grade III–IV IVH). Children were reexamined at 2, 3, 4, and 5 years of age.

Results.—Only 60% of the group with IVH grade III–IV were found to be normal. Multiple regression analysis revealed that duration of hospitalization, VER, and socioeconomic status all have independent effects on the cognitive index. Correlations peformed on predictor variables such as IVH status, VER latency, and socioeconomic status scores with the 5-year neurologic status showed that the relationship between VER latency and neurologic status was reduced with age. Repeated measures of anlysis of variance did not demonstrate a significant time effect.

Conclusion.—Visual evoked reponse latency was not a strong marker, and duration of hospitalization contributed the greatest variance for both cognitive and perceptual outcomes. The Kohen-Raz subscores were significantly correlated with the outcome variables. However, other tests were better predictors.

▶ With the progression of time, we now have a finer grained picture of the effect of intraventricular hemorrhage on the quality of the outcome. As might be expected, infants with shunted hydrocephalus were most affected at 5 years of age. As in past studies (back to the time of Drillen), socioeconomic status continues to have a most significant effect on cognitive status at 5 years. This and other studies should be a major stimulus to include all low-birth-weight infants and their parents in an enriched Head Start program for several years before school begins. Clinical neonatologists will find close reading of this report most helpful.—M.H. Klaus, M.D.

The Health and Developmental Status of Very Low-Birth-Weight Children at School Age

McCormick MC, Brooks-Gunn J, Workman-Daniels K, Turner J, Peckham GJ (Harvard School of Public Health, Boston; Harvard Med School, Boston; Columbia Univ, New York; et al)

JAMA 267:2204–2208, 1992 17–5

Background.—The United States experiences a higher proportion of infants with low birth weights, especially very low birth weight (VLBW), 1,500 g or less, than do other industrialized countries. Outcome studies in older VLBW children have revealed higher levels of less severe disability and health problems other than that of severe disability among children who survived infancy intact. The effect of improved survival of increasingly premature infants was assessed by examining the outcomes at school age in a large group of children born at different birth weights.

Method.—The children were selected from 2 previous multisite cohorts. The cohort of VLBW children had been referred to participating intensive care units, and the heavier low-birth-weight children were drawn from a stratified random sample of births in geographically defined regions. Follow-up information at 8–10 years of age ws obtained by a combination of telephone interviews and home or clinic visits for 65.1% of eligible children. Data concerning 17 specified conditions, alterations in development or limitations in activities of daily living, and

Specific Conditions at School Age by Birth Weight

	Birth Weight, g			
	≤1000 (n=247)	1001-1500 (n=364)	1501-2500 (n=724)	>2500 (n=533)
	≥1 Condition, %			
	71.0	62.5	54.0	51.2*
Odds ratio (confidence interval)	2.33 (1.66-3.27)	1.58 (1.12-2.10)	1.12 (0.89-1.41)	1.00 ...
	% Children Reporting Categories of Conditions†			
Asthma	17.1	18.4	11.7	11.1‡
Neurosequelae associated with prematurity	20.7	16.8	6.4	4.5*
Sensorineural problems	40.9	23.4	23.8	20.3*
Learning problems	24.8	19.0	13.0	10.5*
Intervening central nervous system conditions	6.1	3.3	2.2	0.8*
Other	23.6	23.1	16.3	9.8*

* χ^2 for comparison across 4 birth-weight groups: $P < .0001$.
† More than 1 condition can be reported for any single child.
‡ χ^2 for comparison across 4 birth-weight groups: $P < .005$.
(Courtesy of McCormick MC, Brooks-Gunn J, Workman-Daniels K, et al: *JAMA* 267:2204–2208, 1992.)

both affective and behavioral mental health were collected. In a subset of children, intelligence quotients (IQs) were assessed.

Findings.—Decreasing birth weight was associated with increased morbidity for all measures except affective health. The children who had birth weights of 1,500 g or less were more likely to experience multiple health problems (table). Lower IQs were concentrated among children with birth weights less than 1000 g, and these children were likely to have problems in more than 1 health dimension. Maternal educational attainment did not influence the association of birth weight with morbidity, except for IQ among children whose birth weight was greater than 1,000 g. There were substantial differences in IQ among these children between those with the least and the most educated mothers. Socioeconomic disadvantage appeared to worsen the IQ status of all children irrespective of birth weight.

Conclusion.—Children born at lower birth weights appear to have increased morbidity at early school age. Problems may include specific developmental difficulties, higher levels of distractibility, and more frequent intercurrent illness with school absences and hospitalization. Reducing the prevalence of very premature births and promptly initiating intervention programs may improve outcomes in low-birth-weight infants.

▶ Maureen Hack, M.D., Professor of Pediatrics at Case Western Reserve University, and Director of the Neonatal Follow Up Program at Rainbow Babies and Children's Hospital, notes:

▶ This report is unique in that it uses a multidimensional conceptualization of health status to present information on the outcomes of children of different birth weights. As McCormick notes, "this broader conceptualization of health status is more consistent with the clinical picture presented by many VLBW children, whose management may require attention to specific developmental difficulties, higher level of distractibility, more frequent intercurrent illnesses with school absences and hospitalization." McCormick has recently elaborated on this conceptualization in a recent chapter (1).

The article is furthermore unique in its methodology: 2 existing follow-up cohorts were used to obtain 2 VLBW (< 1,000 g, 1,000–1,500 g) and 2 larger birth weight cohorts (1,500–2,500 g, > 2,500 g). This is an economical way to obtain long-term follow-up information. As the authors note, they would have required a base population of 82,000 births to ensure the same number of VLBW children with at least annual contact and tracing to school age! In general, the outcome of the group with birth weights less than 1,000 g is of concern: 44.8% had disability defined as the presence of a limitation in 1 or more activities of daily living, together with specified conditions or with other health problems. Furthermore, 42% had an IQ less than 85. These children were born during 1976–1978. Since that time, assisted ventilation has been more widely used, and survival has improved dramatically. At best, the school-age outcomes of present survivors will be similar to those reported in this study.—M. Hack, M.D.

Reference

1. McCormick MC: *Clin Perinatal* 20:263, 1993.

Prognostic Reliability of Somatosensory and Visual Evoked Potentials of Asphyxiated Term Infants

Taylor MJ, Murphy WJ, Whyte HE (The Hosp for Sick Children, Toronto)

Dev Med Child Neurol 34:507–515, 1992 17–6

Introduction.—The incidence of birth asphyxia has remained unchanged in recent years, despite advances in prenatal and perinatal management. Prediction of the long-term neurologic outcome in these infants by means of visual evoked potentials (VEPs) has been reliable, but somatosensory evoked potentials (SEPs) were found to be more accurate prognostic measures. The relative accuracies of these measures for pre-

Comparison of Predictive Ability of SEPs and VEPs

	VEP		*SEP*	
	1-3 days (%)	*1-7 days* (%)	*1-3 days* (%)	*1-7 days* (%)
Sensitivity	65	78	87	96
Specificity	100	100	79	88
+ Pred. power	100	100	74	85
− Pred. power	81	87	90	97
Accuracy	86	91	82	91

(Courtesy of Taylor MJ, Murphy WJ, Whyte HE: *Dev Med Child Neurol* 34:507–515, 1992.)

dicting neurodevelopmental outcome in asphyxiated term infants were compared.

Methods.—The study group included 57 infants with an Apgar score of less than 3 at 10 minutes or other signs of asphyxia; 46 survivors were available for follow-up. Both SEPs and VEPs were performed during the first 3 days of life, on day 6 or 7, then weekly until death or discharge. Survivors were followed for a minimum of 18 months and were assessed for hearing, vision, and neurodevelopment.

Results.—Eleven of the infants died, 34 were normal at follow-up, and 12 had severe neurologic sequelae and were mentally retarded. Ultrasound scanning, performed during the first 3 days of life, was a poor predictor of outcome. Of the 30 infants with normal SEPs during the first 3 days of life, 27 had a normal outcome. The other 3 had abnormal SEPs by day 7. Twenty of 27 infants with abnormal SEPs died or were abnormal at follow-up. The accuracy of SEPs was 91% at the end of the first week of life. Thirty-four of 42 infants with normal VEPs during the first 3 days were normal at follow-up. All 15 infants with abnormal VEPs died or had severe disability. At the end of the first week, VEPs also had an accuracy of 91% (table).

Conclusion.—The combination of VEPs and SEPs is a powerful means of predicting outcome in asphyxiated newborns. The measurements are considerably more accurate for this purpose than electroencephalogram, head ultrasound, and CT scans. The use of evoked potentials can aid in the early management of hypoxic-ischemic encephalopathy.

Somatosensory Evoked Potentials and Outcome in Perinatal Asphyxia

Gibson NA, Graham M, Levene MI (Univ of Leicester, England)

Arch Dis Child 67:393–398, 1992 17–7

Introduction.—Perinatal asphyxia remains the single most prominent cause of neurodevelopmental disorders in term infants. Somatosensory evoked potentials (SEPs) for the prognostic assessment of asphyxiated term infants.

Methods.—The SEPs were recorded from the median nerve in 30 term infants who had clinical evidence of perinatal asphyxia. In 16 infants, there were signs of severe encephalopathy. The infants were assessed neurologically at age 12 months.

Results.—All 10 infants who died had severe hypoxic-ischemic encephalopathy. Infants with a normal outcome had normal SEP findings by age 4 days, whereas all 7 with an abnormal outcome had abnormal SEP findings beyond this time. Of the 10 infants who died, 8 had absent cortical SEPs at all times (table). Pattern A is a persistently normal SEP; pattern B, abnormalities at an early stage only; pattern C, abnormal or absent potentials for a variable period; and pattern D, no cortical response at any time. No infants who died of asphyxia had normal SEPs by age 4 days.

Conclusion.—Recording SEPs in term neonates may help predict the outcome when perinatal asphyxia is present.

▶ It is heartening that the conclusions in both reports (Abstracts 17–6 and 17–7) are similar. The observations by M.J. Taylor are more useful because they compare visual evoked potentials (VEPs) with somatosensory evoked potentials (SEPs). Although SEPs appear more reliable in the pediatric intensive care unit (SEPs had an accuracy of 92% compared with VEPs accuracy of 76%) the authors suggest a combination of both be used to assess as-

Relationship of SEP Pattern to Outcome

SEP	*Outcome*				*Total*
	Normal	*Dystonic*	*Cerebral palsy*	*Died*	
A	10	0	0	1*	11
B	2	0	0	0	2
C	1	4	3	1	9
D	0	0	0	8	8

Note: See text for definition of patterns.
* Child with spinal muscular atrophy.
(Courtesy of Gibson NA, Graham M, Levene MI: *Arch Dis Child* 67:393–398, 1992.)

phyxiated neonates. They recommend that VEPs be recorded first; if found to be abnormal, the prognosis is poor and SEPs would not be helpful. However, if the VEPs are normal, the accuracy of a good prognosis can be improved if the SEPs are also found to be normal. For the increased accuracy, they strongly recommend repeat testing at the end of 1 week.—M.H. Klaus, M.D.

Prediction of Neurodevelopmental Outcome in the Preterm Infant: Short Latency Cortical Somatosensory Evoked Potentials Compared With Cranial Ultrasound

de Vries LS, Eken P, Pierrat V, Daniels H, Cesaer P (Wilhelmina Children's Hosp, Utrecht, The Netherlands; Univ Hosp Gasthuisberg, Leuven, Belgium)

Arch Dis Child 67:1177–1181, 1992 17–8

Introduction.—Because the survival of low-birth-weight infants has increased, the number of these children in whom cerebral palsy develops has also increased. An attempt has been made to identify those low-birth-weight newborns who will eventually have neurologic problems, using such novel techniques as somatosensory evoked potentials (SEPs). Somatosensory evoked potentials were used to monitor preterm infants to predict their neurodevelopmental outcome, and SEPs methods were compared with ultrasound in infant neurologic assessment.

Methods.—A total of 126 premature infants with a gestational age of 34 weeks or less entered the study over 26 months and underwent ultrasound examination at least twice a week until discharge. The SEPs examination occurred during the first week in all infants, whereas 69 of the 126 neonates had sequential studies at 40 weeks' postmenstrual age.

Results.—Of the 126 infants, the SEPs demonstrated a normal N1 latency in 107 infants and a delayed N1 latency in 19. Fourteen subjects with a normal N1 latency at 40 weeks' postmenstrual age later had cerebral palsy develop, whereas 11 of 19 infants with delayed N1 latency had this condition develop. Of these 19 neonates, 6 went on to have transient dystonia. The SEPs have a 44% sensitivity and a 92% specificity as a predictor of cerebral palsy development. The ultrasound examination did not correlate with the occurrence of cerebral palsy in infants undergoing both assessments. Ultrasound had a positive predictive outcome of 45% and a negative predictive outcome of 94% for cerebral palsy. For neurodevelopmental outcome, the combination of major ultrasound abnormalities and a delayed N1 latency had a sensitivity of 40%, a specificity of 100%, a positive predictive value of 100%, and a negative predictive value of 78%.

Conclusion.—The use of SEPs of the median nerve in the assessment of preterm infants does not aid in predicting later neurodevelopment of the child. This assessment should not become a routine examination of low-birth-weight infants.

▶ The search continues for a more reliable method to predict the future development of small immature infants. Although SEPs strongly predict the future development of full-term infants asphyxiated at birth, they appear from this large series to have limited value in premature infants. In the hopes of improving sensitivity, the authors are currently studying the SEPs of the posterior tibial nerve and the median nerve together, because the legs of premature infants are more severely involved than the arms.—M.H. Klaus, M.D.

Eight-Year School Performance, Neurodevelopmental, and Growth Outcome of Neonates With Bronchopulmonary Dysplasia: A Comparative Study

Robertson CMT, Etches PC, Goldson E, Kyle JM (Univ of Alberta, Edmonton, Canada; Glenrose Rehabilitation Hosp, Edmonton, Alta, Canada; Royal Alexandra Hosp; Edmonton, Alta, Canada; et al)
Pediatrics 89:365–372, 1992 17–9

Background.—The increasing survival of smaller and smaller infants has resulted in a population with a high incidence of bronchopulmonary dysplasia (BPD). There is much concern about the long-term growth and neurodevelopmental consequences of this condition. Eight-year school performance, neurodevelopmental outcomes, and growth outcomes of neonates with BPD were examined.

Methods.—Three groups of preterm infants with BPD were studied. Group 1 consisted of 21 infants with a birth gestation of 31 weeks or less who were receiving supplemental oxygen until the equivalent of 36 weeks' gestation. Group 2 consisted of 15 infants of the same gestational age receiving supplemental oxygen to 28 days' postnatal age but not to 36 weeks' gestational age. Group 3 contained 11 neonates with a gestation of 32 weeks or more requiring supplemental oxygen for more than 28 days. For each BPD group, there was an individually matched preterm neonatal comparison group and a term peer comparison group.

Findings.—The 3 BPD study groups had similar physical growth and psycho-educational and school performance test scores, with the exception of lower intelligence quotient for those receiving supplemental oxygen for the longest time. Groups 1 and 2 had outcome scores comparable to those of the neonatal comparison group and significantly below those of the peer comparison groups. According to multivariate analysis, 61% of the variance of academic achievement in group 1 was related to lowest recorded pH, father's socioeconomic status, and lowest recorded PaO_2. Even when the disabled children were excluded from analysis, the study groups continued to show academic delay compared with peer groups.

Conclusion.—For the smaller preterm infants in this series, prematurity with and without chronic lung disease along with adverse social factors compromises outcomes for low-birth-weight infants, even after disabled children are excluded from the analysis. For the larger preterm infants, chronic lung disease had an effect.

▶ Maureen Hack, M.D., Professor of Pediatrics at Case Western Reserve University and Director of the Neonatal Follow Up Program at Rainbow Babies and Children's Hospital, makes her annual contribution with this commentary:

▶ This report is a further confirmation of the combined detrimental effects of biological and social risk factors in preterm infants. One problem with this study is the small numbers of infants in each group, which, as admitted by the authors, possibly affected the significance levels. I would have expected that group 1, i.e., those still receiving oxygen at 36 weeks' corrected age, would have had more later health complications, including illnesses requiring medical attention, and rehospitalizations. The results do confirm the high disability rate and need for special help in school for individuals with bronchopulmonary dysplasia, even when those with severe neuromotor disorders are excluded. The authors note that their 8-year-old cohort is very different than the current lower birth weight, lower gestational age, and sicker cohort that currently survives, a group that will most probably have poorer school-age outcomes. I am very concerned about the possible detrimental effects from the current widespread use of steroids to treat bronchopulmonary dysplasia.—M. Hack, M.D.

Neonatal Auditory Brainstem Response Failure of Very Low Birth Weight Infants: 8-Year Outcome

Cox C, Hack M, Aram D, Borawski E (Boston Univ Med Ctr; Rainbow Babies and Children's Hosp, Cleveland, Ohio)

Pediatr Res 31:68–72, 1992 17–10

Introduction.—An increasing number of children are at risk of neurologic, developmental, and language deficits associated with prematurity and very low birth weight (VLBW). Attempts to identify those children who will be handicapped have not been consistently successful.

Methods.—To determine whether predischarge recordings of auditory brain stem reponse (ABR) results are predictive of neurobehavioral development, 56 VLBW children who were born in 1977–1978 and followed up to age 8 years were studied. A battery of intelligence, speech, language, and academic measures was administered at age 8 years.

Results.—Failure of ABR was found in 13 children, in 6 of them bilaterally. These infants failed to respond to stimuli at 30 dB normal hearing level and did not have I–V interpeak latencies within 2 SD of normative data. Nearly half of the failures repeated a grade in school, compared with 16% of those with normal ABR findings. Hearing loss did not correlate closely with neurobehavioral development. Unilatural ABR abnormalities did not appear predictive of subsequent performance, but bilateral abnormalities did.

Conclusion.—Early ABR recordings in very-low-birth-weight infants may help predict their neurobehavioral development.

▶ The authors are appropriately cautious in their conclusions because of the small sample size in each group. Is this correlation between bilateral auditory brain stem responses and subsequent performance on measures of intelligent quotient, language, and reading the result of lesions in the brain or our present inability to educate a child with auditory defects?—M.H. Klaus, M.D.

Effects of Early Intervention on Cognitive Function of Low Birth Weight Preterm Infants

Brooks-Gunn J, Liaw F-r, Klebanov PK (Columbia Univ, New York; Educational Testing Service, Princeton, NJ; et al)

J Pediatr 120:350–359, 1992 17–11

Background.—The benefits of early intervention programs for disadvantaged young children are well recognized. Less is known, however, about the impact of similar programs designed for biologically vulnerable children of low birth weight (LBW). The effects of the Infant Health and Development Program, a randomized clinical trial to test the efficacy of educational and family support services and pediatric follow-up for LBW preterm infants, were studied.

Methods.—Eligible infants were born in 1 of 8 participating medical institutions in 1985. The primary analysis group included 985 infants stratified by clinical site and birth weight (2,000 g or less and 2,001–2,500 g). Children were randomly assigned immediately after hospital discharge to intervention (377) or follow-up (608). Intervention continued until the infant reached 36 months of age; 913 infants completed the intervention or follow-up programs.

Results.—In all 3 cognitive domains—vocabulary, visual-motor skills, and receptive language—children exhibited significant intervention effects at 24 months. The effects were greatest for the visual-motor and spatial skills factor. Intervention was more effective for black children than for white children or Hispanics and for heavier LBW preterm infants than for lighter infants. At 36-month follow-up, intervention had positively affected vocabulary, receptive language, visual-motor and spatial skills, and reasoning.

Conclusion.—Early intervention clearly benefits LBW preterm infants, particularly in the 2 domains in which these children have deficits—language and visual-motor and spatial skills. Educational services for LBW preterm infants should focus on a broad array of cognitive skills. Home-based programs result in health-related gains, but they are less effective than center-based programs in yielding cognitive gains.

▶ I can picture all the members of the Old Guard smiling as they relish the results of this interventional study. All the right buttons are struck, and the concepts have broad populist appeal. How can it not feel right to propose early and comprehensive intervention for an at-risk population? After all, the Robert Wood Johnson–sponsored studies (1) had indicated that the intelligence of the infants could be boosted with a stimulation program. The most vulnerable graduates of the intensive care units frequently are discharged into a non-nurturing home environment. It is almost as if the concept of minimal stimulation, which is so important in the care of the acutely ill, physiologically unstable infant is taken literally when the infant is discharged home.

Although it was encouraging to note gains in all cognitive domains with the intervention program, the duration of follow-up is far too short to press the ecstasy buttons. It remains to be demonstrated whether these advantages will persist when these infants enter school. We will also have the arduous task of convincing the various administrators that these are dollars well invested and that the returns more than justify the investment. If not, the vast majority of infants deprived of a full sojourn in utero will not have the opportunity to realize their true potential. It is my fervent wish to see these interventional programs expanded in scope.

Our imagination is the only limit to what we can have in the future—Charles Kettering

A.A. Fanaroff, M.B.B.Ch.

Reference

1. Infant Health and Development Program. *JAMA* 263:3035, 1990.

18 Epidemiology

Fetal Abnormality: An Audit of Its Recognition and Management

Renwick, M, for the Regional Fetal Abnormality Survey. (Princess Mary Maternity Hosp, Newcastle, England)
Arch Dis Child 67:770–774, 1992 18–1

Objective.—A collaborative mortality survey in the United Kingdom showed that a fifth of all perinatal deaths and a third of later deaths in the first year resulted from fetal abnormality. Accordingly, a survey was undertaken in a population of about 3 million to document all lethal abnormalities. Registered births in the area of study totaled 361,037 between 1982 and 1990.

Findings.—Perinatal mortality declined from 11.7 to 8.1 deaths per thousand births during 1982–1990. The proportion of all perinatal deaths in the region that resulted from congenital malformation decreased from 23% in 1982 to 14% in 1990. Nearly half the decline in perinatal mortality was attributable to a reduction in registered births associated with severe fetal abnormality. Most of the latter decrease reflected an increase in terminations for fetal abnormality (Fig 18–1). An increase in the antenatal recognition of neural tube defects explains only part of the observed decrease in registerable perinatal deaths.

Implications.—It now is possible to monitor the accuracy of ultrasound-based screening and diagnostic efforts in identifying specific fetal abnormalities. As a result, physicians will come to learn how much weight to place on particular antenatal ultrasound findings.

▶ In the 8 years covered in this report, there was a gradual increase in the number of abnormalities discovered. The accuracy varied from duodenal atresia, where a positive diagnosis was as likely to be wrong as right; isolated hydrocephalus, where 10% of the infants were found to be normal at birth; and spina bifida without anencephaly, where 2.5% of the infants were found to be normal at delivery. Accuracy improved with time. As important is the authors' observation that 50% of the improvement in neonatal mortality was the result of fetuses with significant abnormalities being aborted. This will make our statistics look better, but it will not signify that we have improved our ability to care for sick infants.—M.H. Klaus, M.D.

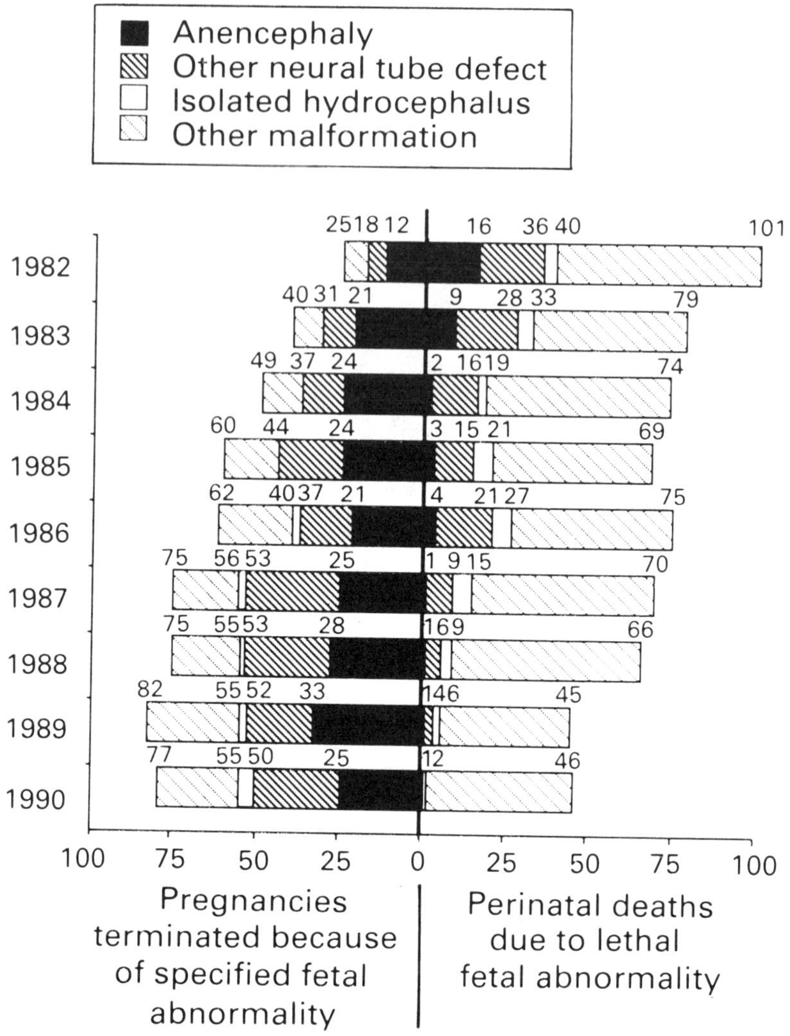

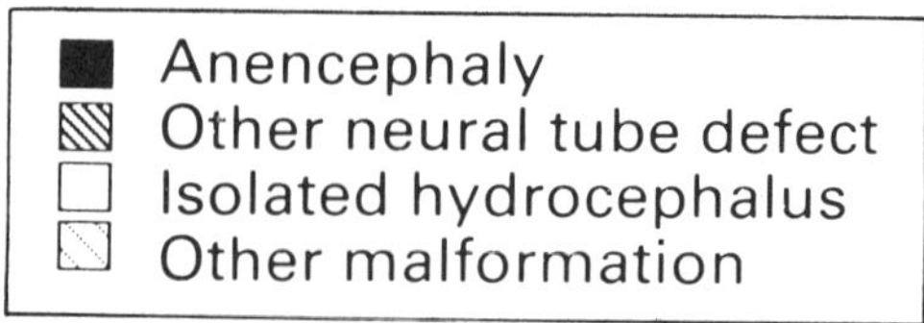

Fig 18–1.—Neural tube defects, congenital hydrocephalus, and other lethal fetal abnormalities in the Northern region 1982–1990, their increasing antenatal recognition, and the impact of this on perinatal mortality. (Courtesy of Renwick M, for the Regional Fetal Abnormality Survey. *Arch Dis Child* 67:770–774, 1992.)

Differences in Hospital Resource Allocation Among Sick Newborns According to Insurance Coverage

Braveman PA, Egerter S, Bennett T, Showstack J (Univ of California, San Francisco)

JAMA 266:3300–3308, 1991 18–2

Objective.—In an earlier study it was suggested that the lack of health insurance was associated with an increased risk of adverse outcomes in newborns. Whether insurance coverage of the newborn is associated with differences in allocation of hospital services was investigated.

Setting.—All civilian hospital discharges for acute care in California for 1987 were analyzed retrospectively. Length of stay, total charges, and charges per day based on insurance status were studied among 29,751 newborns with evidence of serious problems while controlling for race-ethnicity, diagnoses, hospital characteristics (ownership, teaching status, nursery level), and disposition.

Findings.—Uninsured newborns consistently received fewer resources than privately insured newborns with prepaid or indemnity coverage. The resources for newborns with Medicaid coverage were generally greater than those for uninsured newborns and less than those for privately insured newborns. This pattern was observed across all hospital ownership types, race or ethnic group, medical need as indicated by diagnostic categories, and disposition. Length of stay, total charges, and charges per day for uninsured newborns were 16%, 28%, and 10% lower, respectively, than for privately insured newborns; these differences were significant. Both uninsured and Medicaid-covered newborns had more severe medical problems than privately insured newborns.

Implications.—These findings strongly suggest that allocation of hospital resources to sick newborns is influenced significantly by expected reimbursement rather than being determined strictly by medical need. These constitute prima facie evidence of serious inequities that need to be addressed by policy changes.

▶ The terms resource allocation, relative value, diagnostic-related grouping, and others with similar connotations have crept into the hospital jargon. Managed care, Current Procedural Terminology (CPT) codes, and cost containment are daily issues for all hospital personnel. These are complicated matters in changing times.

This abstracted manuscript addresses the subject of resource allocation by insurance coverage and intimates that greater resources are expanded on those with insurance. Instinctively, these findings are at variance with my perceptions of the neonatal intensive care unit. My convictions are that resources are allocated based on need, irrespective of payer class. The California data, however, cannot be lightly regarded but, rather, need to be replicated elsewhere to satisfy other skeptics, like myself. The Clinton Health Care Task Force is in session as this manuscript goes to press. Will the issue of noninsurance become moot when their deliberations have been made public and the new health-care system moves into high gear? In the meantime, those of us in the trenches will strive to provide quality care for all newborns, irrespective of payer class.

He who walks in another's tracks leaves no footprints—Joan Brannon

A.A. Fanaroff, M.B.B.Ch.

Neonatal Therapeutic Intervention Scoring System: A Therapy-Based Severity-of-Illness Index

Gray JE, Richardson DK, McCormick MC, Workman-Daniels K, Goldmann DA (Brigham and Women's Hosp, Boston; Children's Hosp, Boston; Beth Israel Hosp, Boston; et al)

Pediatrics 90:561–567, 1992 18–3

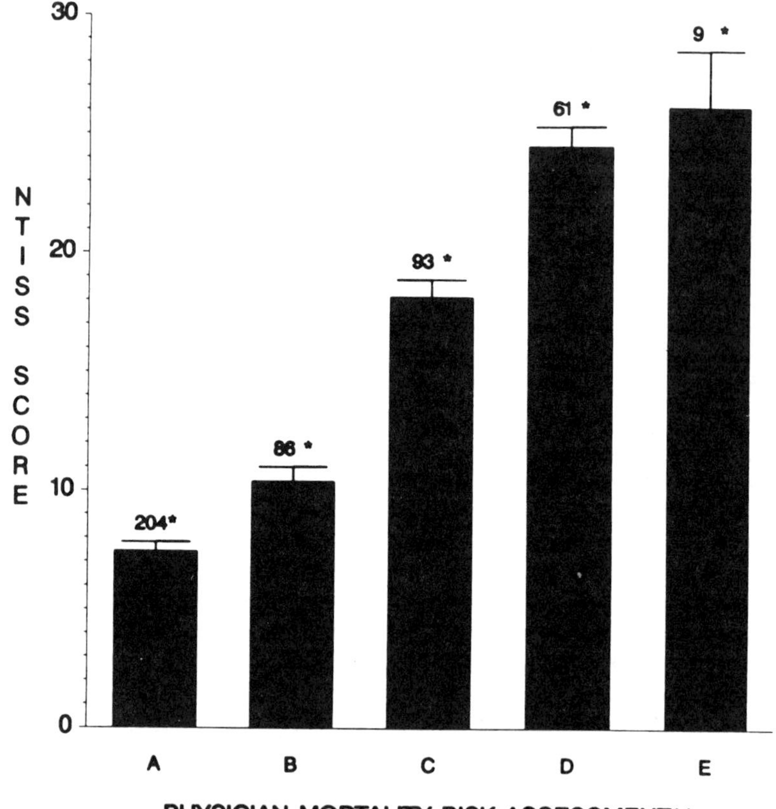

Fig 18–2.—Neonatal Therapeutic Intervention Scoring System (NTISS) vs. physician risk assessment. *Bars* represent standard error. *Equal number of assessments in each risk category. **Risk categories defined as follows: *A*, low risk, except for low-probability catastrophic event; *B*, mildly ill, still at small risk; C, moderately ill, but excellent chance for survival; *D*, extremely ill, but with good chance for survival; *E*, virtually certain death, now or delayed. (Courtesy of Gray JE, Richardson DK, McCormick MC, et al: *Pediatrics* 90:561–567, 1992.)

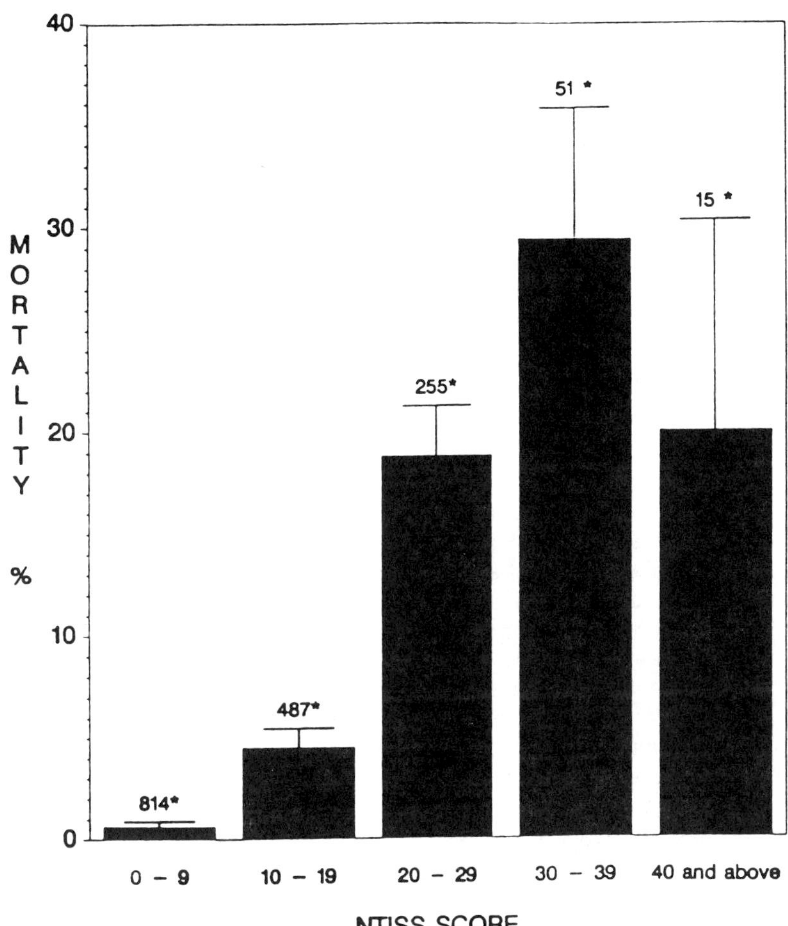

Fig 18–3.—In-hospital mortality rates by NTISS score. *Bars* represent standard error. *Equal number of assessments in each NTISS score category. Moribund patients excluded. (Courtesy of Gray JE, Richardson DK, McCormick MC, et al: *Pediatrics* 90:561–567, 1992.)

Introduction.—Severity-of-illness scales are effective in the evaluation of clinical outcome and resource consumption in adult and pediatric intensive care. This therapy-based approach is less extensively developed in neonatal care.

Setting.—A Neonatal Therapeutic Intervention Scoring System (NTISS) was developed by modifying the adult Therapeutic Intervention Scoring System (TISS). From the original 76 TISS items, 42 were deleted and 28 were added to form the NTISS. The NTISS assigned score points from 1 to 4 based on therapeutic intensity and complexity. The validity of the NTISS was studied among 1,643 newborns admitted to 3 neonatal intensive care units (NICUs) between 1989 and 1990.

Results.—The mean admission-day NTISS score was 12.3 (range, 0 to 47). There was a high degree of internal consistency noted within

NTISS, with an overall α coefficient of .84. The NTISS scores strongly correlated with expected markers of illness severity, including mortality risk estimates by neonatal attending physicians (Fig 18–2), in-hospital mortality rates (Fig 18–3), and a measure of nursing acuity. Furthermore, NTISS scores were predictive of NICU length of stay and total hospital charges among survivors. The NTISS score showed little correlation with birth weight or gestational age.

Conclusion.—The NTISS is a valid measure of therapeutic intensity in the NICU. It is easily and quickly abstracted from medical records, is highly internally consistent, and allows excellent predictions of clinical outcomes and total resource use within 24 hours of admission. The NTISS can be most effectively carried out when used in conjunction with a physiology-based severity-of-illness assessment, such as the Score for Neonatal Acute Physiology.

▶ The alphabet soup of neonatal intensive care unit jargon assumes the consistency of a thick minestrone with the addition of the NTISS and SNAP (Score for Neonatal Acute Physiology) scores (1). These scoring systems are long overdue and represent an attempt to level the playing field when comparing intercenter, interstate, and even international outcome variables. The search for scoring systems has had a long gestation (2), and consumers will soon have a menu to choose from, as Tarnow Mundie in the United Kingdom is rapidly approaching the culmination of his coordinated, multicenter efforts to develop a neonatal scoring system (3). The concept obviously is not unique, and similar scoring systems have been successfully developed for adults and children in the ICU (4).

The scoring systems can be used to define resource needs and predict outcome. Combining the NTISS and SNAP scores presents a better profile of the outcomes and total resource needs. Provision of this data is in concert with the needs of the managed health-care industry, so that the scoring systems for neonates, which once were validated on a broader population, will, in all probability, move to center stage. True resource-based costs will then be generated for various neonatal illnesses. To the delight of some and the distaste of others, we may predict that the reimbursement rates for neonatal intensive care will be stratified on the basis of these scoring systems.

Men stumble over truth from time to time, but most pick themselves up and hurry off as if nothing happened—Sir Winston Churchill

A.A. Fanaroff, M.B.B.Ch.

References

1. Richardson DK: *Pediatrics* 91:617, 1993.
2. Georgieff MK, et al: *Crit Care Med* 17:17, 1989.
3. Tarnow Mundie: *BMJ* 300:1611, 1990.
4. Pollack MM, et al: N *Engl J Med* 316:134, 1987.

Trends in Perinatal Mortality and Cerebral Palsy in Western Australia, 1967 to 1985

Stanley FJ, Watson L (Princess Margaret Hosp for Children, Perth, Australia)

BMJ 304:1658–1663, 1992 18–4

Background.—Interventions aimed at preventing perinatal asphyxia do not appear to have lowered rates of cerebral palsy. The most recent data on trends in perinatal deaths and cerebral palsy in Western Australia were reviewed and related to changes in perinatal care.

Methods.—Perinatal death certificates from 1967 to 1985 were examined to ascertain all stillbirths and neonatal deaths among infants born after 20 weeks' gestation or weighing at least 400 g. Data on cerebral palsy were obtained from the Western Australia cerebral palsy register.

Results.—Both stillbirth rates and early neonatal mortality fell steadily during the study, but the proportion of infants with cerebral palsy remained steady at approximately 2 in 1,000 births. Since 1967, increases have occurred in the percentage of cesarean section deliveries, the use of fetal monitoring and neonatal transport services, and the proportion of live infants weighing less than 1,500 g delivered at centers with access to neonatal intensive care. Death rates fell particularly in low-birth-weight infants, the group in which the rate of cerebral palsy rose significantly (table; Fig 18–4). All spastic categories showed an increase, but spastic hemiplegia and quadriplegia were the main syndromes contributing to the increase in cerebral palsy in low-birth-weight infants.

Conclusion.—The findings suggest that birth asphyxia is no longer a major cause of cerebral palsy. The increase in cerebral palsy in low-birth-weight infants is the result of postnatal complications of immaturity or prenatal damage to the fetal brain, not to deficiencies in obstetric care. This conclusion has implications for malpractice litigation as well as for perinatal care.

▶ These observations are similar to the increasing rates of cerebral palsy in low-birth-weight infants recently reported in Sweden, the United Kingdom, Ireland, and Finland and discussed in previous YEAR BOOKS. The proportion of all cerebral palsy that occurred in low-birth-weight infants (< 1,000 g) increased from 1.3% in 1975–1978 to 7.3% in 1983–1985. The earlier series of cerebral palsy reported in the 1970s noted that most of the infants had mild spastic diplegia and, often, a normal intellect. In the recent studies, the increase in the incidence of cerebral palsy is in all the spastic syndromes, and it is often associated with other severe handicaps. Significantly, the very experienced senior author believes that "a considerable contribution must be coming from the postnatal complications of extreme prematurity."—M.H. Klaus, M.D.

Rates of Cerebral Palsy per 1,000 Neonatal Survivors According to Birth Weight, Western Australia, 1975–1985

	<1000	1000-1499	1500-1999	2000-2499	≥2500	Unknown	All
1975-78							
Neonatal survivors	56	261	741	2,839	74,467	3,243	81,607
Cerebral palsy	2	7	25	19	104	1	158
Rate	35.71	26.82	33.74	6.69	1.40		1.94

1979-82							
Neonatal survivors	93	363	857	3,062	79,992	637	85,004
Cerebral palsy	7	13	17	19	105	-	161
Rate	75.27	35.81	19.84	6.21	1.31		1.89
1983-85							
Neonatal survivors	113	358	761	2,545	64,680	68	68,525
Cerebral palsy	11	27	11	17	84	-	150
Rate	97.35	75.42	14.45	6.68	1.30		2.19

(Courtesy of Stanley FJ, Watson L: *BMJ* 304:1658–1663, 1992.)

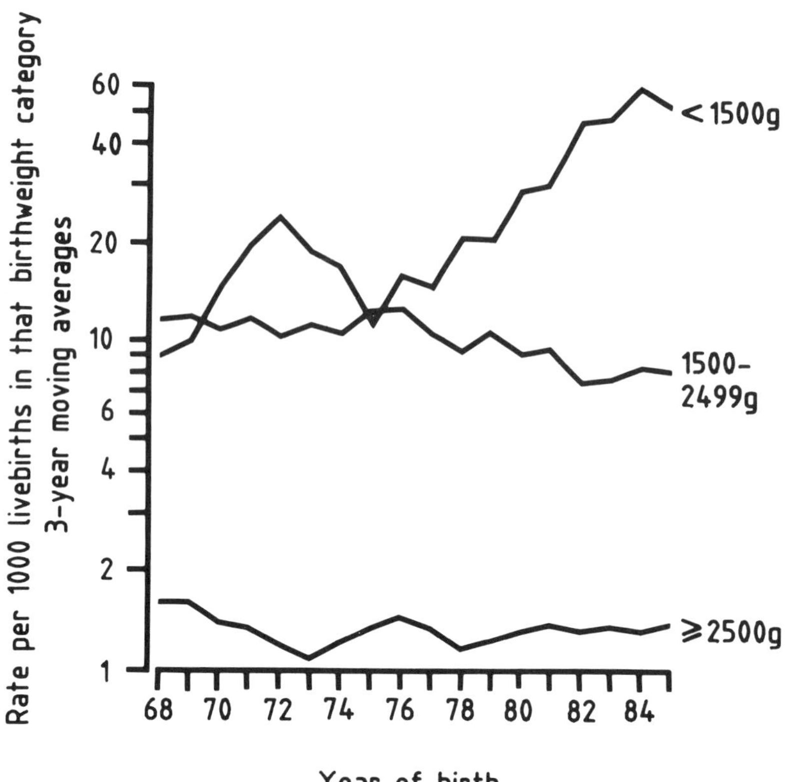

Fig 18–4.—Rates of cerebral palsy in very-low-birth-weight (less than 1,500 g), low-birth-weight (1,500–2,499 g), and normal-birth-weight (at least 2,500 g) infants per 1,000 live births in Western Australia in 1975–1985. (Courtesy of Stanley FJ, Watson L: *BMJ* 304:1658–1663, 1992.)

Supplemental Reading List

The Fetus

Capeless EL, Kelleher PC, Walters CP: Elevated maternal serum fetoprotein levels and maternal risk factors: Their association with pregnancy complications. *J Reprod Med* 37:257–260, 1992.

Huisman TWA, Stewart PA, Wladimiroff JW: Ductus venosus blood flow velocity waveforms in the human fetus: A Doppler study. *Ultrasound Med Biol* 18:33–37, 1992.

Patriquin H, Fontaine S, Michaud J, et al: Development of the fetal brain in the second trimester: An anatomic and ultrasonographic demonstration. *Can Assoc Radio* 43:131, 1992.

Genetics and Teratology

Bower C, Stanley FJ: Periconceptional vitamin supplementation and neural tube defects: Evidence from a case-control study in Western Australia and a review of recent publications. *J Epidemiol Community Health* 46:157–161, 1992.

Tsipouras P, Mastro R, Sarfarazi M, et al: Genetic linkage of the Marfran syndrome, ectopea lentis, and congenital contractural arachnodactyly to the fibrillin genes on chromosomes 15 and 5. *N Engl J Med* 326:905–909, 1992.

Medical Complications of Pregnancy

Antepartum Fetal Surveillance

Shaw GM, Malcoe LH: Residential mobility during pregnancy for mothers of infants with or without congenital cardiac anomalies. *Arch Environ Health* 46:310–312, 1991.

Wilhelm J, Morris D, Hotham N, et al: Epilepsy and pregnancy: A review of 98 pregnancies. *Aust NZ Obstet Gynaecol* 30:290, 1990.

Labor and Delivery

Infectious Diseases and Developmental Immunology

Bingen E, Denamur E, Lambert-Zechovsky N, et al: Analysis of DNA restriction fragment length polymorphism extends the evidence for breast milk transmission in *Streptococcus agalactiae* late-onset neonatal infection. *J Infect Dis* 165:569–573, 1992.

Faix R: Invasive neonatal candidiasis: Comparison of *albicans* and *parapsilosis* infection. *Pediatr Infect Dis J* 11:88–93, 1992.

Francis BM, Gilbert GL: Survey of neonatal meningitis in Australia: 1987–1989. *Med J Aust* 156:240–243, 1992.

Lester P, Partridge JC, Cooke M: Postnatal human immunodeficiency virus antibody testing: The effects of current policy on infant care and maternal informed consent. *West J Med* 156:371–375, 1992.

Noel GJ, Kreiswirth BN, Edelson PJ: Multiple methicillin-resistant *Staphylococcus aureus* strains as a cause for a single outbreak of severe disease in hospitalized neonates. *Pediatr Infect Dis J* 11:184–188, 1992.

Waites KB, Crouse DT, Cassess GH: Antibiotic susceptibilities and therapeutic options for *Ureaplasma urealyticum* infections in neonates. *Pediatr Infect Dis J* 11:23–29, 1992.

Follow-Up and the Nervous System

Christie FB, Stirrups DR, Mackenzie JS, et al: An orthodontic evaluation of 16-year-old males with an original complete unilateral cleft lip and palate problem repaired during the neonatal period. *Br J Plast Surg* 44:557–561, 1991.

Cox C, Hack M, Aram D, et al: Neonatal auditory brainstem response failure of very low birth weight infants: 8-year outcome. *Pediatr Res* 31:68–72, 1992.

Elliman A, Bryan E, Elliman A: The growth of low-birthweight children. *Acta Paediatr* 81:311–314, 1992.

Ellison PH, Petersen MB, Gorman WA: A comparison of neurological assessment scores from two cohorts of low-birthweight children evaluated at age four years: Dublin and Copenhagen. *Neuropediatrics* 23:68–71, 1992.

Nicholson A, Alberman E: Cerebral palsy: An increasing contributor to severe mental retardation. *Arch Dis Child* 67:1050–1055, 1992.

Park TS, Owen JH: Surgical management of spastic diplegia in cerebral palsy. N *Engl J Med* 326:745–749, 1992.

Ramey CT, Bryant DM, Wasik BH, et al: Infant health and development program for low birth weight, premature infants: Program elements, family participation, and child intelligence. *Pediatrics* 89:454–465, 1992.

Saigal S, Rosenbaum P, Szatmari P, et al: Non-right handedness among ELBW and term children at eight years in relation to cognitive function and school performance. *Dev Med Child Neurol* 34:425–466, 1992.

Sham PC, O'Callaghan E, Takei N, et al: Schizophrenia following pre-natal exposure to influenza epidemics between 1939 and 1960. *Br J Psychiatry* 160:461–466, 1992.

Vannucci RC, Yager JY: Glucose, lactic acid, and perinatal hypoxic-ischemic brain damage. *Pediatr Neurol* 8:3–12, 1992.

Veelken N, Stollhoff K, Claussen M: Development and perinatal risk factors of very-low-birthweight infants. Small versus appropriate for gestational age. *Neuropediatrics* 23:102–107. 1992.

Yu VYH, Gomez JM, McCloud, PI: Survival prospects of extremely preterm infants: A 10-year experience in a single perinatal center. *Am J Perinatol* 9:164–169, 1992.

Behavior and Pain Management

Gastroenterology and Nutrition

Adamkin DH, McClead RE, Desai NS, et al: Comparison of two neonatal intravenous amino acid formulations in preterm infants: A multicenter study. *J Perinatol* 11: 375–382, 1991.

Beeby PH, Jeffery H: Risk factors for necrotizing enterocolitis: The influence of gestational age. *Arch Dis Child* 67:432–435, 1992.

Brown AK, Seidman DS: Jaundice in healthy, term neonates: Do we need new action levels or new approaches? *Pediatrics* 89:827–828, 1992.

Butte NF, Wong WW, Garza C: Prediction equations for total body water during early infancy. *Acta Paediatr* 31:264–265, 1992.

Cashore WJ: Hyperbilirubinemia: Should we adopt a new standard of care? *Pediatrics* 89:824–826, 1992.

Dewey KG, Heinig MJ, Nommsen LA, et al: Growth of breast-fed and formula-fed infants from 0 to 18 months: The DARLING study. *Pediatrics* 89:1035–1041, 1992.

Gutcher GR, Farrell PM: Intravenous infusion of lipid for the prevention of essential fatty acid deficiency in premature infants. *Am J Clin Nutr* 54:1024–1028, 1991.
Jones AW: Alcohol in mother's milk. (editorial) N *Engl J Med* 326:766–767, 1992.
Leaf AA, Leighfield MJ, Costeloe KL, et al: Factors affecting long-chain polyunsaturated fatty acid composition of plasma phosphoglycerides in preterm infants. *J Pediatr Gastroenterol Nutr* 14:300–308, 1992.
Sibbons PD, Spitz L, Velzen D: Necrotizing enterocolitis induced by local circulatory interruption in the ileum of neonatal piglets. *Pediatr Pathol* 12:1–14, 1992.
Sievers E, Oldigs HD, Dorner K, et al: Longitudinal zinc balances in breast-fed and formula-fed infants. *Acta Paediatr* 81:1–6, 1992.
Wilson DC, Tubman R, Bell N, et al: Plasma manganese, selenium and gluthatione peroxidase levels in the mother and newborn infant. *Early Human Development* 26:223–226, 1991.

The Respiratory Tract

Almog R, Goldkrand JW, Saulsbery RA, et al: Prediction of respiratory distress syndrome by a new colorimetric assay. *Am J Obstet Gynecol* 166:1827–1834, 1992.
Ashton MR, Postle AD, Hall MA, et al: Phosphatidylcholine composition of endotracheal tube aspirates of neonates and subsequent respiratory disease. *Arch Dis Child* 67:378–382, 1992.
Atkinson JB, Poon MW: ECMO and the management of congenital diaphragmatic hernia with large diaphragmatic defects requiring a prosthetic patch. *J Pediatr Surg* 27:754–756, 1992.
Dubin SB: The laboratory assessment of fetal lung maturity. *Am J Clin Pathol.* 97:836–849, 1992.
Guntheroth WG, Spiers PS: Sleeping prone and the risk of sudden infant death syndrome. *JAMA* 267:2359–2362, 1992.
Price MR, Galantowicz ME, Stolar CJH: Mechanical forces contribute to neonatal lung growth: The influence of altered diaphragm function in piglets. *J Pediatr Surg* 27:376–381, 1992.

The Heart and Blood Vessels

Backer CL, Zales VR, Idriss FS, et al: Heart transplantation in neonates and in children. *J Heart Lung Transplant* 11:311–319, 1992.
Charache S, Nelson L, Saw D, et al: Accuracy and utility of differential white blood cell count in the neonatal intensive care unit. *Am J Clin Pathol* 97:338–344, 1992.
Denjean A, Bridley F, Praud JP, et al: Accuracy of measurements of HbF with OSM3 in neonates and infants. *Eur Respir* 5:105–107, 1992.
Edwards AD, Brown GC, Cope M, et al: Quantification of concentration changes in neonatal human cerebral oxidized cytochrome oxidase. *J Appl Physiol* 71:1907–1913, 1991.
Ford EG, Stanley P, Tolo V, et al: Peripheral congenital arteriovenous fistulae: Observe, operate, or obturate? *J Pediatr Surg* 27:714–719, 1992.
Golberg SJ, Dawson BV, Johnson PD, et al: Cardiac teratogenicity of dichlorethylene in a chick model. *Pediatr Res* 32:23–26, 1992.
Hosseinzadeh T, Tchervenkov CI, Quantz M, et al: Adverse effect of prearrest hypothermia in immature hearts: Rate versus duration of cooling. *Ann Thorac Surg* 53:464–471, 1992.

Konduri GG, Theodorou AA, Mukhopadhyay A, et al: Adenosine triphosphate and adenosine increase the pulmonary blood flow to postnatal levels in fetal lambs. *Pediatr Res* 31:451–457, 1992.

Murray DJ, Forbes RB, Mahoney LT: Comparative hemodynamic depression of halothane versus isoflurane in neonates and infants: An echocardiographic study. *Anesth Analg* 74:329–337, 1992.

Rubay JE, Sluysmans TH, Alexandrescu V, et al: Surgical repair of coarctation of the aorta in infants under one year of age. *J Cardiovasc Surg* 33:216, 1992.

Skinner JR, Milligan DWA, Hunter S, et al: Central venous pressure in the ventilated neonate. *Arch Dis Child* 67:374–377, 1992.

The Blood

Batton DG, Goodrow D, Walker RH: Reducing neonatal transfusions. *J Perinatol* 11:152–155, 1992.

Endocrine and Metabolic Disorders

Kaiserman I, Siebner R, Kletter G, et al: A ten-year temporal analysis of primary congenital hypothyroidism in Israel. *Early Human Development* 26:193–201, 1991.

Newman K, Randolph J, Anderson K: The surgical management of infants and children with ambiguous genitalia. (From the Departments of Surgery and Pediatrics, Children's National Medical Center, and George Washington University Medical School, Washington, DC.)

Hart PS, Hymes J, Wolf B: Biochemical and immunological characterization of serum biotinidase in profound biotindase deficiency. *Am J Hum Genet* 50:126–136, 1992.

Developmental Pharmacology and Toxicology

Arnon S, Grigg J, Nikander K, et al: Delivery of micronized budesonide suspension by metered dose inhaler and jet nebulizer into a neonatal ventilator circuit. *Pediatr Pulmonol* 13:172–175, 1992.

Bhatt-Mehta V, Johnson CE, Schumacher RE: Gentamicin pharmacokinetics in term neonates receiving extracorporeal membrane oxygenation. *Pharmacotherapy* 12:28–32, 1992.

Volpe JJ: Effect of cocaine use on the fetus. N *Engl J Med* 327:399–407, 1992.

Miscellaneous Topics

Bell JE, Fryer AA, Collins M, et al: Developmental profile of plasma proteins in human fetal cerebrospinal fluid and blood. *Neuropathol Appl Neurobiol* 17:441–456, 1991.

Chessare JB: Circumcision: Is the risk of urinary tract infection really the pivotal issue? *Clin Pediatr* 31:100–104, 1992.

Gardiner HM, Duncan AW: Radiological assessment of the effects on splinting on early hip development: Results from a randomized controlled trial of abduction splinting vs. sonographic surveillance. *Pediatr Radiol* 22:159–162, 1992.

Millis MB, and Share JC: Use of ultrasonography in dysplasia of the immature hip. *Clin Orthop* 274:171, 1992.

Postnatal Growth and Development

Epidemiology

Berge LN, Rasmussen S, Dahl LB: Evaluation of fetal and neonatal mortality at the University of Tromso, Norway, from 1976–1989. *Acta Obstet Gynecol Scand* 70:275–282, 1991.

Braveman PA, Egerter S, Bennett T, et al: Differences in hospital resource allocation among sick newborns according to insurance coverage. *JAMA* 266:3300–3308, 1991.

Collins JW, Jr: Disparate black and white neonatal mortality rates among infants of normal birth weight in Chicago. *J Pediatr* 120:954–960, 1992.

Overpeck MD, Hoffman HJ, Prager K: The lowest birth-weight infants and the US infant mortality rate: NCHS 1983 linked birth/infant death data. *Am J Public Health* 82:441–444, 1992.

Robertson PA, Sniderman SH, Laros RK, et al: Neonatal morbidity according to gestational age and birth weight from five tertiary care centers in the United States. *Am J Obstet Gynecol* 166:1629–1645, 1992.

Bilirubin

Gartner LM: Management of jaundice in the well baby. *Pediatrics* 89:826–827, 1992.

Johnson L: Yet another expert opinion on bilirubin toxicity! *Pediatrics* 89:829–831.

Merenstein GB: 'New' bilirubin recommendations questioned. *Pediatrics* 89:822–823, 1992.

Newman TB, Maisels MJ: Evaluation and treatment of jaundice in the term newborn: A kinder, gentler approach. *Pediatrics* 89:809–818, 1992.

Newman TB, Maisels MJ: Response to commentaries evaluation and treatment of jaundice in the term newborn: A gentler, kinder approach. *Pediatrics* 89:831–833, 1992.

Obinata K, Nittono H, Yabuta K, et al: 1B-hydroxylated bile acids in the urine of healthy neonates. *J Pediatr Gastroenterol Nutr* 15:1–5, 1992.

Poland RL: In search of a 'Gold Standard ' for bilirubin toxicity. *Pediatrics* 89:823–824, 1992.

Vales T: Bilirubin Toxicity: The problem was solved a generation ago. *Pediatrics* 89:819–820, 1992.

Wennberg RP: Bilirubin recommendations present problems: New guidelines simplistic and untested. *Pediatrics* 89:821–822, 1992.

Subject Index

A

B

C

D

E

F

G

H

J

K

L

M

N

O

P

S

T

U

V

W

Author Index

A

B

C

H

I

J

K

L

Q

R

S

The Year Books–
The best from 236,287 journal articles.

At Mosby, we subscribe to more than 950 medical and allied health journals from every corner of the globe. We read them all, tirelessly scanning for anything that relates to your field.

We send everything we find related to a given specialty to the distinguished editors of the **Year Book** in that area, and they pick out the best, the articles they feel every practitioner in that specialty should be aware of.

For the 1993 **Year Books** we surveyed a total of 236,287 articles and found hundreds of articles related to your field. Our expert editors reviewed these and chose the best, the developments you don't want to miss.

The best articles–condensed and organized.

Not only do you get the past year's most important articles in your field, you get them in a format that makes them easy to use.

Every article that the editors pick is condensed into a concise, outlined abstract, a summary of the article's most important points highlighted with bold paragraph headings. So you can quickly scan for exactly what you need.

Personal commentary from the experts.

If that was it, if all our editors did was identify the year's best articles, the **Year Book** would still be a great reference to have. (Can you think of an easier way to keep up with all the developments that are shaping your field?)

But following each article, the editors also write concise commentaries telling whether or not the study in question is a reliable one, whether a new technique is effective, or whether a particular trend you've heard about merits your immediate attention.

No other abstracting service offers this expert advice to help you decide how the year's advances will affect the way you practice.

No matter how many journals you subscribe to, the Year Book can help.

When you subscribe to a **Year Book**, we'll also send you an automatic notice of future volumes about two months before they publish. If you do not want the **Year Book**, this convenient advance notice makes it easy for you to let us know. And if you elect to receive the new **Year Book**, you need do nothing. We will send it upon publication.

No worry. No wasted motion. And, of course, every **Year Book** is yours to examine FREE of charge for thirty days.